Ethical Challenges
in Health Care

Vicki D. Lachman, PhD, MBE, APRN, is a Clinical Associate Professor in the College of Nursing and Health Professions at Drexel University in Philadelphia, PA. In her role at the university, she primarily teaches ethics to master's and doctoral nursing students and acts as the track coordinator for the Innovation and Intra/Entrepreneurship in Advanced Nursing Practice MSN.

Dr. Lachman is a frequent presenter on ethical topics at national conferences. She writes the quarterly Ethics, Law and Policy column for *MEDSURG Nursing: The Journal of Adult Health.* Dr. Lachman also serves on the American Nurses Association Center for Ethics and Human Rights Advisory Board and often advises executives on organizational ethics and front-line staff on end-of-life ethical issues. Her book, *Applied Ethics in Nursing,* was published by Springer Publishing Company in November 2005.

Ethical Challenges in Health Care

Developing Your Moral Compass

Vicki D. Lachman, PhD, MBE, APRN

Springer Publishing Company, LLC
11 West 42nd Street
New York, NY 10036
www.springerpub.com

Acquisitions Editor: Allan Graubard
Production Editor: Barbara A. Chernow
Cover design: David Levy
Composition: Agnew's, Inc.

Ebook ISBN: 978-0-8261-1090-9

14 15 / 9 8 7

The author and the publisher of this Work have made every effort to use sources believed to be reliable to provide information that is accurate and compatible with the standards generally accepted at the time of publication. The author and publisher shall not be liable for any special, consequential, or exemplary damages resulting, in whole or in part, from the readers' use of, or reliance on, the information contained in this book. The publisher has no responsibility for the persistence or accuracy of URLs for external or third-party Internet Web sites referred to in this publication and does not guarantee that any content on such Web sites is, or will remain, accurate or appropriate.

Library of Congress Cataloging-in-Publication Data

Lachman, Vicki D.
  Ethical challenges in health care : developing your moral compass /
Vicki D. Lachman.
    p. ; cm.
  Includes bibliographical references and index.
  ISBN 978-0-8261-1089-3 (alk. paper)
  1. Medical ethics. 2. Corporate culture. I. Title.
  [DNLM: 1. Ethics, Medical. 2. Delivery of Health Care—ethics. 3. Morals.
4. Organizational Culture. 5. Patients. 6. Safety. W 50 L138e 2009]
  R724.L23   2009
  174.2—dc22
                                                              2009015443

Printed in the United States of America by Gasch Printing

This book is dedicated to all healthcare professionals, managers, and executives who have the moral courage to "speak up" and advocate for patients and their families.

Contents

Section IV: Organizational Opportunities for Moral Courage

Section V: Further Opportunities for Moral Courage

Preface

Courage is something we all respect. When asked to describe courage, however, many of us will conjure up an image of a soldier in battle or a firefighter running into a burning building, or possibly even of a fictional hero, of Superman or Spiderman, saving the day. Certainly, such images of courage are prevalent in our media, including the local hero who dives into a rushing river to save a child from drowning. Yet all these images exemplify individuals who demonstrate *physical* courage.

This book, however, will focus on *moral* courage. In our society, we use the phrase "courage of my convictions" to describe moral courage—the courage demonstrated when individuals "take action," especially when others looked away or chose to do nothing. This is the courage we note when an individual holds onto his or her values when faced with disapproval, humiliation, loss (for example, of job), or isolation from peers.

I commend to your reading Rushmore Kidder's (2005) book, *Moral Courage,* which speaks articulately for the courage to be ethical and do right. This book is designed to speak to the mind, heart, and soul of healthcare professionals and leaders. The focus of the examples, cases, and successes described by Kidder come primarily from the trials and tribulations endured in the healthcare environment.

Here, in this book now in your hands, my goal is clear: to help individuals and organizations not only triumph over the fear that stops many from exercising moral courage, but to also feel the personal and professional gratification it offers. Developing moral courage may be difficult. Fortunately, we have many role models, and I will use their examples and quotations throughout the book. One such archetype, the great South African civil rights leader Nelson Mandela, said, "I learned that courage was not the absence of fear, but the triumph over it. The brave man is not he who does not feel afraid, but he who conquers that fear."

For healthcare providers and leaders to demonstrate the needed action at difficult times, they need to understand their obligations, be skillful in assertiveness and negotiation, and manage this fear that Mandela refers to. "Standing up for what you believe in, even if it means standing alone" requires having the strength to do the right thing when faced with moral decisions involving patient safety, patient confidentiality, and the patient's autonomous right to know the truth about his or her diagnosis, prognosis, and risk of recommended treatment.

In the hope of instilling or increasing the healthcare professional's moral courage, this book will provide knowledge, strategy, and encouragement. Each of its five sections features case examples from actual healthcare providers and leaders to illustrate skills or opportunities. Tables and figures will provide readers with succinct points to remember as they develop their moral compass.

Multiple helpful ideas from the book *Crucial Conversations* (2002) by Kerry Patterson, Joseph Grenny, Ron McMillan, and Steven R. Covey will be sprinkled throughout the pages to come.

The first section of the book focuses on the personal development of moral courage and on existing opportunities for professionals in health care to demonstrate moral courage. After a brief review of the origin of the concept of moral courage, Section I spotlights the knowledge and skills necessary for "standing up and speaking out." For example, the reader will learn the values they are expected to honor as healthcare professionals—values that are nonnegotiable obligations in the professionals' Code of Ethics that society expects us to respect. Perspectives on how to manage the risk and our fear of speaking up, as well as helpful information on how to deliver bad news to patients, coworkers, and leaders, are also included here.

Sections III and IV focus on leaders and leadership in healthcare organizations. Section III examines the four arenas in which leaders need to center their attention if they want to build an organizational culture that supports moral courage. The significance of ethical culture, executive leadership "walking the walk," accountability, and human resource policies that permanently hardwire the organization for integrity and excellence are discussed. Section IV opens with chapters on the supports required for moral courage, such as organizational and clinical ethics committees and a culture of patient safety. Chapter 18 specifically discusses the problem of disruptive physicians in preventing a civil culture where all voices can be heard to prevent and resolve patient safety and quality concerns. In Chapter 19 on leadership development, strategies are taken from successful organizations, such as Baptist Health Care and Disney and the companies in Jim Collins's *Good to Great* (2001). These organizations can provide leaders with guidance to finely tune their moral compasses. This chapter also frames the duty of a healthcare organization to develop future ethical leaders who can be exemplars in moral courage for the staff.

Section V ends the book with the one unresolved national healthcare issue that impacts all healthcare providers and leaders on a daily basis—46 million uninsured people. This tragedy will require the moral courage of our politicians and the intellect of many in economics, health care, and business to resolve. My hope is that as the code of silence ends, apathy will lift and healthcare professionals and leaders will demonstrate the moral courage necessary to tackle this heartbreaking problem.

Vicki D. Lachman, PhD, MBE, APRN

Ethical Challenges
in Health Care

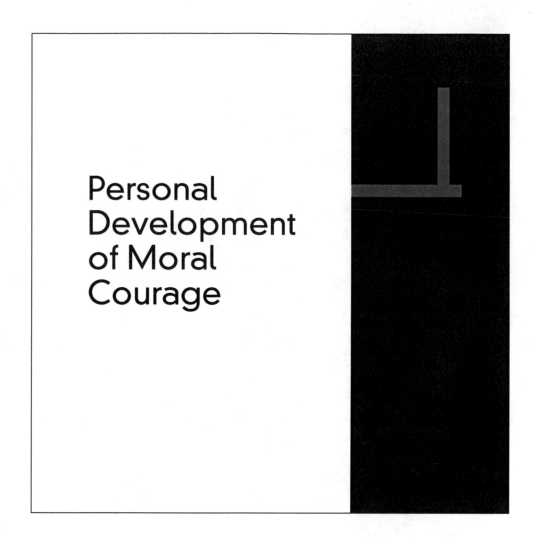

Personal Development of Moral Courage

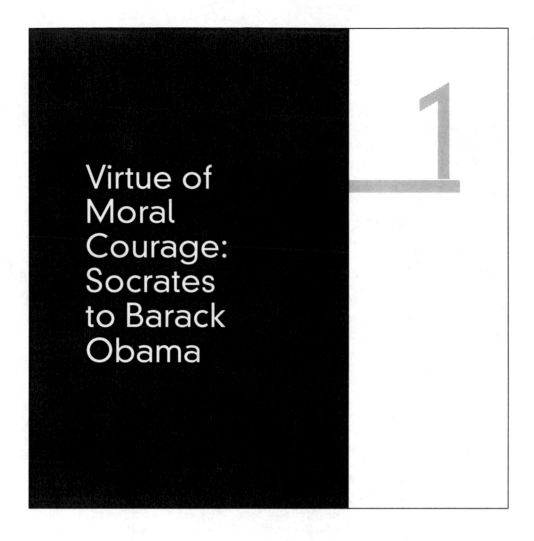

Virtue of Moral Courage: Socrates to Barack Obama

The world is a dangerous place, not because of those who do evil, but because of those who look on and do nothing.

—Albert Einstein, a great scientist and humanitarian

It is only fitting that our discussion of ethical challenges in health care begins with the founding fathers of philosophy—Socrates, Plato, and Aristotle. They agree more than they disagree on the subject, but their differences are helpful to our understanding of the importance of moral courage. Their influence has continued through the centuries, as can be seen in the lives of two healthcare professionals born in the nineteenth century—Florence Nightingale and Albert Schweitzer, both of whom epitomize the virtue of moral courage.

Although this book highlights the contributions of many people who have exhibited an exemplary commitment to the health and well-being of others, this chapter concludes with stories of moral courage outside the healthcare environment, beginning with holocaust rescuers. These individuals are included because they exemplify the everyday person's willingness to do his or her part to right a wrong, and I hope they will serve as an inspiration to healthcare professionals, who also need to right the wrongs—the wrongs inflicted on patients who are vulnerable, such as those dying in ICUs, those at risk for patient errors, and those who are uninsured. Finally, the chapter highlights the philosophy of Barack Obama, who was recently elected president of the United States. May you have his audacity to hope for a safer and more just healthcare system, a system that honors your voice as you speak out for the patients you serve.

Trio of Famous Philosophers: Socrates, Plato, and Aristotle

The emergence of philosophy and science in Athens began with Socrates, who was born in 470 BC. His approach to drawing out the truth became known as the Socratic method. By asking his students and listeners a series of penetrating questions, he tried to help them achieve greater clarity of thought. But, his method sometimes revealed that respondent's ideas were not particularly logical. As a result, he was not a favorite of many politicians. In 399 BC, a jury of 500 fellow citizens charged Socrates with immorality. He was sentenced to death by a margin of six votes but was offered the chance to save his life by paying a small fine for his impiety. He cast off the option. He also rejected the pleas of Plato and other students, who had a boat waiting for him at Piraeus, to flee to freedom. Socrates simply refused to break the law. He asked, "What kind of citizen would I be if I refused to accept the judgment of the jury? No citizen at all." He spent his last days with his friends before he drank the fatal dose of hemlock. We shall return to the question of whether his decision and action reflect moral courage.

Socrates lectured mostly to the sons of well-to-do aristocrats, one of whom was Plato, born in 428 BC. He was 28 years old when Socrates was put to death. At the age of forty, Plato established a school, the Academy, for the education of Athenian youth. His students were most likely aristocrats, and they discussed all subjects, including politics, economics, science, philosophy, mathematics, and morality. Plato's ideas are set out in the *Republic* in the form of a dialog that discusses the physical, mental, and spiritual development of the individual that is necessary to produce a perfect society (Aristotle, trans. 2004). Plato argued that reality is known only through the mind because our senses may deceive us. He therefore believed in a higher world, a world of Ideas or Forms that define what is unchanging, absolute, and universal. In today's world, many people see few absolutes, as moral relativism permeates our culture. Moral relativists maintain that moral disagreements arise because what is right for one is not necessarily right for another. However, as you shall see, some absolutes are outlined in our codes of ethics.

The third member of this trio, Aristotle, was born in 384 BC. At the age of 18, Aristotle came to Athens to study at Plato's Academy, and he stayed until Plato's death in 348 BC. He agreed with Plato that the highest human faculty was reason and that its supreme activity was contemplation. In addition to studying metaphysics and mathematics, Aristotle thought it was also very important to study the world around him—from physics and mechanics to biology. Perhaps being raised in the house of a physician had given him an interest in living things. What he achieved in those years in Athens was the beginning of a school of organized scientific inquiry on a scale exceeding anything that had preceded him.

Plato and Aristotle agreed that the world is the product of rational design and that the only true knowledge is that which is irrefutable. The essential difference between them is well known: Plato considered *mathematical reasoning* as the means to reveal truth, while Aristotle believed that *detailed empirical investigations* of nature were essential if humans were to understand their world. And there, in the space of just a few decades, we have the essence of the two philosophical traditions that have dominated the Western intellectual tradition for the past 2500 years: Rationalism—knowledge is *a priori* (comes before experience)—and Empiricism—knowledge is *a posteriori* (comes after experience).

What, then, were the differences between Plato and Aristotle? Plato suggested that people were born with knowledge, and Aristotle argued that knowledge comes from experience. Aristotle had little patience with Plato's higher world of Forms. Aristotle argued that there were universal principles, but that they are derived from experience.

Views on the Virtue of Courage

After reading contemporary analyses of these founding fathers of our intellectual tradition, they clearly should be included in our analysis of the virtue of moral courage. Literally, a virtue is a desirable quality, a quality we would expect to find in a person of merit. Virtue theory focuses on the character of the person rather than on the person's decision-making process. Virtue theory holds that a person of good moral fiber will make the right decision, regardless of the process.

All three philosophers argued that education is the key in shaping an individual's character. Plato, however, emphasized the importance of story telling, particularly when the main character demonstrates a desired virtue. Aristotle, however, further believed that character is also the result of habit. If the individual repeatedly strives for excellence, this habit will yield an excellence of character.

Of course, the initial writings of the trio focused on courage on the battlefield. This should not surprise us, as they lived during the dismantling of the Athenian Empire as a result of the Peloponnesian War, with its many legendary battles. In his *Nicomachean Ethics,* for example, Aristotle's discussion of courage centers on dying on the battlefield, which was considered noble, unlike dying from disease.

The distinction between physical and moral courage, however, is not as straightforward as it might seem. In our own history, we can distinguish between soldiers who have physical courage, as required by their commanders in war, and those who, like Martin Luther King, Jr., have both moral and physical courage. King displayed both as he died fighting for the moral principles in which he believed. His war was not a military battle. Rather it focused on winning the battle against the enemy of racism (King, 1963).

Dr. King knew that he was always in danger of assassination, as do many who seek to change the injustices of their times. Socrates knew it. Galileo knew it. Joan of Arc knew it. In *Laches,* Socrates and his discussion partners determined that physical acts without the knowledge of good and bad (morality) can never be courageous (Plato, trans. 2004, pp. 195c–197b). If the individual speaking out does not understand that he is speaking against an established wrong, the person can not receive credit for moral courage.

Courage is one of the four cardinal virtues in the lasting tradition of moral character described by Plato. The other qualities are temperance, justice, and wisdom. These four virtues have been accorded a pivotal status in moral life from ancient times to the present day.

Will is introduced as an executive function between the impulses (appetites) and rational aspects of human experience. Will is the result of education in the physical, mental, and spiritual realms. Socrates and Plato both believed that management of mind over body was the *only* way that human actions could become virtuous. Temperance contained the appetites with good judgment (wisdom) by focusing on justice (fairness for all, as opposed to self-centeredness). Courage manifests as the ability to manage the hardships that conflicts bring, along with an ability to endure adversity or suffering.

Aristotle's further refined his view of courage by focusing not on cardinal virtues, but on virtue of thought and virtue of character. Virtue of thought is increased through education, and virtue of character is advanced through habit. But, you might ask, could not habit also lead to the development of a vice?

Aristotle believed that courage was the balance (mean) between the extremes of cowardice and rashness. Therefore, a person might rush headfirst into danger either because he is blinded by rage (as a terrorist might be) or because he is oblivious (if intoxicated) to the hazards that lie ahead. According to Aristotle, courage is defined as having rational control of emotion and passion—the person is expected to have control over fear and other emotional states. He supposed that both deficiency and excess of a virtue could be catastrophic. Aristotle writes in *Nichomachean Ethics,* "he is courageous who endures and fears the right things, for the right motive, in the right manner, and at the right time and who displays confidence in a similar way" (Aristotle, trans. 2004, Book III7, pp. 1115b15–20). Aristotle was resolute in his belief that a virtue, like courage, could only be used for honorable ends. From a slightly different perspective, Plato would say that courage for wicked ends was a lack of the cardinal virtue of wisdom.

Aristotle believed that virtuous individuals are so desirous of doing good that they struggle to make moral decisions (Roberts, 1984). Therefore, such persons do not require will power or courage to motivate them to do what is right. However, most of us face moral struggles, and Roberts (1984) helps us differentiate between an assessment based on "purity of heart" and an assessment based on being a "hero." According to Roberts, an internal struggle bolstered by will power enables an individual to choose the virtuous action. The eighteenth-century German philosopher Immanuel Kant (1788/1996) sees the choice of virtuous action as a result of moral reasoning. However, Kant's focus is on duty or obligation, whereas virtue focuses on character. Aristotle's focus was the importance of acting, not just reasoning. He said that "one must not only know what to do, but he must also be able to act accordingly" (Aristotle, trans. 1954, Book VII, pp. 1152a5–10).

Through the centuries, many people have shown moral courage in different fields and different situations. Here are a few examples of people with the moral courage to live by and fight for their values.

Florence Nightingale: More Than a Lady With a Lamp

Born in 1820, Florence Nightingale was an English hospital reformer credited with fighting for improved sanitary practices in hospitals, public health facilities, and formal training for nurses. Unlike medicine, nursing did not evolve from a craft guild tradition. As a result, there was little formal training.

Florence Nightingale was acquainted with the lives of the ancient Greeks and read and translated the works of Plato. Her notion of God suggests the Platonic ideal of good character as founded on objective knowledge. A person of good character is one who knows clearly and completely what is good and invariably chooses according to that knowledge. Nightingale also equates doing what is right with happiness (Calabria & Macrae, 1994). These ideas are in accord with Plato's, as argued in the *Republic,* that virtue is knowledge and is the grounding of human flourishing and happiness.

Nightingale's conception of nursing is also similar to Plato's conception of public service, appropriate for what he called guardians. Plato believed that the purpose of education for guardians was to form moral character and not to teach technical expertise (Le Vasseur, 1998). Platonic education aimed to turn talented people into leading citizens, who would care for the good of the community. Nightingale's use of her talents, education, and connections to crusade for healthcare reform points to a broad political function concerned with a societal good.

Nightingale's goal of a healthy world is only possible through leadership and global action. In *Florence Nightingale Today: Healing, Leadership, Global Action* (Dossey, Selanders, Beck, & Attewell, 2004), the authors use interpretive biographical methodology and synthesize essential patterns from Nightingale's writings to link her teachings to contemporary nursing theory. Nightingale's many undertakings to better public health resulted in decreasing the death rate during the Crimean War, collecting groundbreaking evaluative statistics, establishing the first secular nursing school, and improving sanitation in Great Britain. The authors also describe her as a mystic, theorist, researcher, teacher, author, leader, activist, and visionary. They advise that if nurses would use Nightingale for inspiration, each could make a difference in the state of health on the microscopic and macroscopic levels.

Letters depicting Florence Nightingale as an ambitious meddler who went over doctors' heads show a spirit that nurse leaders in the profession consider necessary, a strength I find is still needed. Her efforts clearly reflect her evidence-based framework, ranging from Nightingale's first work after her return as a heroine from the Crimean War in 1856 to a later attempt to influence social policy with a proposal for a chair in "social physics" at Oxford University in 1891. Nightingale also fought for a woman's right to do purposeful work outside the home.

Other health professionals, such as Elizabeth Blackwell, the first female physician, were also staunch advocates of nursing education. Another outspoken English nurse reformer, Ethel Bedford Fenwick, championed nursing registration and founded the *British Journal of Nursing* in 1893. Her American colleague, Lavinia Lloyd Dock, author of *Materia Medica for Nurses,* wrote one of nursing education's first textbooks. Both were prominent advocates of women's suffrage. All of these women, like Nightingale, demonstrated moral courage as advocates for better patient care over the objections of doctors, politicians, and popular opinion. Much of what they advocated is now considered common knowl-edge, but it was revolutionary in its day.

Dr. Albert Schweitzer: He Lived His Argument

Like Nightingale, Schweitzer had always felt a powerful longing toward direct service to humanity and, like Nightingale, his moment of direction came sud-denly. Born in 1875, Schweitzer was a medical missionary, theologian, and philoso-pher with ties to France and Germany. In 1904, he read an article in the Paris Missionary Society's publication signifying a pressing need for physicians in the French colony of Gabon in Africa. Hundreds of young men and women read this piece, but few were as affected as Albert Schweitzer. When he had completed the article, he put the magazine away and quietly began his work. But his search was over. He saw his time and place and future; his life took clear shape (Ives & Valone, 2007).

Again, like Nightingale, Schweitzer did not receive support from family and friends for his calling. Despite this resistance, he began medical studies at the age of 30, receiving his degree, with a specialization in tropical medicine and surgery, some eight years later. What he had failed to anticipate was the Paris Missionary Society's refusal to employ his services. Today, we would character-ize the Paris Missionary Society's view of Albert Schweitzer as a person who was "politically incorrect," just like Nightingale. Both were considered radical in their time. Both were people of convictions with the moral courage to do for their patients what they needed done.

In March 1913, Dr. and Mrs. Schweitzer, a trained nurse, left for Africa to build their own hospital at Lambaréné in the French Congo, now Gabon. They focused on developing bonds of trust between hospital personnel and the local population. He treated thousands of people suffering from severe illnesses, such as malaria, sleeping sickness, skin sores, leprosy, dysentery, venereal diseases, and heart failure. Apart from occasional fund-raising visits to Europe, he con-tinued his medical work in Africa for the rest of his life.

Dr. Schweitzer was known to have repeatedly said that "everyone must find his own Lambaréné" and that "My life is my argument." In his Nobel Prize ac-ceptance speech in 1954, he spoke about the importance of rejecting war for ethical reasons, stating that war makes us guilty of the crime of inhumanity. He spoke about the importance of nurturing the human spirit so that humanity will have the moral courage to stand up against war. He said:

> The spirit is not dead; it lives in isolation. It has overcome the difficulty of hav-ing to exist in a world out of harmony with its ethical character. It has come to realize that it can find no home other than in the basic nature of man. The in-dependence acquired through its acceptance of this realization is an additional asset.
>
> It is convinced that compassion, in which ethics takes root, does not assume its true proportions until it embraces not only man but every living being. To the old ethics, which lacked this depth and force of conviction, has been added the ethics of reverence for life, and its validity is steadily gaining in recogni-tion. . . . Once more we dare to appeal to the whole man, to his capacity to think

and feel, exhorting him to know himself and to be true to himself. We reaffirm our trust in the profound qualities of his nature (Nobelprize.org).

What is most remarkable about this man was his unbelievable passion for learning and his energy for diverse experiences and work. He held doctorates in three major subjects—theology, philosophy, and medicine—and was a gifted organist and world authority on Bach. Schweitzer was not a philosopher of the abstract variety. He wrote many times that "he lived his argument," and his actions certainly prove this. He is one of the great humanitarians of the twentieth century. His biography reveals a man willing to stand up for his convictions for the sake of his patients and for humanity (Brabazon, 2000).

Let us turn now to everyday people who demonstrated the moral courage that many lacked during World War II.

Lessons From the Holocaust Rescuers

The three "participant" categories of the Holocaust are commonly identified as murderers, victims, and bystanders. But there were also rescuers, as discussed in *Rescuers: Portraits of Moral Courage in the Holocaust* (Block & Drucker, 1992). These courageous individuals provide firsthand accounts that help us understand an unfathomable time, that give us a sense of what it felt like to live under a brutal government or occupation. For *Rescuers,* Rabbi Malka Drucker interviewed 21 individuals who rescued from a few to hundreds of Jews from the death camps. What character traits did these individuals share? They showed compassion, empathy, an intolerance of injustice, and an ability to endure risk beyond what any of us can or wants to imagine. Just as we cannot forget the Holocaust, we must never forget those courageous individuals whose humanity transcended it.

Despite the diverse background of the rescuers, they shared one significant characteristic. Drucker stated "it wasn't so much that I was in the presence of exceptionally virtuous 'good' people; in fact, they were quite ordinary people" (http://www.malkadrucker.com/right.html). It was more what Eva Fogleman has described as "the ability to transcend fear . . . and the ability to tolerate risk." As one rescuer said when asked if she had been afraid, "At such times it is normal to be afraid." Once the rescuers knew what was happening to the Jews, they felt compelled to help. Chapters 2 and 3 will discuss how to increase our tolerance of fear and to become better risk takers.

Most of the rescuers objected to being seen as heroes or saints. They saw themselves as people called to do what was right. They saw what the necessary moral action was, and they helped young and old survive. Today, they can stand as a reminder to all of us to ask ourselves, "For what moral issue will I stand up and be counted?"

Barack Obama: A Politician With Moral Courage

In July 2004, Barack Obama electrified the Democratic National Convention with a speech that spoke to the hearts of citizens across United States. He spoke with optimism about our future, an optimism he called the "audacity of hope." Today, as we listen to his presidential speeches, we begin to believe that maybe, just maybe, we can again believe in goodness of America.

Like Plato, President Obama believes in public service. He spent years quietly toiling in Chicago's inner city, helping churches and underfunded community groups deliver services to the poor. And although he was elected the first African-American President of the *Harvard Law Review* in the journal's 104-year-history, he opted to turn down prestigious judicial clerkships and high-paying law firm jobs to return to Chicago to advocate for the poor and disenfranchised. To me, that spoke volumes about his commitment to public service. He received the education necessary to turn a talented person into a leading citizen. He, like Socrates, believes that an "unexamined life is not worth living." One need only read *Dreams from My Father* (2004) and *Audacity of Hope* (2006) to see the depth of his critical self-reflection.

Like Nightingale, President Obama has a sense of mission and a sense of commitment to social justice. In the *Republic,* Plato sketches the attributes of those who would lead a perfect political community. His "philosopher kings" are empowered to make decisions in the best interests of the community on the basis of reason, understanding of the common good, and a lifetime of gathering information through learning. According to Plato, the true political function is that of a guardian. Both Nightingale and Obama have shown a strong sense of duty to society and a fervor for reform. For both, it was not enough to know what was the good and right thing to do. Like Aristotle, they saw a need to put their beliefs into action. As I review Socrates' actions in Athens, Nightingale's letters to Sidney Herbert from the Crimea, and Obama's Web site messages, it is clear that they believe they were put on the planet for a greater service to God (LeVasseur, 1998; Vicinus & Nergaard, 1990; Obama, 2007a). The role of the Platonic guardian is to know the good and make proper decisions with all things considered. I believe our nation is now desperate for such a guardian.

But, specifically to the point of this book, what is Obama's plan for health care? It is both a plan for the United States and a plan for global action. It is not unlike Nightingale's plan for Britain and other parts of the world. Take one example. During Nightingale's life, sanitation issues stood front stage; today, the AIDS pandemic is a key issue in world health. Forty million people across the planet are infected with HIV/AIDS. Obama plans to create a National Health Insurance Exchange and to be a global leader in the fight against AIDS. The exchange is part of a larger program to provide all Americans with health insurance and improved health care.

As he said in a Speech in Iowa City on May 29, 2007:

> *We now face an opportunity—and an obligation—to turn the page on the failed politics of yesterday's health care debates . . . My plan begins by covering every American. If you already have health insurance, the only thing that will change for you under this plan is the amount of money you will spend on premiums. That will be less. If you are one of the 45 million Americans who don't have health insurance, you will have it after this plan becomes law. No one will be turned away because of a preexisting condition or illness (Obama, 2007b).*

But Barack Obama more generally epitomizes moral courage by acknowledging the multiple moral problems in which we find ourselves rather than turning away from them. What makes him morally courageous is that his behavior is consistent with his beliefs regardless of public opinion. He stood among only 22 of 100 senators in opposition to the decision to authorize the Iraq war. He sees the need for America to stand and accept the greatest responsibility to lead in the arena of environmental policy, as we are the world's largest producer of greenhouse gases. Like the Holocaust rescuers, he is motivated in his actions by justice and compassion. He has demonstrated Plato's cardinal virtues. He believes, as Aristotle did, that we must practice using courage and demonstrate this virtue to our young. He is not only a role model for African-American children, but for all children. He is facing the moral dilemmas—the question is will he be able to seize that moment and begin the world anew.

Conclusion

Moral courage is a virtue; a virtue that puts into action the reasoning and wisdom acquired through education and experience. We need to ask ourselves the penetrating questions Socrates would ask. We need to recognize our fears without letting them stop us from being the patient advocates we are obligated to be as healthcare professionals. The next five chapters focus on developing the skills healthcare professionals and administrators need to "speak up" for our patients, for our community, and for the changes needed in our healthcare system.

Key Points to Remember

1. Our discussion of moral courage begins with the founding fathers of philosophy—Socrates, Plato, and Aristotle. All three argue that education is the key to shaping an individual's character.
2. Socrates and his discussion partners determined that physical acts without the knowledge of good and bad (morality) can never be courageous.
3. Courage is one of the four cardinal virtues in the lasting tradition of moral character described by Plato.
4. Aristotle further refined his view of courage by focusing not on cardinal virtues, but on virtue of thought and virtue of character.
5. Martin Luther King, Jr., displayed both moral and physical courage as he died fighting for the moral principles in which he believed.
6. Nightingale's use of her talents, education, and connections to crusade for healthcare reform points to a broad political function concerned with a societal good.
7. Schweitzer spoke about the importance of nurturing the human spirit so that humanity will have the moral courage to stand up against war.
8. Holocaust rescuers saw themselves as people called to do what was right.
9. President Obama has a sense of mission and a sense of commitment to social justice.
10. Moral courage is a virtue that puts into action the reasoning and wisdom acquired through education and experience.

References

Aristotle. (trans. 1954). *Nichomachean ethics*. Ross, D. (Trans.). London: Oxford University Press.

Block, G., & Drucker, M. (1992). *Rescuers: Portraits of moral courage in the holocaust*. Teaneck, NJ: Holmes & Meier. Retrieved June 3, 2008, from http://www.holocaustrescuers.com

Brabazon, J. (2000). *Albert Schweitzer: A biography*, 2d ed. Syracuse, NY: Syracuse University Press.

Calabria, M.D., & Macrae, J.A. (Eds.) (1994). *Suggestions for thought by Florence Nightingale: Selections and commentaries*. Philadelphia: University of Pennsylvania Press.

Dossey, B., Selanders, L.C., Beck, D.M., & Attewell, A. (2004). *Florence Nightingale today: Healing, leadership, global action*. Silver Spring, MD: American Nurses Publishing.

Ives, D., & Valone, D.A. (2007). *Reverence for life revisited: Albert Schweitzer's relevance today*. Cambridge: Cambridge Scholars Publishing.

Kant, I. (1788/1996). *Practical philosophy*. Gregor, M.J. (Trans./Ed.) New York: Cambridge University Press.

King, M.L. (1963). *I have a dream* (speech). Retrieved June 3, 2008, from http://www.school formoralcourage.com/kingdream.html

LeVasseur, J. (1998). Plato, Nightingale, and contemporary nursing. *Journal of Nursing Scholarship, 30*(3), 281–285.

Obama, B. (2007a). *Barack Obama on faith*. Retrieved June 3, 2008, from http://www.barack obama.com/pdf/ObamaonFaith.pdf

Obama, B. (2007b). *Plan for healthy America* (speech). Retrieved June 3, 2008, from http://www .barackobama.com/issues/healthcare/

Obama, B. (2006). *The audacity of hope*. New York: Crown Publishing.

Obama, B. (2004). *Dreams from my father*. New York: Crown Publishing.

Plato (trans. 2004) (trans.) *Laches*. Jowett, B. (Trans.). Retrieved June 3, 2008, from http://www .classicreader.com/booktoc.php/sid.8/bookid.2084/

Plato (trans. 2004) *The Republic*. Jowett, B. (Trans). Retrieved June 3, 2008, from http://www .constitution.org/pla/republic.htm

Roberts, R. (1984). Will power and the virtues. *Philosophical Review, 93*(2), 227–247.

Schweitzer, A. (1954). *Nobel Prize acceptance speech*. Retrieved June 2, 2008, from http:// nobelprize.org/nobel_prizes/peace/laureates/1952/schweitzer-lecture-e.html

Vicinus, M., & Nergaard, B. (Eds.) (1990). *Ever yours, Florence Nightingale: Selected letters*. Boston: Harvard University Press.

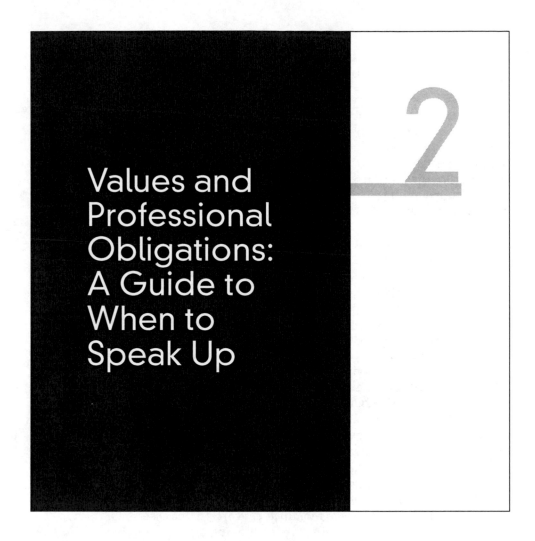

Values and Professional Obligations: A Guide to When to Speak Up

The best way to speak the truth is to know it clearly, believe it implicitly, love it sincerely, live it courageously, and proclaim it zealously.
　　　　　　　—Clifton J. Allen, author of numerous books on the Bible

A key component of the moral compass for healthcare professionals is the code of ethics that each field has created for its practitioners. These codes contain concrete principles and guidelines that create a nonnegotiable contract of ethical behavior between healthcare professionals and the society they serve.

This chapter presents four of these codes, including a summary of the explicit and implicit similarities in all. Based on this review, 12 ethical obligations clearly apply to all healthcare professionals across all fields. To fulfill these obligations, healthcare professionals have the responsibilities outlined that follows.

Values and Values Clarification

Values are the concepts, ideals, and significant themes that give meaning to our personal lives. They evolve from a person's life experiences and are shaped by family, education, religious beliefs, occupation, gender, culture, political orientation, and social system. We internalize these values into a pattern of behavior that reflects our attitudes toward people and ideas. Based on these values, we express and stand up for what we believe to be true. In some situations, however, fear can interfere with our ability to choose freely from our established values—pressuring us to espouse a cause in which we do believe to protect ourselves from such consequences as conflict with superiors at work or school.

Values are organized into hierarchical structures. This ordering across a continuum reflects the importance of the values. When one value (for example, honesty) competes with another value (for example, caring), the individual must determine which outranks the other; in other words, which is more important? The level of commitment to a value is measured by the allocation of time, energy, and resources necessary to support the value. To ensure that a person consciously chooses a value rather than simply accepts the values of family or profession, the individual needs to engage in values clarification.

Values clarification makes us conscious of our values and the underlying motivations that guide our actions. It is a process that involves choosing, prizing, and acting. Personal values guide our decisions, whether we are aware of them or not. Therefore, if our actions are to flow from our words, we must take the time to examine if we are living life in the way we truly value.

When inconsistencies between our value system and our actions occurs, known as a dissonance, it needs to be resolved. For example, a nurse who values his family above all other values is required to work because of a disaster. As a result, his sick child has to remain at daycare. In this case, the nurse is likely to experience an internal conflict. After this incident is over, he may further clarify his values by considering if he should change jobs to avoid the situation in the future or make alternative plans for his family's care in a way that satisfies his values. The answers at the end of values clarification are not right or wrong. Rather, they are resolutions of any conflicts experienced by that individual.

Professionals must always be conscious of their personal values, which may sometimes be in conflict with the professional values of their discipline or other referent groups. For example, a physician assistant who believes in telling a patient the truth (honesty) may be in conflict with the supervising physician, who consistently avoids giving bad news by being overly optimistic about a patient's prognosis. Another example is a physical therapist who places a high value on educating patients to prevent reoccurrences of low back pain, but finds that he or she is practicing in a facility that earns its money mainly by managing such pain.

Although nurses are taught to focus on the entire patient as a holistic being, they often work in institutions that emphasize the medical model of specialization, which focuses on the patient's specific problem or complaint. This becomes especially problematic in an understaffed hospital or agency, where the focus tends to shift toward task completion. In this situation, a nurse can experience both a personal and professional value conflict because he or she is not meeting the responsibilities outlined in the Code of Ethics for Nurses (American Nurses Association, 2001).

Professional Codes of Ethics

A major responsibility of professional organizations is to create and execute a code of ethics that guides the profession in regulating the conduct of its members. Codes are part of a profession's commitment to the society it serves. Such codes define expected behaviors and responsibilities, thereby providing a set of benchmarks by which members can evaluate their own professional conduct. They also guide the professional development of all students.

The Code often requires a higher level of ethical behavior than is specified in the legal requirements for the profession, which are usually seen in the regulatory requirements of state boards. Professional licensing boards protect the health, safety, and welfare of the public from fraudulent and unethical practitioners.

American College of Healthcare Executives

The American College of Healthcare Executives (ACHE) also has several ethical polices, covering such issues as ethical decision making for executives and how to create an ethical environment for employees. Two of the eight code guidelines require that executives demonstrate the importance of ethics to the organization through their professional behavior and by supporting organizational mechanisms for ethical resolution of conflicts (American College of Healthcare Executives, 2007). Chapter 13, which focuses on executive leadership, offers an in-depth discussion of this Code of Ethics.

Medical Code of Ethics: Historical Background

The Code of Hammurabi was the first known code of laws; it covered all professions, including for physicians. Because it was specific to the Babylonian culture of the eighteenth century BC, it is not practical for today's society. However, the Hippocratic Oath, which dates from the fourth to fifth century BC, has survived. That oath, which physicians still take on graduation from medical school, sets out general principles to protect the patient. Its distinctive features emphasize beneficence toward the patient, the physician's obligation to maintain competence, and practices to limit admission to the profession to qualified individuals (Hippocrates, trans. 1964).

Maintaining the tradition of Hippocrates and subsequent Greek philosophers, the profession of medicine has allied itself with the values of the Christian, Jewish, and Islamic religions, as well as many smaller religious groups. As such, the physician is seen as an instrument of God's power to heal. In addition to prayer, for example, the medieval rabbi-physician Maimonides suggested that a close connection existed between health and obedience to God by following the ten commandments. One had to be physically healthy to follow God's commandments, for it was "impossible during sickness to have any understanding or knowledge of the Creator." In fact, the Talmud, seeking to sustain the spiritual connection between God and humans, prohibited Jews from living in a city without a physician (Burns, 1977).

In 1803, an English physician named Thomas Percival published his *Code of Medical Ethics,* which focused on virtues, such as temperance and professional etiquette (Leake, 1927). At its first meeting in 1847, the American Medical Association (AMA) adopted a code of ethics based primarily on Percival's code. In broad terms, the code remained the same until the beginning of the twenty-first century.

The Judicial Council of the AMA, which is now called the Council on Ethical and Judicial Affairs, is the body responsible for the *Code of Medical Ethics.* This code contains the statement of core principles and "current opinions," which include the application of specific ethical issues along with reports on these issues. The most recent revision was in 2001, and the principles in this code can be seen in Exhibit 2.1 (American Medical Association, 2001).

The most significant changes in principles from the 1980 AMA Code to the 2001 Code are the following added comments:

1. Change to II. "That physician must uphold the standards of the profession and report physicians not meeting these standards to the appropriate entities."
2. Added to V. "maintain a commitment to medical education"
3. Added to VII. "improvement of community and betterment of public health"
4. Added "A physician shall, while caring for a patient, regard responsibility to the patient as paramount."
5. Added "A physician shall support access to medical care for all."

These changes support lifelong learning, betterment of public health, access to medical care for all, and support for standards that place the patient at the center of a physician's concerns.

Professional Nursing Ethical Codes

The creation of nursing ethics is generally credited to Florence Nightingale and the nursing ideals embodied in her Nightingale Pledge. Although this pledge is often quoted to signify the requirement that nurses obey the instructions of physicians, Nightingale never called for blind obedience. Her primary consideration was always the needs of the patient. Since the 1970s, the focus of medical and nursing codes has shifted from an emphasis on the final authority and power of the physician to client advocacy, which emphasizes the autonomy of the patient.

Although the International Council for Nurses (ICN) revised its *Code of Ethics for Nurses* in 2005 (published in 2006), the essence of the original document remained untouched. Primary changes include the addition of a new major element to the code, entitled "Nurses and Society," along with several sentences focusing specifically on this topic in other areas of the code. The phrase "research-based" was also added to the nurse's responsibility to continue acquiring professional knowledge. The most significant change was the inclusion of a helpful section at the end on how to help nurse practitioners, managers, educators, and researchers integrate the code into practice. All of the changes in language and format help the reader to understand the ethical obligations of nurses. As I found nothing in this document that was not also in the ANA Code, the focus here will remain on the ANA Code.

The original *Code of Ethics for Nurses* was developed in 1950, revised in 1976, 1985 and then again in 2001. This present Code with the interpretative state-

2.1 Principles of Medical Ethics

Preamble

The medical profession has long subscribed to a body of ethical statements developed primarily for the benefit of the patient. As a member of this profession, a physician must recognize responsibility to patients first and foremost, as well as to society, to other health professionals, and to self. The following Principles adopted by the American Medical Association are not laws, but standards of conduct which define the essentials of honorable behavior for the physician.

Principles of medical ethics

I.   A physician shall be dedicated to providing competent medical care, with compassion and respect for human dignity and rights.

II. A physician shall uphold the standards of professionalism, be honest in all professional interactions, and strive to report physicians deficient in character or competence, or engaging in fraud or deception, to appropriate entities.

III. A physician shall respect the law and also recognize a responsibility to seek changes in those requirements which are contrary to the best interests of the patient.

IV. A physician shall respect the rights of patients, colleagues, and other health professionals, and shall safeguard patient confidences and privacy within the constraints of the law.

V.   A physician shall continue to study, apply, and advance scientific knowledge, maintain a commitment to medical education, make relevant information available to patients, colleagues, and the public, obtain consultation, and use the talents of other health professionals when indicated.

VI. A physician shall, in the provision of appropriate patient care, except in emergencies, be free to choose whom to serve, with whom to associate, and the environment in which to provide medical care.

VII. A physician shall recognize a responsibility to participate in activities contributing to the improvement of the community and the betterment of public health.

VIII. A physician shall, while caring for a patient, regard responsibility to the patient as paramount.

IX. A physician shall support access to medical care for all people.

Reprinted with permission from American Medical Association. (2001). *Code of medical ethics*, Chicago, IL: AMA. Retrieved July 1, 2008, from http://www.ama-assn.org/ama/pub/category/2512.html

ments can be seen in Exhibit 2.2. The emphasis on client advocacy and caring remains a central focus of this Code.

Physical Therapist Code of Ethics

This *Guide for Professional Conduct* (Guide), shown in Exhibit 2.3, was written to help physical therapists understand the Code of Ethics (Code) of the American Physical Therapy Association, particularly in matters of professional behavior (American Physical Therapy Association, 2004). This Guide is subject to

2.2 Code of Ethics for Nurses With Interpretive Statements (2001)

Nine Provisions With Interpretive Statements

1. The nurse, in all professional relationships, practices with compassion and respect for the inherent dignity, worth, and uniqueness of every individual, unrestricted by considerations of social or economic status, personal attributes, or the nature of health problems.
   - Respect for human dignity
   - Relationships to patients
   - The nature of health problems
   - The right to self-determination
   - Relationships with colleagues and others
2. The nurses' primary commitment is to the patient, whether an individual, family, group, or community.
   - Privacy of the patient's interest
   - Conflict of interest for nurses
   - Collaboration
   - Professional boundaries
3. The nurse promotes, advocates for, and strives to protect the health, safety, and rights of the patient.
   - Privacy
   - Confidentiality
   - Protection of participants in research
   - Standards and review mechanisms
   - Acting on questionable practice
   - Addressing impaired practice
4. The nurse is responsible and accountable for individual nursing practice and determines the appropriate delegation of tasks consistent with the nurse's obligation to provide optimum patient care.
   - Acceptance of accountability and responsibility
   - Accountability for nursing judgment and action
   - Responsibility for nursing judgment and action
   - Delegation of nursing activities
5. The nurse owes the same duties to self as to others, including the responsibility to preserve integrity and safety and to maintain competence, and to continue personal and professional growth.
   - Moral self-respect
   - Professional growth and maintenance of competency
   - Wholeness of character
   - Preservation of integrity
6. The nurse participates in establishing, maintaining, and improving health care environments and conditions of employment conducive to the provision of quality health care and consistent with the values of the profession through individual and collective action.
   - Influence of the environment on moral virtues and values
   - Influence of the environment on ethical obligations
   - Responsibility for the health care environment

2.2 **Continued**

7. The nurse participates in the advancement of the profession through contributions to practice, education, administration, and knowledge development.
   - Advancing the profession through active involvement in nursing and in health care policy
   - Advancing the profession by developing, maintaining, and implementing professional standards in clinical, administrative, and educational practice
   - Advancing the profession through knowledge development, dissemination, and application to practice
8. The nurse collaborates with other health professionals and the public in promoting community, national, and international efforts to meet health needs.
   - Health needs and concerns
   - Responsibilities to the public
9. The profession of nursing, as represented by associations and their members, is responsible for articulating nursing values, for maintaining the integrity of the profession and its practice, and for shaping social policy.
   - Assertion of values
   - The profession carries out its collective responsibility through professional associations
   - Intraprofessional integrity
   - Social reform

Reprinted with permission from American Nurses Association (ANA). (2001). *Code for ethics for nurses with interpretative statements.* Silver Spring, MD: American Nurses Publishing. Retrieved July 5, 2008, from http://www.nursingworld.org

monitoring and timely revision by the Ethics and Judicial Committee of the association, as is the AMA code.

Physician Assistant Code of Ethical Conduct

The physician assistant (PA) profession has revised its code of ethics several times. However, the fundamental principles underlying the ethical care of patients have not changed. Four bioethical principles directed the development of these guidelines: autonomy, beneficence, nonmaleficence, and justice. The "Statement of Values" within this document defines the fundamental values that the PA profession strives to uphold. These values provide the foundation on which the guidelines rest (see Exhibit 2.4) (American Academy of Physician Assistants, 2007).

Obligations Existing Across All the Codes for Healthcare Professionals

Codes are nonnegotiable contracts that healthcare professionals have with the general public. They represent an understanding of the practitioners' commitment

2.3 Code of Ethics of the American Physical Therapy Association

PREAMBLE

This Code of Ethics of the American Physical Therapy Association sets forth principles for the ethical practice of physical therapy. All physical therapists are responsible for maintaining and promoting ethical practice. To this end, the physical therapist shall act in the best interest of the patient/client. This Code of Ethics shall be binding on all physical therapists.

PRINCIPLE 1
A physical therapist shall respect the rights and dignity of all individuals and shall provide compassionate care.

PRINCIPLE 2
A physical therapist shall act in a trustworthy manner towards patients/clients, and in all other aspects of physical therapy practice.

PRINCIPLE 3
A physical therapist shall comply with laws and regulations governing physical therapy and shall strive to effect changes that benefit patients/clients.

PRINCIPLE 4
A physical therapist shall exercise sound professional judgment.

PRINCIPLE 5
A physical therapist shall achieve and maintain professional competence.

PRINCIPLE 6
A physical therapist shall maintain and promote high standards for physical therapy practice, education, and research.

PRINCIPLE 7
A physical therapist shall seek only such remuneration as is deserved and reasonable for physical therapy services.

PRINCIPLE 8
A physical therapist shall provide and make available accurate and relevant information to patients/clients about their care and to the public about physical therapy services.

PRINCIPLE 9
A physical therapist shall protect the public and the profession from unethical, incompetent, and illegal acts.

PRINCIPLE 10
A physical therapist shall endeavor to address the health needs of society.

PRINCIPLE 11
A physical therapist shall respect the rights, knowledge, and skills of colleagues and other health care professionals.

Reprinted with permission from American Physical Therapy Association. (2004). *Code of ethics and guide for professional conduct.* Retrieved June 4, 2008, from http://www.apta.org/AM/Template.cfm ?Section=Ethics_and_Legal_Issues1&Template=/TaggedPage/TaggedPageDisplay.cfm&TPLID =48&ContentID=41162

2.4 Physician Assistant Statement of Values

AAPA Guidelines for Ethical Conduct for the PA Profession

Statement of Values of the PA Profession

1. PAs hold as their primary responsibility the health, safety, welfare, and dignity of all human beings.
2. PAs uphold the tenets of patient autonomy, beneficence, nonmaleficence, and justice.
3. PAs recognize and promote the value of diversity.
4. PAs treat all persons who seek care equally.
5. PAs hold in confidence the information shared in the course of practicing medicine.
6. PAs assess their personal capabilities and limitations, striving always to improve their medical practice.
7. PAs actively seek to expand their knowledge and skills, keeping abreast of advances in medicine.
8. PAs work with other members of the healthcare team to provide compassionate and effective care of patients.
9. PAs use their knowledge and experience to contribute to improvement in the community.
10. PAs respect their professional relationship with physicians.
11. PAs share and expand knowledge within the profession.

Reprinted with permission of American Academy of Physician Assistants (2007). *Guidelines for ethical conduct for physician assistants*. Retrieved June 4, 2008, from http://www.aapa.org/manual/22 .EthicalConduct.pdf

to society. I have examined all the codes mentioned and found twelve similarities, either explicit or implied. The following are succinct statements of these shared ethical obligations.

1. Respect for the human dignity and rights of each individual.
2. Responsibility to the patient is supreme.
3. Duty to maintain confidentiality.
4. Honesty in all interactions.
5. Report illegal or unethical practice to appropriate authorities.
6. Seek changes in polices and laws that oppose the best interests of the patient.
7. Commitment to lifelong learning and evidence-based practice.
8. Advance the profession through knowledge development.
9. Collaborate with other healthcare professionals.
10. Participate in activities that improve the health of the community, nation, and world.
11. Right to free and informed choice; right to self-determination.
12. Compassionate care toward patient.

We can now begin to determine what responsibilities these individuals must assume to meet these 12 ethical obligations. Our most important conversations with patients, family members, and each other will focus on these responsibilities.

They are the crux of the examples used throughout this book, because, in many instances, speaking out about these requirements will necessitate moral courage. It is our duty to protect a patient's rights and advocate for them. Below is a list of the 11 duties that I believe evolve from these obligations:

1. Honor a patient's advance directive, even when the family threatens legal sanctions.
2. Provide palliative care for all patients at end-of-life, regardless of their location in healthcare system.
3. Only share information about a patient with those who have "a need to know."
4. Do not allow incompetent healthcare professionals to care for patients, regardless of the cause of their incompetence.
5. Develop and implement evidence-based protocols to improve the efficiency, effectiveness, and safety of patient care, as well as to increase the empowerment of front-line healthcare professionals.
6. Conduct and/or participate in quality improvement and/or research and write about findings to increase knowledge of best practices.
7. Assertively communicate and cooperate with all members of the interdisciplinary team as if the patient's life depended on it.
8. Compassionately tell the truth to all patients and/or their families about diagnosis, prognosis, and treatment alternatives to assure informed consent.
9. Continuously improve professional's expertise by engaging in lifelong learning.
10. Be involved in activities that support the health of the human race at local, national, and/or global levels.
11. If a patient's rights (e.g., confidentiality, informed consent) are being violated and resolution is not possible with the individuals involved or through present organizational systems, then call an ethics consultant. If patient rights are still being violated, report to an outside regulatory or licensing body.

These obligations and duties will be repeatedly referenced throughout this book. The professional code for each discipline is nonnegotiable. It is a compact healthcare professionals have made with society, and these obligations must be met through moral courage.

Conclusion

Values clarification makes us aware of which values guide our actions. It is an ongoing process involving choosing, prizing, and acting on values. However, when you enter a profession, there may be obligations and duties outlined in the relevant code of ethics that are counter to your personal values and beliefs. In these situations, you need to engage in values clarification.

The four codes in this chapter have more similarities than differences and result in the summary of 11 professional responsibilities listed above. These obligations guide all healthcare professionals to the required actions necessary to advocate for the patient. To act on values and speak out against unethical conduct, a healthcare professional must know his or her obligations. As Aristotle said, education helps reasoning, and action is necessary when one knows the moral action to take. The next chapter focuses on how to soothe one's internal fears to facilitate behavior that reflects moral courage.

Key Points to Remember

1. Values are the concepts, ideals, and significant themes that give meaning to our personal lives. Based on these values, we express and stand up for what we believe to be true.
2. Values clarification makes us conscious of our values and the underlying motivations that guide our actions.
3. Although nurses are taught to focus on the entire patient as a holistic being, they often work in institutions that emphasize the medical model of specialization, which focuses on the patient's specific problem or complaint.
4. A major responsibility of professional organizations is to create and execute a code of ethics that guides the profession in regulating the conduct of its members.
5. Since the 1970s, the focus of medical and nursing codes has changed from an emphasis on the final authority and power of the physician to client advocacy, which emphasizes the autonomy of the patient.

References

American Academy of Physician Assistants. (2007). *Guidelines for ethical conduct for physician assistants.* Retrieved June 4, 2008, from http://www.aapa.org/manual/23-EthicalConduct.pdf

American College of Healthcare Executives. (2007). *Ethical decision making for healthcare executives.* Retrieved July 1, 2008, from http://www.ache.org/policy/decision.cfm

American Medical Association. (2001). *Code of medical ethics.* Chicago, IL: AMA. Retrieved July 1, 2008, from http://www.ama-assn.org/ama/pub/category/2512.html

American Nurses Association (ANA). (2001). *Code for ethics for nurses with interpretative statements.* Silver Spring, MD: American Nurses Publishing. Retrieved July 5, 2008, from http://www.nursingworld.org

American Physical Therapy Association. (2004). *Code of ethics and guide for professional conduct.* Retrieved June 4, 2008, from http://www.apta.org/AM/Template.cfm?Section=Ethics_and_Legal_Issues1&Template=/TaggedPage/TaggedPageDisplay.cfm&TPLID=48&ContentID=41162

Burns, C.R. (1977). *Legacies in ethics and medicine.* New York: Neale Watson Academic Publications.

Hippocrates. (1964). *The theory and practice of medicine.* New York: Philosophical Library.

The International Council for Nurses (ICN). (2006). *Code of ethics for nurses.* Retrieved June 4, 2008, from http://www.icn.ch/icncode.pdf

Leake, C. (1927). *Percival's medical ethics.* Baltimore, MD: Williams and Wilkins.

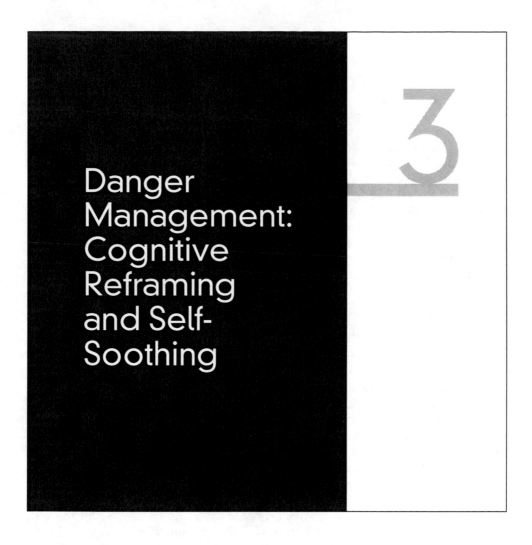

Danger Management: Cognitive Reframing and Self-Soothing

3

Freedom is what you do with what's been done to you.
—Jean-Paul Sartre, French writer and philosopher

Case 3.1

Susan, a registered nurse (RN), and Howard, a physical therapist (PT), have been arguing at the nursing station over the treatment of a stroke patient. As their voices become louder, they realize they are not acting professionally. Howard attempts resolution first by taking a deep breath (self-soothing), recognizing that he has gotten into an either/or stance (cognitive reframing), and says, "I am sorry. Can we start over in our discussion about the strategy to care for Mr. Anders?" Susan realizes that she is raising her voice because she believes the young PT is trying "to boss her around" (her story). She accepts Howard's invitation to start the conversation over because she realizes there are multiple ways to resolve the problem (cognitive reframing).

To demonstrate moral courage, you need to have many kinds of crucial conversations about patients. In fact, in *Crucial Conversations,* the authors define these discussions about tough issues. According to the authors, these conversations have three components: (1) opinions differ, (2) stakes are high, and (3) emotions are strong (Patterson, Grenny, McMillian, & Switzler, 2002). Examples of these dialogs are giving a supervisor feedback about his or her controlling behavior, talking to a team member who violated patient safety standards, or talking with a physician who is notoriously abusive. All of these are potentially dangerous situations. The results of these conversations could have a huge impact on a person's professional and personal life. In this and subsequent chapters, I will provide strategies for standing up and speaking up in these crucial conversations that require moral courage. I will begin with an overview on how the mind processes difficult situations, with a special focus on the many ways that your perception of events influences your conduct.

How the Mind Processes Difficult Situations

To cope effectively with the stress of a difficult situation, you must acknowledge your feeling of fear, but still act rationally. For example, well-trained professionals will not yell at patients, students, or staff when they make mistakes, even though those errors could cause injury to themselves or others. Although you have a right to be scared and even angry at their behavior, you fulfill your responsibility to uphold policies and standards by dealing assertively, but professionally, with the problem. Learning danger management strategies enables you deal with the stress of the situation by choosing an appropriate response, rather than by reacting emotionally.

You should remember that stress is not what happens to you, but the way you handle what happens to you (Greenberg, 2006; Olpin, Hesson, & Cole, 2006). For one person, a difficult problem may be an exciting challenge, whereas another may find it a terrifying threat. Your interpretation of an event determines whether you experience anxiety (stress) or excitement. Between stimulus and response, there is always a space. In that space, you have the freedom to choose your response.

The perceptual and cognitive functions of your brain determine how you perceive an event. Suppose, for example, you had some difficult interactions with a resident physician because he has not been managing a patient's pain effectively. After this resident walks by without saying hello, the patient's attending physician asks to see you because of a problem. The way you interpret these events could create an anticipatory stress reaction. If, for example, you think the call means the attending physician is displeased with you, you are likely to trigger your fear or anger response. If, on the other hand, you take these events to mean that the attending physician must be preoccupied with last-minute preparations for a conference and actually wants to discuss the poster you are presenting together, you will not experience stress. Your choice of response to any event depends on what you perceive and how you interpret your perception.

Your perception of patients, colleagues, executives, and physicians affects how you relate to them. Remember the example of the nurse who viewed the PT as being "bossy." If you see physicians as unfeeling, your colleagues as passive, executives as out of touch with realities of practice, and the patient with pain as demanding, then you will relate to them with those adjectives screening incoming data. Because you tend to screen out all data that do not fit "your descriptive adjectives," you begin to make certain decisions about these people. These decisions are based on your perception of them as interpreted through these screens, or frames.

Frames are cognitive timesavers that help make sense of complex information. They help us comprehend the world around us through selective simplification. As such, frames profoundly affect how we perceive and understand the world. They help us control multifaceted phenomena by dividing them into logical and comprehensible categories. These frames of reference are often subconscious. Therefore, we see problems and delineate solutions based on these underlying cognitive structures often without an awareness of what motivates our decisions. Because our frames are built on individual beliefs, values, and experiences, other people may often build frames that significantly differ from yours.

When emotions affect these frames of reference, your perception can become distorted. You may distort the importance of patient problems by minimizing or maximizing the situation. In our opening example, Susan realized that she was maximizing potential problems with the PT's recommendations because of the recent death of a patient. What you perceive depends on your senses and your frame of reference; how you interpret the data depends on your value system and your cognitive processes. Cognitive processes involve thinking, decision making, and problem-solving. Your perception affects your professional judgment—therefore, some understanding of perception and the ways it interacts with emotions is important.

Perception Principles

Exhibit 3.1 lists the principles of perception. Although many more recent articles exist, no one has summarized these principles better than Kolivosky and Taylor (1973). These principles profoundly affect your perception and, therefore, your response in a difficult situation.

As you can see, a number of variables affect why you see, hear, and experience what you do. These variables also affect your behavior. For instance, if your self-image is negative, you would be likely to interpret criticism more harshly than if your self-image is positive. Your behavior would be defensive, since criticism is threatening to your already low self-esteem. Your image of yourself affects how you relate to others.

Unsatisfactory relationships with others are a major source of stress. Therefore, an important stress-reduction technique requires that you become aware of how your perceptions of yourself and others create communication problems. Begin to notice peoples' different perceptions. Notice how your own perceptions vary with your moods. The need to be "right" in your perceptions of others is often the cause of communication difficulties (Patterson et al., 2002).

Finally, perceptions are the mainspring of motivation. If you have not spoken up about a patient safety issue, your attention will return to this uncompleted task. Your obsession will motivate you to complete the assignment, as

3.1 Perception Principles

No two people see things the same way.

A person's self-image influences how he or she sees the world.

A person's image of the other colors his or her relationship with the other.

A person sees things in terms of his or her own past experiences.

A person sees things differently at different times.

A person learns to see things as he or she does.

A person sees things in terms of his or her own values.

A person tends to see things largely as they were seen before.

A person sees what he or she wants to see.

A person's feelings color what he or she sees.

A person tends to complete those things which appear to be incomplete.

A person tends to either simplify or complicate those things that are not understood.

A person first sees an object as a general pattern, and then focuses attention on a particular part of it.

A person tends to remember the first and last items in a series of things.

A person learns new perceptions only through new experiences.

Reprinted with permission from Kolivosky, M.E. & Taylor, L.J. (1973). *Why do you see it that way? Principles of perception: Most applicable principles for guidelines in interpersonal relationships.* Hillsdale, MI: Hillsdale College, p. 12.

otherwise it will increase your level of distraction. It is difficult to deal with the present when your mind is on the past or future.

Your perception process is thus affected by numerous variables, only one of which is stress. Thinking about a problem is a complex process that begins with perception and ends with a decision. During times of stress, your mind may become confused or distracted. As a result, the natural process of perception, thinking, and reaching a decision is blocked. Many errors in thinking occur because this normal thought process is affected by emotions.

The authors of *Crucial Conversations* (2002) offer suggestions on how to gain control over your emotions and perceptions by understanding the story you create and how this affects your actions. This storytelling occurs so quickly that we may be unaware of it. These stories make a problem our fault or the other person's fault or may even lead us to conclude that we are powerless to change the situation at all. If we are to control our emotions, we need to control the stories we tell ourselves.

The authors of *Crucial Conversations* suggest a process for reversing the automatic path most people take. It begins with noticing behavior and then asking yourself if this behavior is going to achieve the outcome you desire. Most people justify their actions based on their stories. For example, you need to speak up about a problem, but justify your inaction by saying "it will do no good." In reversing this pattern, it becomes obvious that nothing will change if you remain silent. The authors help us focus on change by recommending that people ask themselves, "Am I in some form of silence or violence?" (Patterson et al., 2002).

Not speaking up and screaming at someone are just the flipside of each other. Neither will help motivate others to change behavior. Your story is often based on your perceptions and conclusions rather than on facts gained in dialog with the other person, a dialog in which a shared meaning of the situation can be created. There can be a number of cognitive distortions in your own thinking that falsely increase the perceived danger in a given situation.

Errors in Thinking

Albert Ellis (2001), the founder of a theory and therapy called rational emotive therapy, describes several common errors in thinking. Dr. David Burns, a protégé of Dr. Aaron Beck, is probably the best-known popular author on how to conquer these cognitive distortions (Burns, 1999). More recent authors (Attwood, 2007; Greenberg, 2006) echo this initial focus on changing these distortions, as they halt the action necessary for moral courage. Common errors in thinking include the following.

1. *Dichotomous thinking.* "I either work or stay home." This is either/or, black/white thinking. Your mind naturally does either/or thinking when you initially consider a problem, but critical thinking requires greater depth and breath. People who operate mainly in this mode are seen as inflexible; under stress, they attempt to screen out stimuli. This type of thinking accomplishes just that.
2. *Reliance on another's judgment.* "What you think about me or what you think is the right answer is more important than what I think." Sometimes this type of thinking is useful when dealing with authoritative types—such as police officers. Otherwise, recognize that others may dislike you or not agree with you for completely irrational reasons (e.g., because you remind them of someone). If "what will they think of me?" runs your life, you will be especially interested in the section on "guilt" later in this chapter.
3. *Overgeneralizing.* "All doctors are egomaniacs." "Nursing is a dead-end street." "University hospitals are the only place to work." Overgeneralizations are vague and indefinite. The hospital looks very different when you think all doctors do the best they can, rather than generalize negatively about them.
4. *Stereotyping.* "Pediatric nurses all love children," "Psychiatric nurses are all neurotic." Both of these statements create mental pictures. Stereotyping is fixing an image, either positive or negative, in your mind. "Category X persons are . . ." is the standard form of stereotyping. By stereotyping, you divide the world into categories, and each category is associated with a permanent set of qualities or characteristics. In the end, you respond to the category rather than to the individual or the situation. For instance, create a picture of a "hippie," a "drug user," and a "feminist"; each of these words create images in your mind. It is a very convenient way to deal with the world—you do not have to think. Ellis does not say this, but I suggest that overgeneralization leads to stereotyping. If you make vague, indefinite statements about someone or something long enough, you begin to believe it yourself.
5. *Catastrophizing.* "I made a medication error last week, I am obviously not cut out to be a nurse." "This day has started badly—the whole day will be terrible." Catastrophizing is viewing events as 100 percent bad.

These errors in thinking raise your stress level by preventing effective problem-solving. Remember that your perception and interpretation of events plays a large role in coping with stress. If you begin to notice how you perceive events, without a judgmental attitude, you will begin to unblock your perceptual apparatus. Observe yourself as you launch into one of your erroneous thinking patterns. The way to change these patterns is to become aware, stop your pattern when you notice it, and change it to a thinking pattern that focuses on the present situation and needs.

Other psychologists have called this the internal dialog or self-talk. When everything you say to yourself about yourself is negative, you believe you deserve to feel guilty. If you congratulate yourself for your successes and treat your mistakes as learning experiences, then your self-talk will be more positive.

"I am what I think I am" is the simple basis for the idea of positive self-talk. Saying to myself, "I am a coward," which is exactly the same thing as thinking I am coward, will create a self-image of cowardliness. I may then behave passively in fulfillment of this self-image. Through self-talk, you can become what you tell yourself you are, and you can become what you think you are.

This concept of negative self-talk can also be applied to a group of people, such as healthcare professionals, "We don't have the power to change the administration or the power to make a difference in how this country's healthcare system works. No, we are powerless. There is nothing we can do." This negative group self-talk is perpetuated when each member gives up trying to make a difference. Being willing to stand up and be heard comes from positive self-talk. Sound like a political rally? Perhaps it is—a rallying call for each healthcare professional to take charge of personal and professional power by changing the way he or she thinks about self-image.

Cognitive Reframing

Cognitive reframing consists of strategies to facilitate cognitive reorganization. This often involves confronting individuals with information different from, or at odds with, their expressed views, attitudes, or self-images. This is designed to provoke cognitive dissonance (Festinger, 1957). The fundamental idea behind cognitive dissonance theory is that people do not like to have discordant cognitions. As a result, when someone experiences two or more conflicting thoughts, the individual attempts to eliminate the dissonance. This gives us an opportunity for reframing and reorganizing the way we think.

The following example of cognitive distortions shows how they can lead to dysfunctional responses and symptoms. It also offers an illustration of the reframing process.

Stressor	Advance directive of terminally ill patient is being violated with PEG tube.
Distorted thought	If I speak up, I will not be heard and will be ridiculed for taking a stand.
Realistic thought	I will call the ethics committee to take a stand with me so that I am not the lone voice.

In this situation, the healthcare professional did not engage in "catastrophizing," but instead thought about what resources were available to help them take a stand. We have to reprogram ourselves and remember that it is not what happens to us that hurts us. In fact, our most difficult experiences become the crucibles that forge our character and develop our internal powers. It is the way we let the situation act on us, instead of acting to make the best of that situation, which leads to our downfall.

Psychological signs and symptoms block us from effective expression and action in issues requiring moral courage. They result from ineffective handling of one's emotions and distorted thinking patterns. In the case at the beginning of the chapter, both Howard and Susan were caught up in their emotional responses until they stepped back and saw the distortion in their thinking. Therefore, the ability to reframe how we look at a situation and self-soothe our emotional state becomes crucial. If we are looking at a situation through a black-or-white lens, we may choose an action based on fear rather logic. Danger management strategy requires that we gain control over our emotions.

Understanding and Coping With Emotions

Understanding and accepting your responses to situations in life is the crucial first step in managing danger. The second step is to recognize the methods that work best to keep your mind in a more relaxed thinking state. The third step is to consistently and repeatedly practice workable methods. Remember that changing mental response patterns is a lifelong learning process, a process that requires having patience with yourself.

Keep in mind that our stress response is actually the fight-or-flight response, which involves feelings of anger and fear. Both are legitimate feelings, but research has proved that with practice we can actually change our responses (Begley, 2007).

Anxiety as a Stress Symptom

Anxiety is the most prominent symptom of a stress reaction, as well as of psychosomatic disorders. An individual who experiences anxiety is so emotionally troubled that he or she is often unable to think clearly. Further, symptoms of anxiety are also associated with the other prominent psychological illness—depression.

Anxiety is not in itself pathological. In fact, to a certain extent, it is unavoidable. Anxiety is considered normal when its intensity and character are appropriate to a given situation (MacKay, Davis, & Fanning, 2007). A person can be more alert, sensitive, and perceptive about a situation when moderately anxious. People actually seek a rise in tension through movies, spy novels, and competitive sports. The key is that the anxiety must not be too intense or last too long.

The type of anxiety discussed in this chapter is not the pleasure of excitement, but the nervous tension you experience when responding to a threat, whether real or imagined. Your body may feel electrified with tension or tied in knots, as your muscles contract for fight or flight.

You experience anxiety when you see a need to assume an offensive or defensive position against a threat. In preparing for an anxious situation, you may rehearse the anticipated danger so that when it finally materializes, your response strategy is already in place. Healthcare professionals can surely remember instances in which anticipating a problem prevented you from being overwhelmed by a sense of helplessness or powerlessness.

Psychological symptoms occur when you become overwhelmed to some degree by anxiety, which is considered pathological when:

1. There is no adequate justification for the anxiety—when it is exaggerated, unduly prolonged, gives rise to defensive maneuvers that interfere seriously with the enjoyment and the effectiveness of your life (Lazarus & Folkman, 1984).
2. It is diffused in hyperactivity, is repressed, or causes you to lose spontaneity.
3. You engage in impulsive and aggressive acts.

All these behaviors will create some disorganization in your interpersonal relationships and usually require counseling.

In plain words, you experience some degree of anxiety when you are afraid. You may or may not know what you fear, but the degree of tension you experience determines your level of anxiety. In the case at the beginning of the chapter, both Susan and Howard were able to contain their anxiety and resolve their differences.

Anxiety affects your thinking in one of three ways.

1. Your mind feels as if it is racing—thoughts stream by so quickly you cannot concentrate on any one of them.
2. Your mind tries to follow a single thought, but you find yourself suddenly unable to complete the thought sequence. Your mind has reached a dead end, and either you cannot come to a conclusion or the conclusion does not seem sensible. This is called confusion.
3. You go blank. You were thinking (and sometimes you were talking) and all of a sudden, nothing—no words and no thoughts. Often, much to your embarrassment, you lose your train of thought, and your mind goes blank.

Whether your mind races, you get confused, or you go blank, anxiety is affecting your thinking. Any of these signs can be both a cause and effect of the stress you experience in a situation you labeled dangerous.

Anger and Fear as Stress Symptoms

Anger is the emotion that accompanies the realization that someone or something is not changing in accordance with your desires. Although you may think anger is caused by someone else's self-centered, ignorant, and inconsiderate actions, the truth is that you create your own anger. Your feeling results from the meaning you give to the event, not from the event itself. (Patterson et al., 2002).

Feeling a feeling is not the same as acting on a feeling. You may sometimes feel anger because of how you interpret a situation, but you can take control of your emotions and not act on your anger. Neither aggression nor violence equals anger. There is a difference among feeling a feeling of anger, expressing a feeling of anger, and acting on a feeling of anger (e.g., throwing a chart). Instead of responding with anger, a healthy expression of anger would be, "I feel angry. You may not like what I said to you. You may not scream at me."

Fear is an emotion that accompanies the contemplation of the unknown. It is often described as anxiety in the presence of danger, which is perceived as a threat to your emotional or physical survival. As discussed, what scares you varies with what your internal thoughts tell you about a situation or person. The extremes of fear—terror and panic—are overwhelming feelings that can paralyze you or lead to frantic, aimless activity.

People are conditioned to fear certain situations. If your mother—and then a nervous instructor—constantly say, "be careful," you can make yourself nervous by repeating the thought internally. Similarly, if either of these people attacks you in emotional outbursts, you learn to live in fear of those outbursts. When a patient takes a turn for the worse, you may feel scared. When you have a new responsibility or role you have never performed, you may feel scared. When you are confronted with an unknown situation or a new person, one of the emotions that you could manifest is fear. Fear can be a normal human response when faced with uncertainty; it is important to understand what triggers your fears.

Identifying what triggers your anger and fear is an important part of learning to control your response. Because these feelings are most often associated with the fight-or-flight responses in difficult situations, controlling them allows you to make better choices in response to stressors. When you have control over your emotions, you are better able to show moral courage in difficult situations. Ask yourself, "What am I telling myself, and what images am I creating (the story)?" If you can repeatedly observe your own behavior, you will begin to understand and change your internal and, therefore, your external responses.

People who feel their anger is justified may find it difficult to modify their anger responses. It is no easy task to persuade a person to replace angry responses with an understanding of how he or she created the anger through internal thoughts. To take charge of your stress response, you need to develop an awareness of what triggers your reactions.

Observing your own anger responses is an ongoing assignment. Its purpose is to learn about yourself, not to feel guilty or judge yourself based on your actions. Guilt does not occur when you "watch" yourself. It does, however, stop you from thinking and learning because you focus on your "mind chatter" rather than on problem-solving.

The same is true for many of your fear responses. Begin the process of overcoming fear by identifying what scares you. You can choose to avoid certain people or situations, but as a professional you can not avoid your moral obligations. Your fears limit you if avoidance becomes your major coping technique. In understanding fear, you need to remember that it is a protective response each of us has.

To change, look at what you really fear and what support you need to face that fear. To understand further, do the following exercise. Picture a situation in which you are fearful of speaking up and answer the following questions.

1. What is scaring you—fear of failure, disapproval, or retaliation? What are you afraid of?
2. What are you afraid of if this fear is realized?

3. If that happens, what are you afraid of next?
4. If that fear is realized, then what do you fear will happen?

Continue this line of questioning until nothing more comes to your mind. It is important that you begin to understand the root of your fear, so that you can take steps to self-soothe or reframe the situation. For example, deciding to speak up about an ethical issue of concern to your manager or supervising physician can create anxiety. Believing they will ridicule you or fire you could arouse fears strong enough to paralyze you. Your fear of speaking up may be basically a fear of criticism or a fear of losing control when criticized. Once you have identified your fear, you can develop skills in a step-by-step process to minimize it.

Identifying what triggers your anger and fear will help you gain some degree of control over your emotions. Three other emotions that affect your behavior are disappointment, hurt, and guilt. All involve unfulfilled expectations of self or of another. You can gain control over these emotions as well.

Disappointment

Disappointment is the feeling you have when plans or hopes are unrealized because your or another's lack of effort or perhaps just fate. Most often your disappointment comes not because others have failed to keep their promises, but because your expectations of yourself and of others are different from your/their performance.

Disappointment over foiled plans is a common emotional experience. An alternative to sitting and sulking over a disappointment is to decide, "OK, now what?" The key to treating disappointment is to look at your choices. For instance, you expect healthcare providers to honor the hand-washing policy, but you see a physician assistant and a nurse both touch a patient's dressing without first washing their hands. You could complain to others about your disappointment or you could determine how to tactfully approach the situation.

Perhaps you know people who are almost always disappointed. They continually visualize how they want their work to be, but they do not take action to create the desired situation. They just expect it to "just happen." Expecting others to know your needs is expecting them to be mind readers. In reality, people are too occupied with their own lives to divine the expectations of others. To expect them to do so means setting yourself up for disappointment and hurt. Instead, identify and ask for what you want. Getting something without asking for it should be the icing on the cake, not the cake itself. Learn that imagining and hoping are not equivalent to planning and acting assertively. What will you ask for today to improve patient quality or safety?

Hurt

Hurt, like disappointment, often arises out of unfulfilled expectations. "I feel hurt because she didn't show appreciation for the fact that I worked overtime." "I feel hurt because Dr. Jones didn't recognize the benefits of PT for his patient's recovery." Each of these statements has a built-in set of expectations that another person should have behaved differently.

To hurt is to cause physical or emotional injury, damage, or pain to another. Hurt is often thought of in relation to injuring someone's feelings. Although these definitions view hurt as generated by another person, hurt is really self-generated mental distress. Reducing your self-made hurts will help you deal with the harm (intentional or unintentional) inflicted by others.

I see hurt as a combination of anger and sadness. Anger because you feel taken advantage of, abused in some way, or treated unfairly by someone of importance. Sadness occurs because of the loss of trust that accompanies being hurt. To heal the hurt, it needs to be acknowledged and dealt with so that the truth can be reestablished. If it is not resolved, the hurt festers. This creates stress and destroys relationships, particularly as years of accumulated hurt create resentment. In our case, Susan or Howard could have held on to hurt feelings. Instead, they spoke directly and resolved the situation.

The hurt that comes from unfulfilled hopes and expectations often can be dealt with internally. It is important not to blame others with the standard reaction, "You should have known I felt . . . I wanted . . . I expected. . . ." When you assume that people will "mind read" your hopes and your expectations, you are setting yourself up to feel hurt. Clearly expressing your needs will go a long way toward reducing the damage you could create in your relationships if you blame others.

Guilt

Guilt is the feeling you experience when you have done "wrong" according to some legal or ethical value system. Not living up to your expectations of yourself and not acting according to your value system creates guilt. It reflects a discrepancy between what you think you should do and what you have done. The distance between your ideal self and your real self (who you are now) determines your degree of guilt. The closer you are to who you think you should be, the less anxiety and guilt you will experience. Guilt can be abated by closing the gap between who you think you should be (your value system) and who you are. The possibility of feeling guilt will sometimes stop healthcare professionals from speaking up.

Albert Ellis (2001) sees guilt as a consequence of telling yourself you are bad for not doing what you ought to have done. This is especially important to remember when a patient is dying. Healthcare professionals have essentially the same range of reactions to death as do laypeople—the more unexpected the event, the more difficult it is to deal with. While we share our emotions of grief and loss with others over the event, when a patient dies we often add on guilt.

The guilt is caused by the persistent idea that we can defeat death. No matter how progressive we are and no matter how hard we try to purge it, that idea is still lurking in some dark corner of our preconscious. So every time a patient dies, a small voice from within informs us that if only I had tried harder, or intervened sooner, or knew more, that person would still be alive.

That voice needs to be addressed. If not, you will torture yourself. Perhaps talking to your oncology or hospice colleagues would help, since their job many times is to help a patient die with dignity.

It is important to learn the difference between rightful and unreasonable expectations of yourself. Take a look at the values and principles that guide your life. Are they truly yours or are they the prescriptions of parents, friends, and society?

Worry: Problematic Self-Talk Strategy

Worry is thinking about and feeling anxious over some future event that could be a catastrophe. It can certainly hinder moral courage. But, in fact, how often have you worried about a possible tragedy that never occurred? All that wasted strategizing self-talk depletes your energy and makes you anxious.

Imagine what you could have done with all that time—watching those sunsets, smelling beautiful flowers, and sharing time with a close friend. When you worry about how to prevent your adolescent daughter from becoming pregnant or how to deal with a surgeon's ego, you are missing a lot. I am certainly not against planning, as planning to manage risk is important, but worrying and planning are not the same. Continuous strategic planning is not necessary. When you develop the attitude that you can handle almost anything that happens—a pregnant adolescent or a screaming doctor—you will begin to worry less and have more courage. You need to control your response to situations, not your responses to other people.

Art of Self-Soothing to Manage Danger

The term "self-soothing" comes from self-psychology, a school of thought founded by Heinz Kohut (Siegel, 1996). The goal of self-soothing is to comfort yourself emotionally in the face of stressful encounters by doing things that are pleasant. These techniques calm and relax the body and the mind. By engaging in self-soothing, you take deliberate steps to calm yourself while facing a difficult situation that triggers fear (Domar & Dreher, 2001).

Self-soothing is the natural result of the simple effort to attend to ourselves by focusing on the present. Inner calm essentially arises from connecting with our genuine experience in the moment. In reality, it means finding the courage to embrace ourselves as we are, no matter how we feel about ourselves.

Calmly attending to your "bodily-felt" world creates space between events and your immediate reactions to them. This provides an important opportunity to see what's really happening inside ourselves, so that we do not act out familiar patterns that are hurtful to ourselves and others. This acceptance of yourself is at the heart of self-soothing (Fiore, 2006).

Self-soothing is essential not only for peace of mind, but also for developing satisfying relationships. Unless we have a way of dealing with the feelings that arise within us in relationships, we may react with fear or blame when things do not go our way. We may judge or attack others to protect ourselves from unpleasant experiences, such as the fear of abandonment, the shame of being insulted, or the fear of being wrong. Instead of speaking out to solve the problem, we may attack or withdraw (McKay, Wood, & Brantley, 2007).

Dr. Mark Dombeck and Dr. Jolyn Wells-Moran offer an array of self-soothing options at MentalHealth.net. Some of these are traditional stress management techniques, such as relaxation, deep breathing, journaling, distraction, or healthy self-talk. The ideas and techniques listed below are only a starting point. Everyone has to find what works for them. Think of soothing each of your five senses.

1. *Vision*—Observe what you see, find soothing things upon which to look.
   Notice the play of light on the wall. Enjoy the pattern of colors reflected on the floor. Look out the window and watch the birds glide, the sun casting shadows, or the efficient movement of passing people.
2. *Hearing*—Mentally focus on what you can hear.
   Listen to delightful, relaxing, or revitalizing music. Pay attention to sounds of nature (e.g., waves crashing, birds chirping, leaves rustling). Sing your favorite songs. Hum a soothing tune. Learn to play an instrument. Be mindful of any sounds that come your way, letting them go in one ear and out the other. Notice how sounds on the unit feel different at various times of day.
3. *Smell*—Be aware of the memories that smell can bring.
   Notice the scent of your soap and shampoo while showering. Try to find brands of deodorant, lotion, and other things that have a soothing smell to you. Sit quietly for a few minutes and try to identify all of the smells that you notice. Enjoy the smell of your meals in the dining room. See if you can smell each type of food individually. Savor the smell of popcorn, and remember other times in your life when you have enjoyed popcorn.
4. *Taste*—Carefully savor the flavors that the day brings you.
   Have a good meal; enjoy your dessert. Have a favorite soothing drink, such as herbal tea or hot chocolate. Treat yourself to a favorite snack from the canteen. Suck on a piece of peppermint candy. Chew your favorite gum. Really taste the food you eat. Eat one thing at a time mindfully.
5. *Touch*—Find comfort in touch.
   Take a bubble bath. Savor the feeling of crisp, clean sheets on the bed. Soak your feet. Soften your skin with lotion. Put a cold compress on your forehead. Brush your hair for a long time. Place your hand on a smooth, cool surface. Enjoy the feeling of a favorite piece of clothing, or clean clothes. Notice the comforting warmth of clothing that is fresh from the dryer. Experience whatever you are touching and notice touch that is soothing.

Conclusion

Self-soothing and cognitive reframing are the key skills in managing fear. Without these skills, your perceptions, thinking, and decision-making can become distorted and erroneous. This chapter offers strategies to contain emotion and avoid overreacting to situations. Once these cognitive distortions are eliminated, healthcare professionals can accurately perceive the situation, logically analyze it, and take the necessary action for resolution. Healthcare professionals need to learn these necessary strategies if they are to show moral courage. Another strategy, to which we now turn, is risk management.

Key Points to Remember

1. To demonstrate moral courage, you need to have many kinds of crucial conversations. These conversations have three components: (1) opinions differ, (2) stakes are high, and (3) emotions are strong.
2. To cope effectively with a stressful situation, you must acknowledge your feeling of fear, but still act rationally.
3. Stress is not what happens to you, but the way you handle what happens to you.
4. Your perception of your patients, colleagues, executives, and physicians affects how you relate to them.
5. Frames are cognitive timesavers that help make sense of complex information. They help us comprehend the world around us through selective simplification.
6. What you perceive depends on your senses and your frame of reference; how you interpret the data depends on your value system and your cognitive processes.
7. Cognitive processes involve thinking, decision making, and problem-solving.
8. Common errors in thinking include dichotomous thinking, reliance on another's judgment, overgeneralizing, stereotyping, and catastrophizing.
9. You experience anxiety when you see a need to assume an offensive or defensive position against a threat.
10. Anger is the emotion that accompanies the realization that someone or something is not changing in accordance with your desires.
11. Fear is an emotion that accompanies the contemplation of the unknown.
12. Disappointment is the feeling of being made unhappy by the failure of one's hopes or expectations.
13. Hurt often arises out of unfilled expectations.
14. Guilt is the feeling you experience when you have done "wrong" according to some legal or ethical value system.
15. Worry is thinking about and feeling anxious over some future event that could be a catastrophe.
16. The goal of self-soothing is to comfort yourself emotionally in the face of stressful encounters by doing things that are pleasant.

References

Amodeo, J. (2001). Self-Soothing: A foundation for authentic love. *Personal Excellence, 7,* 8–10. Retrieved July 5, 2008, from http://theselfpages.tripod.com/id21.html

Attwood, T. (2007). *Exploring feelings: Cognitive behavior therapy to manage anxiety, sadness, and anger.* Lynchburg, VA: Studio Horizons. (DVD).

Begley, S. (2007). *Train your mind, change your brain: How a new science reveals our extraordinary potential to transform ourselves.* New York: Ballantine Books.

Burns, D. (1999). *Feeling good: The new mood therapy.* New York: Avon.

Dombeck, M., & Wells-Moran, J. (2006). *Self-soothing techniques: Venting and journaling.* MentalHealth.net. Retrieved July 5, 2008, from http://www.mentalhelp.net/poc/view_doc.php?type=doc&id=9758&cn=353#

Domar, A.D., & Dreher, H. (2001). *Self-nurture: Learning to care for yourself as effectively as you care for everyone else.* New York: Penguin.

Ellis, A. (2001). *Overcoming destructive beliefs, feelings, and behaviors: New directions for rational emotive behavior therapy.* Amherst, NY: Prometheus Books.

Festinger, L. (1957). *A theory of cognitive dissonance.* Palo Alto: Stanford University Press.

Fiore, N.A. (2006). *Awaken your strongest self.* New York: McGraw-Hill.

Greenberg, J. S. (2006). *Comprehensive stress management.* New York: McGraw-Hill.

Kolivosky, M.E., & Taylor, L. J. (1973). *Why do you see it that way? Principles of perception: Most applicable principles for guidelines in interpersonal relationships.* Hillsdale, MI: Hillsdale College.

Lazarus, R.S., & Folkman, S. (1984). *Stress, appraisal and coping.* New York: Springer Publishing.

McKay, M., Davis, M., & Fanning, P. (2007). *Thoughts and feelings: Taking control of your moods and your life.* New York: New Harbinger Publications.

McKay, M., Wood, J.C., & Brantley, J. (2007). *Dialectical behavior therapy workbook: Practical DBT exercises for learning mindfulness, interpersonal effectiveness, emotion regulation, & distress tolerance.* New York: New Harbinger Publications.

Olpin, M., Hesson, M., & Cole, B. (2006). *Stress management for life: A research-based experiential approach.* Florence, KY: Brooks Cole.

Patterson, K., Grenny, J., McMillian, R., & Switzler, A. (2002). *Crucial conversations: Tools for talking when the stakes are high.* New York: McGraw-Hill.

Siegel, A. (1996). *Heinz Kohut and the psychology of the self.* New York: Routledge.

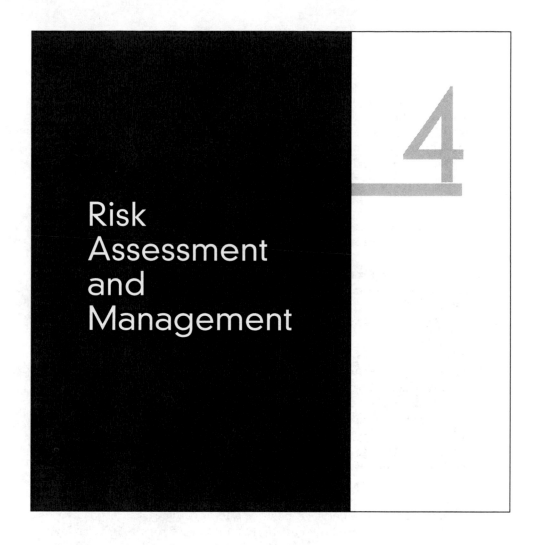

4

Risk Assessment and Management

No noble thing can be done without risks.
—Michel de Montaigne, French Renaissance thinker

When we think of the word *risk,* most of us conjure up images of danger with its chance of loss or injury. This loss could be status, money, job, or pride. The injury could be a physical, but it is more likely a social or emotional injury. Risk is often experienced when you are about to do something you have not done before— when you are entering unfamiliar territory. Your strength, courage, and faith in yourself or someone else may be required to meet this new challenge.

At the same time, risk taking can open up new ideas and experiences, creating an opportunity to discover your talents and dreams. Instead of waiting for things to happen, you make them happen. In effect, every time you take a risk, you are saying, "This is what I choose; this is who I am." Each risk teaches what you can or cannot do—the more risks you take, the more you will learn about yourself.

Generally, you take a risk because you believe that what you will gain is better than what you have. You are willing to put yourself on the line in some way because the outcome will be rewarding, significant, and worth the effort. For example, if you speak to a colleague about her lack of attention to detail in physical assessment, you will be able to sleep better at night knowing the patient is receiving quality care. Certainly, this is better than what you felt before the conversation, which was frustration and fear.

Risk tolerance is the degree of uncertainty that you can handle with regard to a possible negative result. All of us have some uneasiness with the idea of risk. Some individuals have a high tolerance for physical risk, but a low level of open-mindedness when it comes to emotional risk. Others adore learning new skills or information and will risk looking stupid or inept in the hope of enriching their lives. Still others are unable to risk any level of self-disclosure regardless of the outcome.

All communication risks fall into the self-disclosure category because you are making private information public. When you admit to a patient an error or tell someone you are angry at their demeaning behavior, you are taking a risk. As we will see in Chapter 5, you can not be assertive without accepting the risk of self-disclosure.

One of the paradoxes of life is that security requires risk taking (Treasure, 2003). Self-confidence comes from a deliberate expansion of who you are. To become self-actualized, you must sacrifice security. Deliberate expression and action to improve patient care requires stepping on some toes, not hard enough to cause backlash, but hard enough to motivate change. Risk takers recognize that hostile responses are part of the process of change. Criticism is weathered by self-soothing and cognitive reframing. Healthcare professionals with an adequate self-definition are willing to rock the boat at work and in their personal relationships. They understand that they are not defined by their personal or professional titles.

What is the difference between positive and negative risks? A positive risk gives you the chance to stretch yourself; it is a risk that results in your feeling proud, regardless of the outcome. A negative risk usually involves acting thoughtlessly or hastily. You may be trying to prove something to yourself or others, you may want attention, or you may want to feel important or seek vengeance. The question is not, "Am I taking enough risks?," but, "Am I taking enough risks of the right kind—the kind that promotes your professional and personal growth or the growth of others?"

Similarities of All Risks

We are a nation founded by pioneers who took extraordinary risks and faced many uncertainties. We admire people who take risks, whether they are constructive, such as those taken by Martin Luther King, Jr., and astronaut John Glenn, or just entertaining, such as those undertaken by the daredevil Evel Knievel. But whether they are promoting positive change or are empty risks, they share the following commonalities (Treasure, 2003) (see Exhibit 4.1).

1. *All risk taking involves choice.* A healthcare professional must pick from alternatives. For example, do you allow an impaired colleague in the operating room or do you report that person to your supervisor? We have options, but

4.1 Similarities of All Risks

1. All risk taking involves choices
2. All risk taking requires an investment (e.g., time, money, energy, etc.)
3. All risk taking cannot succeed
4. All risk taking requires the person to put himself/herself on the line in some way
5. All risk taking is accompanied by feelings of stretching oneself
6. All risk taking carries important emotional rewards
7. Virtually all risk taking sparks feelings of excitement, often disguised as fear

Treasure, W. (2003). *Right risk: 10 powerful principles for taking giant leaps with your life.* New York: Berrett-Koehler.

the individual with moral courage understands that the code of ethics offers only one choice — to protect the patient and get your colleague to take the first step in recovery.

2. *All risk taking requires an investment (e.g., time, money, energy).* When a nurse intervenes on a patient's behalf because he knows the patient does not understand the consent form she has signed, he is investing time. It requires courage to call the surgeon and time to listen to the informed consent process and then debrief the patient, particularly if the patient has been dealing with a surgeon who is upset. It takes energy to muster the courage and possibly more time to follow through with the next shift to ensure that informed consent has occurred. The physician and physician assistant may be sacrificing reimbursement (money) when they choose to take time from their schedules to fully inform the patient about options.

3. *All risk taking cannot succeed.* Even the best laid plans are not always successful. Skill is important and knowledge is important, but sometimes the patient will remain on life support until necrosis occurs. No matter how tactfully and assertively the healthcare professional speaks and how many organizational layers are involved, a patient will needlessly suffer. However, if more individuals speak up, the more system will tip toward change.

4. *All risk taking requires the person to put himself/herself on the line in some way.* In the end, the individual healthcare practitioner or executive/manager has to deal with the consequences of his or her actions. The kinds of situations we are discussing require that the individual take risks in ways some of us find normal. But to many, the risk is monumental and the ridicule devastating to their self-esteem. One can never judge the courage of another; only the individual knows the fear he or she has conquered.

5. *All risk taking is accompanied by feelings of stretching oneself.* Individuals must mature to meet increasing challenges. When they shrink from their professional obligations, they lose their elasticity and begin the dive into maintaining the status quo or, worse, into burnout and apathy. Individuals with resilience know confidence and courage come from doing things they thought they could not do. Resilience is the result of stretching ourselves when we believe we have no hope, no ability, no skill. When a resident physician speaks truth-

fully to a father about his 17-year-old son's terminal prognosis, she is demonstrating risk taking. She is willing to say the truth compassionately, regardless of what the father prays he will hear.

6. *All risk taking carries important emotional rewards.* These rewards could be feelings of pride in speaking up or the satisfaction of knowing that this patient spent his last two weeks of life at home, rather than in a critical care bed, because you told the truth about his prognosis. The reward could have been an appreciation of your seemingly instinctive skills at diagnosis, even though your attending physician disagreed. It could be the reward that a nurse experiences when her sensitivity to a patient's unexpressed thoughts leads her to ask the question, "Are you feeling suicidal?" With this one question, the nurse helped save a patient's life.

7. *Virtually all risk taking sparks feelings of excitement, often disguised as fear.* There is no physiological difference between the roller-coaster rider who experiences terror and the one who experiences excitement. The difference is in the cognitive framing of the situation. The same is true for the physical therapist who lets go of a patient to see if he or she can walk alone. They have done their due diligence in assessment, but at some point all healthcare professionals have to let go and see if the patient can regain his or her independence.

The Difference Between Risks That "Make a Difference" and Empty Risks

In health care, we have seen meaningless risks, such as taking Phase I clinical trial results as indicative of probable cures, following resuscitation orders on a 90-year-old patient with metastatic carcinoma of the breast, or fulfilling a PEG tube order on a patient with severe dementia. Empty risk taking is sparked by the desire to avoid feeling helpless and liable and by not wanting to deal with sad or angry patients and families. The surge of "doing something" dulls these feelings for a while, but these actions are only illusory gestures devoid of appropriate substance. They will not make a difference in the quality or possibly even the length of the patient's life. Empty risks also can jeopardize a patient's safety, such as the risk involved in not doing a read-back of a verbal order.

The risks that make a difference have a positive effect on the risk taker and receiver. Our character is the result of the decisions we make, so the risks we take shape our lives. When we assume responsibility for honoring a patient's privacy or giving a patient an accurate prognosis, we influence their lives and our own. We may not make a major difference here, as Mother Theresa or Gandhi did, but we can exert a significance influence on the projectory of a patient's life. We can, for example, offer hospice care as an option should a patient's condition call for it. When we tell the truth, we promote our emotional development, as well as an organizational culture that honors truth, regardless of consequences. When we back away from the risk of telling the truth, we fail to develop as a person and a professional. We take a step backward from self-actualization.

Risks in healthcare communication are expected of professionals to protect patients, but less than 10% of physicians, nurses, and other clinicians confront colleagues who skip standard infection control procedures or see an individual act incompetently in practice (VitalSmarts, 2005). Therefore, those who do confront such colleagues are courageous. Given these results, it becomes obvious that speaking up in the situations identified involved risk taking. For example, in our litigious society, disclosing medical errors requires courage. Never underestimate the bravery required to voice the truth.

Guiding Principles for Improving Chance of Success in Risk Taking

The guiding principles for improving risk taking include (1) improving the odds of success; (2) reducing the exposure to loss; and (3) reducing uncertainty. Improving the odds of success requires five steps in the decision-making process. The following is an example of a nurse who wants to have a surrogate decision-maker's voice heard for a critical care patient.

Improve the Odds of Success

1. *Identify the stakeholders.* Stakeholders are persons or a group of persons who share a direct interest, involvement, or investment. For example, in caring for a critically ill patient who is unconscious and terminally ill, all direct caregivers (e.g., nurses, physicians, including consultants on the case, and residents) and family members are the stakeholders.
2. *Clarify stakeholders' objectives and values.* Any one of these individuals could desire to maintain the status quo. Supporting the family's surrogate voice requires understanding the differences in values among all these stakeholders.
3. *Identify and evaluate alternatives.* Once you have identified the desired outcome, such as having the family's voice seriously considered in the treatment decision, examine your options for attaining the outcome. Would it be better to coach and role play with the family member, call social work to help orchestrate a family meeting, or call an ethics consultant?
4. *Assess your risk-taking bias.* If you were to choose a metaphor to assess your own risk-taking bias, would it more likely be "better safe than sorry" or "nothing ventured, nothing gained?" People with a risk-avoidance pattern have a tendency to overrate uncertainties and underrate the probability of realizing desired outcomes. Risk-preference pattern people are the opposite (Kindler, 1999). Avoiders are more likely to be pessimistic, while risk-preference pattern people are optimistic and enjoy the excitement of change. If you lean toward risk avoidance, you often postpone decisions. However, in this example,

4.2 **Guiding Principles**

1. Improve the odds of success.
2. Reduce the exposure to loss.
3. Reduce uncertainty.

you must meet your ethical obligation to the family. Deciding how to increase your chance of success needs to be your focus.

5. *Choose a change strategy.* When more than one voice is involved in confronting a problem, the chance of changing the status quo improves. There is merit in the old saying "safety in numbers." Building alliances with other healthcare professionals reduces risk. For this reason, an ethics consultant is often helpful, as this individual has the time to allow all voices to be heard. Such a meeting helps clarify the conflict between the values of peaceful death desired by family and the desire to continue treatment by the medical staff physician. Therefore, in the case above, the nurse could improve her odds of success in having the family's voice heard by accessing organizational support for moral courage.

In this scenario, change is required quickly, but in other cases, an incremental change strategy could be very effective. Incremental change is a series of small, often planned, modifications. An example is how our healthcare system is changing to cover the most vulnerable patients, rather than to take the higher risk of universal health care for all citizens. In our case scenario, a transformational change would be mandating that the quality benchmark of a family conference be held within 72 hours of admission for all patients in critical care units (Curtis, 2004).

Reduce the Exposure to Loss

Loss could be a lost opportunity, in which the outcome is less favorable than you would have liked or leaves you worse off than before you took the risk. Loss can come from action or inaction. Individuals who are risk averse often fear looking foolish and have anxiety over confrontations or changes. They lose opportunities because they are so concerned about security that they lose the positive self-esteem that comes with the courage to take risks. Risk-averse individuals tend to focus on the risks as opposed to the rewards. They punish themselves for losses, rather than turn the experience into a lesson learned.

You should try discussing the situation with individuals who have less emotional attachment to the outcome than you do. They can provide a fresh perspective on the reward/risk ratio. Perhaps, they would even be willing to role play the conversation involved in the risk. Role playing helps ease anxiety as your mind has now been through a dry run of the necessary dialog.

This conversation could also focus on the "worst case scenario." If you cannot cope with the worst possible outcome, then you need to tackle that problem first. Maybe further analysis of the stakeholders and alternatives is necessary before any action is taken.

Even for the individual who enjoys risk, the action should not be thoughtless or impulsive. That is why the decision process outlined above has five steps. Sometimes individuals try to prove themselves rather than focus on the situation to be resolved. The individual's rational mind becomes clouded with what Aristotle called rashness or arrogance. Both will lead to vulnerability and loss.

For both avoiders and risk takers, checking assumptions is crucial. An assumption is a proposition that is taken for granted and is treated for the sake of a given conversation as if it were true. Healthcare environments are filled with them. They include, "That is not the way we do things," "Do not give bad news," and "Rocking the boat will only lead to trouble." Remember that people actually presume these statements are true, so any violation of them creates a risk. But assumptions must be tested and evaluated just as rigorously as evidence. This reaffirms the need to understanding the values of the stakeholders, discuss the situation with those not emotionally involved, and share the risk through alliances with others.

Reducing Uncertainty

Since certainty is perfect knowledge, what in our world is certain other than death? Under what possible circumstances could you be without any doubt? The French philosopher Voltaire wrote, "Doubt is not a pleasant condition, but certainty is absurd." Uncertainty means you have limited knowledge, so describing future outcomes exactly is impossible. Ambiguity tolerance is the ability to accept ambiguity in information and behavior in a neutral and open way. This attitude opens the door to gathering as much reliable information as time allows to gain control over the situation. If timing is not urgent, patterns will emerge and the appropriate course of action often becomes recognizable.

Information can reduce uncertainty by addressing questions of magnitude, probability, and exposure. The more you stand to lose or gain, the larger the magnitude of the problem and the more you want reliable information. Determining the likelihood that you will incur a gain or loss is probability. Because you cannot prevent all losses, the question surrounding exposure is how can you lessen the impact? Without a crystal ball, the next best solution is the ability to see patterns of actions and behavior based on what the person has done in similar situations.

For example, in the above scenario, if the attending physician is open to your opinion and dialogue, then maybe an ethics committee consultation is unnecessary. But if you have repeatedly met with resistance when the words palliative care and hospice are mentioned, then the probability is that an ethics consultation is needed. In fact, the ethics committee consultation could help all "save face," thereby lessening a negative impact.

Understanding and Managing Our Fears

This discussion would not be complete without addressing fear in further depth. The odds are that you pass up taking risks because you are afraid. Fear is biologically programmed in each of us. Only in fiction are heroes seemingly fearless. Remember, moral courage involves acting despite the feeling of fear.

Chapter 3 offered some strategies to deal with fear caused by your perception of your life story and/or your distorted thinking. You make this the type of fear worse by negative self-talk. In this chapter, I focus on the key situational fears you are likely to encounter as you demonstrate moral courage. The steps may sound simplistic (see Exhibit 4.3), but when you are experiencing "fight or flight," you need to keep it simple.

When a healthcare professional encounters a difficult situation that they feel unprepared to manage, they are likely to experience situational fear. Sometimes

4.3 How to Act in Response to the Fear

1. Identify the risk you want to take.
2. Identify the situational fear you experience.
3. Determine the outcome you want and what you have to do to achieve it.
4. Identify resources accessible to you.
5. Take action.

the fear is cleverly disguised as anger, but do not be fooled by this "fight-or-flight" response. Many fears exist; I will mention the four main ones I see blocking moral courage over and over again.

Fear of Disapproval

Fear of disapproval originates in the low self-esteem of many. When what others think of you is more important than what you think of yourself, your self-worth is fragile. If your desire to please dominates your behavior, you will eventually lose yourself and not remember your professional values and obligations. Your need for approval becomes more and more indiscriminant. Real heroes, like Martin Luther King, Jr., and Florence Nightingale, realized that disapproval does not invalidate the reliability of an idea. You may desire to be liked, but do not please others at the risk of losing your personal or professional identity.

Fear of Rejection

Fear of rejection can dominate a person's persona to the point that he or she takes a back seat in all interactions. This is particularly sad, because there is certain randomness in who accepts or rejects you. Catch a person on a good day and all is well; catch the same person on a bad day and, no matter what you do, nothing will gain you acceptance. Some people judge all others harshly, so it is an error to allow your view of yourself to rest on their pessimistic view of the world. Great writers suffer many rejections, as did social activists such as Elizabeth Cady Stanton and Susan B. Anthony. Fortunately, both continued to champion women's rights.

Fear of Failure

Fear of failure is another fear associated with low self-esteem. The list of individuals who first failed and then went on to accomplish great acts for humanity is endless—Abraham Lincoln, Benjamin Franklin and Dorothea Dix. You can choose to quit, or you can choose to be tenacious in your pursuit of patient safety and quality care. The fear of being wrong is a close cousin of the fear of failure, because both make you too cautious to make a choice with significant consequences. This desire for certainty is a pointless chase. Failure is a great learning opportunity.

Fear of Confrontation

An individual who fears confrontation may easily be taken advantage of in life. After all, confrontation simply means bringing a person face to face with a situation. This means confrontation is an exchange of information. You will always learn something about yourself and the other person when you speak out and attempt to "clear the air." Often, individuals with this fear are conflict avoidant, as will be discussed in Chapter 5.

Conclusion

When you venture into the unknown, you learn to face a challenge that may demand strength, courage, and faith in yourself or another. Tolerating risk and managing risk are necessary skills if you are to break your silence and refuse to tolerate disrespect to patients, families, colleagues, and yourself or the breaking of rules that jeopardize patient safety. To be successful in your risk taking, use the three guiding principles and strategies presented—improve the odds of success, reduce the exposure to loss, and reduce uncertainty. The four primary sources of fear must be mastered if you are to regain your voice and dialog with other healthcare professionals and executives/managers to eliminate the barriers to quality care and a quality work environment.

Happy experimenting.

Key Points to Remember

1. A positive risk gives you the chance to stretch yourself. A negative risk usually involves acting thoughtlessly or hastily.
2. The risks that make a difference have a positive effect on the risk taker and receiver.
3. The guiding principles for improving risk taking include (1) improving the odds of success; (2) reducing the exposure to loss; and (3) reducing uncertainty.
4. The four primary sources of fear must be mastered if you are to regain your voice and dialog with other healthcare professionals and executives/managers to eliminate barriers to quality care and a quality work environment.

References

Curtis, J. (2004). Communicating about end-of-life care with patients and families in the intensive care unit. *Critical Care Clinics, 20*(3), 363–380.

Kindler, H.S. (1999). *Risk taking: A guide for decision makers.* Menlo Park, CA: Crisp Publications.

Treasure, W. (2003). *Right risk: 10 powerful principles for taking giant leaps with your life.* New York: Berrett-Koehler.

VitalSmarts. (2005). *Silence kills: The seven crucial conversations for healthcare.* Retrieved July 5, 2009, from http://www.silencekills.com/Download.aspx

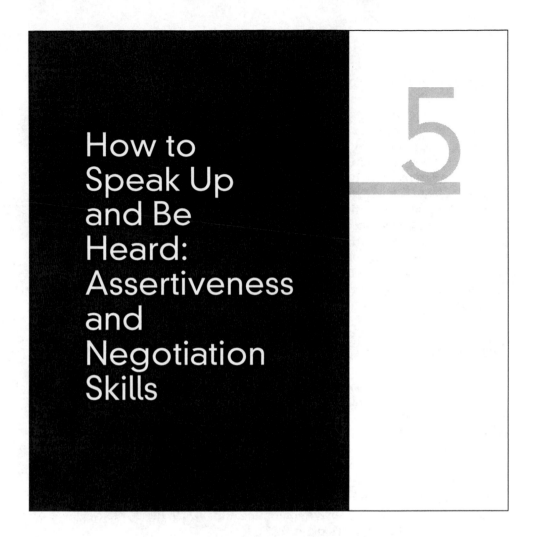

How to Speak Up and Be Heard: Assertiveness and Negotiation Skills

5

When we have the courage to speak out—to break our silence—we inspire the rest of the "moderates" in our communities to speak up and voice their views.

—Sharon Schuster, an internationally recognized photographer

Moral courage requires that you understand your professional obligation to trigger the motivation that encourages you to take necessary risks. A successful outcome, however, requires excellent communication skills, including listening, assertiveness, and negotiation. These crucial skills will help you deal with the hostility, defensiveness, side-stepping debates, and other tactics people will use to scare you into silence.

Chapter 3 discussed the importance of self-soothing and cognitive reframing in controlling your emotional responses during a conflict. To deal with emotional upsets, you need to recognize that person or event that triggered your reaction, as well as understanding what you tell yourself about the occurrence (self-talk or your story). For instance, if you are dealing with someone who has a false sense of self-importance, you become upset only after you call that person arrogant in your mind and believe that action is required. When you become emotionally upset, first look at yourself—not to find fault, but to truly understand what is upsetting you. Once the cause of your reaction is identified, change your self-talk and determine what options are available for remedying the situation. Select the best choice and act (Patterson, Grenny, McMillian, & Switzler, 2002). Remember, first you must *identify* what you are telling yourself about the situation or person. *Listen* to your self-talk, and *change* it to helpful, supportive talk. This self-soothing behavior will help you remain calm, so that you can think clearly and choose an appropriate response. The goal is assertive behavior, not aggressiveness or passivity.

A 2005 study, conducted by VitalSmarts and the American Association of Critical Care Nurses, listed the following seven categories of crucial conversations that healthcare professionals failed to discuss (Maxfield, Grenny, Patterson, McMillan, & Switzler, 2005): (1) broken rules; (2) lack of support; (3) mistakes; (4) incompetence; (5) poor teamwork; (6) disrespect; and (7) micromanagement. These seven categories will be used in examples throughout this chapter.

Assertiveness

Assertiveness is acting confidently; it is stating your position with assurance. Your goal is to protect your legitimate rights or the rights of a patient without violating the rights of anyone else (Clark, 2003; Leebov, 2003). Assertive behavior is an honest, direct, and appropriate expression of one's thoughts, feelings, and opinions. Appropriate expression means that you chose the right place and the right time to state your case. Assertiveness focuses on solving a problem, which often requires that another person change his or her behavior. It communicates respect for the other person, but not necessarily for that person's behavior. An example of assertive communication is, "Dr. Block, please glove-up before you touch the patient's dressing."

In contrast, the goal of aggressive behavior is to humiliate, dominate, and put the other person down (Benun, 2006). It is an attack on the person, rather than on the problem. The person stands up for his or her rights, but in such a way that the other person's rights are violated. An example of aggressive communication is, "Dr. Block, you know you have to put on gloves before touching dressing. Are you that arrogant that you think the rules don't apply to you?"

Nonassertive behavior allows others to have their way—it allows your rights or the rights of patients to be violated. This passivity lets others make the decision, because you passively submit to their point of view. An example of a non-assertive communication is complaining to someone else that Dr. Block did not glove-up when changing dressings on a new post-op.

There are three primary barriers to assertive behavior (Benun, 2006; Bishop, 2006). First, the person does not believe he or she has the *right* to speak up. Gender, culture, or role does not entitle him or her to a voice in this situation. In fact, the healthcare provider, notwithstanding these reasons, has an obligation to speak up when, as in the example above, an infection control rule was broken. Second is the *anxiety or fear* the individual experiences when choosing to speak. This addresses the importance of self-soothing and cognitive reframing. *Lack of skills,* which is the third barrier, is the focus of this chapter.

This discussion will use the following formula to give you a model of behavior that requires less work for your frontal cortex, which is already busy managing the danger of speaking. Using this simple formula will help you organize your response:

> When you do X, I feel Y because of Z, and what I'd
> like instead is [request behavior change].

For example, when a physician refuses to discuss the condition of a terminal patient with a family, it could take this form:

> When you refuse to talk to the family *(X)* I feel
> upset *(Y)* because they now believe he will be going
> home *(Z)*. I would like you to spend the time with
> them and help them understand that will not
> happen [the behavior change].

When dealing with someone who is disrespectful toward you, name the behavior that disturbs you:

> I feel angry *(X)* when you are arrogant *(Y)*. The Y
> part needs to name the behavior, not judge it.

The assertive communication paradigm is thus a four-part message:

1. A disclosure of the asserter's feelings.
2. A nonjudgmental description of the behavior to be changed.
3. A clarification of the concrete and tangible effect of the other person's behavior on the asserter, patient, family, or someone else.
4. A statement of the desired behavior change or solution you want or an invitation to problem solve (Dryden, 2005).

The last item may simply mean talking about the behavior, but you may also request that the person think about the consequences of his or her behavior. The "I'd like . . ." part of your statement informs the person of your preferences. You may choose to delete this part until you have heard the other person's response to your assertive statement. An example of an assertive statement that deals with lack of teamwork is, "When I ask you to cover my patients when I go to lunch, and I return to find neither of the two meds I asked you to give have been given and another patient is in pain *(X)*, I feel frustrated *(Y)* because I thought I could rely on you for this teamwork. I would like to understand what happened."

Unfortunately, sending an assertive message does not guarantee that the other person will respond positively. Even the best message may trigger a defensive response because the other person often feels threatened. For example, a defensive response to the above assertion might be, "Well, at least you got lunch. I am a good nurse and do not appreciate your insinuation that I am not." People often feel uncomfortable being told that they have a negative effect on others. Consequently, the next section focuses on handling the five most problematic responses to your assertive statement: (1) defensiveness, (2) hostility, (3) side-stepping, (4) tears, and (5) withdrawal.

Defensiveness

People become defensive when they feel threatened. Defensiveness is a self-protective response (Pfeiffer, 2003; Small, 2006). *Pause* before replying to a defensive response, as this gives you time to self-soothe and avoid responding in kind. Reflect the emotion you see neutrally with statements such as "I can tell this makes you upset." Nonverbal behaviors can help validate the other person. These include good eye contact, facial expressions that are neutral or indicate thoughtfulness, body orientation indicating that you are engaged in the conversation, and vocal volume, pitch, and rate that is low and slow. Avoid troubling phrases, such as "you should . . .", and "yes, but. . . ." Finally, paraphrase your understanding of what the other person is saying. Examples of reflective listening responses include, "You feel that I don't understand" or "If I understand you, you see the situation differently." Many times a defensive response is the result of a false interpretation of your assertive statement, as in the example above where the nurse *heard* that she was not a good nurse.

Hostility

Antagonistic and argumentative responses may appear angry, but they are often fueled by fear. It is important to create a safe environment for your conversation, so the dialog can be open (Patterson et al., 2002). For this reason, your first response should emphasize areas of agreement. Connect the agreement and the disagreement with the word "and." Avoid using the word "but" in the middle of a sentence, as it negates everything that preceded it. For example, if you say to someone, "I hear your point, but . . . ," what you are really saying is, "I do not like your point" or "I disagree with your point."

To respond positively, you need to self-soothe and listen to hear where you agree, then, you can appropriately clarify your message. If the individual's response appears to indicate that your words were misinterpreted, ask for clarification by saying, "What did you hear me say?" It is crucial to keep your voice free of sarcasm or judgment.

Suggestions for dealing with both defensiveness and hostility can be found in *Crucial Conversations* (Patterson et al., 2002). The authors repeatedly emphasize that all participants are responsible for creating a conversational space that is safe for dialog. If you, as the asserter, have made a mistake that has hurt others, begin the conversation with an apology that conveys genuine regret. You may surrender a bit of your ego by admitting your error, but what you gain in good will is well worth it. The authors further suggest you use the communication strategy known as contrast (don't/do statements) when others misinterpret either your purpose or your intent. A "don't" statement addresses concerns that you do not respect them or that you have a malicious aim. The "do" statement verifies your respect and makes clear your real purpose. This technique addresses the threat to the safe environment and allows you to return to the issue under discussion. For example, in a "lack of support" example, you might say, "The last thing I would want you to conclude is that I do not want to help you. I want you to know I value you as a member of our team. Unfortunately, when you asked for my help I was on the way to give stat medications to a very sick patient. How can I help you now?" Sometimes people misinterpret negative aspects of your assertive behavior. Contrasting helps put your negative message or comments in the context of the larger picture by first explaining what you did not mean.

Sidestepping

Let's return to the example of the physician who was not making time to speak to the family about the patient's prognosis. In this case, two examples of side-stepping responses might be "Since you seem to have the time to badger me, why don't you have the conversation?" or "The conversation will be had by the resident when he discusses the DNR order."

The first example is a question flavored with sarcasm; the second diverts the discussion away from your request. Both are examples of tangential transactions and are not central to your request. A good response would be to restate your request.

Tears

Tears are an effective way to dodge an assertive confrontation. You may be uncertain how to continue the discussion while recognizing the tears, which could either be a natural reaction to the situation or a form of manipulation designed to divert your attention to soothing the person. The best strategy is to empathically respond with, "I can see you are upset. I'd like to continue to solve the problem. Are you willing to do that?" This acknowledges the emotion and the problem, while giving the individual the choice to continue or postpone the discussion. Some can cry and solve the problem simultaneously; others may become so upset that they need time to bring their emotions under control. If a person cannot continue, set a specific time that day or the next to continue the conversation.

Withdrawal

Another person may remain silent in your presence or actually walk away without responding to your statement. In this case, provide space for that person to think about an appropriate response by being silent yourself (Fred Pryor Seminars, 2006). However, if the person does not respond after a minute, then try to interpret his or her body language and reassert your desire to solve the problem. You might say, "Your silence and your looking away suggest that you do not want to continue this conversation. Are you willing to make an effort to solve this problem?" During the minute of silence, you can be self-soothing, but maintain eye contact with the person, even if he or she is looking away. If the person continues to remain silent, it is probably best to say, "I take your silence to mean that you do not want to talk about this and you will meet my request (doing what ever you asked for originally)."

If the individual truly walks away, you need to decide if you should follow them and reassert your statement. Most of the time, it is more effective to approach the person and continue the conversation the next time you meet. It is a second test of your moral courage not to let the issue die. If you do, then you are essentially saying that your initial request was not relevant. You need to strike a balance between backing the person into a corner and accepting a mutually agreed-on solution.

Finally, a few additional suggestions may increase your chances for success. First, catch the slightest nuance of an offered solution. Sometimes people stumble over their words or offer tentative solutions. Second, do not insist that the person be cheerful about meeting your request. We all have to do things in life we find distasteful. Third, always remember to paraphrase the solution back to the other person if you encounter any of the barriers mentioned above. Too often the solution gets lost in the heat of the moment. Finally, end the conversation with a polite thank you. After all, you surely are appreciative that the problem has been resolved.

Other Assertiveness Techniques

Additional assertiveness techniques can help you cope with the fear of being criticized. The following examples reflect ways you might respond assertively if you are the person responsible for a problem.

Negative Inquiry

The technique of *negative inquiry* is used to clarify or make vague criticisms more specific. For example, when a respiratory therapist says, "You are an incompetent nurse," and you have no idea why, you could respond by saying, "What did I do or say that made me look incompetent?" Here, you are attempting to clarify the root of the judgmental comment, rather than simply responding defensively. You are probing the negative comment while keeping the communication open.

Negative Assertion

In the second assertiveness technique, *negative assertion,* you agree with the truth in the criticism. For instance, a colleague says to you, "Your manager's criticism is you are always late to the meeting." You respond to the grain of truth in that statement, as you want to agree assertively with the negative statement: "You are right. I have been late to the last two meetings and I have been on time to the other five." This exemplifies a negative assertion. The technique can be seen as a way to accept responsibility or as a way to dismiss the feedback. Your critics will expect you to become defensive. When you do not, the emotional tone of the interaction diminishes. Both of these techniques direct the person to the content of the criticism rather than to your emotional response.

Fogging

Fogging is a third assertiveness technique that is related to the concept of "fog." Just as fog does not resist as you move through it, this technique requires that you let criticism flow past you. This is an effective strategy if you want to stop the conversation because you are feeling baited to argue (Clark, 2003). However, it does cut off dialog about the negative feedback. Consider the following example:

Patient: "Nurses here don't spend enough time with patients."
Nurse: "I can see why you would feel that way today."
Patient: "You, Nurse Hopkins, are unavailable to me."
Nurse: (having spent most of the morning in a meeting) "I understand why you feel that way."

The nurses' response to this comment could have also used the technique of negative assertion. In that case, the nurse would say, "You are right; I have spent most of the morning in meetings."

These three techniques are additions to your assertiveness toolkit. By avoiding a defensive reaction to criticism, you improve work and social relationships. To have moral courage, you need an assortment of assertiveness skills to deal with a variety of interpersonal situations.

Saying No and Setting Limits

"Saying no" is also considered a skill because it involves an empathetic understanding of the other person's position, as well as the use of assertive communication skills (Mayer, 2006). "No" can be said in an assertive, but tactful, way. When the nurse asked Dr. Block to glove before changing dressings, she was setting limits. When healthcare professionals voice to their preceptors that they do not feel ready to do a certain procedure because they have never seen it done, they are setting limits. For that reason, setting effective boundaries is a required skill for moral courage.

You may hurt someone's feelings with an assertive "no," but the hurt will heal. Other behavior, such as passive-aggressive (talking behind their back) or aggressive (sarcastic, abusive language) techniques, cuts much more deeply—and the cut heals very slowly, if ever. Empathetic assertion enables you to say no while still maintaining your self-respect. Greater self-respect makes it easier to say "no."

Many times, you feel uncomfortable saying "no," and we almost never like hearing "no." "No" means we do not get "our way," and we usually want "our way." Do you remember your developmental psychology courses? Do you remember the stress placed on the importance of saying "no" in raising children? Children need limits; therefore, adults need to say "no." You may be thinking, "I did not like 'no' as a child, and I do not like it much more now." The only difference between a two-year old's response and your adult response as a healthcare provider is that you have been socialized into believing that throwing a temper tantrum is selfish, rude, and certain to create posttantrum embarrassment.

Saying no is important in setting limits in moral issues (Raiffa, 2005; Raiffa, Richardson, & Metcalfe, 2007). However, saying yes can also define your limits. For instance, you may say no to serving on a committee for designing a patient fall prevention program, but say yes to committees to improve the working relationships among hospital departments. In this way, you are defining your own limits.

Expanding your limits by venturing out of your comfort zone for a challenging task or a new way of responding brings some rewards. Without some monetary, verbal, or intrinsic rewards, the task will seem burdensome. Saying "no" to an organizational culture norm that does not require "time outs" before the incision is made in the operating room could take you out of your comfort zone.

When anyone says "no," conflicts can arise. Being able to resolve such conflicts frequently requires the skill of collaborative problem-solving, or negotiation (Shell, 2006). Of course, negotiation is not always possible. Nor is it always the correct strategy. But many times negotiation is part of a strategy to resolve the numerous ethical problems that arise in health care.

Negotiation for Conflict Resolution

Collaborative problem-solving and win-win conflict resolution are other terms for negotiation (Lewicki, Barry, & Saunders, 2006; Lewicki & Hiam, 2006). All involve resolving disagreements through discussion and compromise. Negotiation involves two or more parties with common and conflicting interests, who come together to put forth and discuss explicit proposals for the purpose of reaching agreement (Fisher, Ury, & Patton, 1997). Negotiation is relevant when the need for satisfaction is important for all sides. If there is no need for a win-win solution, negotiation is not necessary. The win/win approach is about changing the conflict from adversarial attack or deference to cooperation. Simply, this approach means, "I want to resolve this conflict so that both of us feel like winners." What skills would a person need to achieve this outcome?

Successful negotiators share seven traits (Aquilar & Galluccio, 2007; Karrass, 1994) (See Exhibit 5.1).

Planning Skills

The first is planning skills. Just as you would not ask your supervisor for a raise without doing significant investigation and planning, you need to take great care in negotiating with the chief of surgery who is not enforcing "time out" before the first cut of surgery. You want to have the answers to questions such as, "How extensive is the problem? Are there system problems that create significant bar-

5.1 The Seven Traits of Successful Negotiators

1. Planning skills
2. Ability to think clearly under stress
3. Ability to use common sense
4. Verbal ability
5. Content knowledge
6. Personal integrity
7. Ability to perceive and use power

Karrass, G.L. (2003). *Effective negotiating workbook and discussion guide.* Beverly Hills, CA: Karrass.

riers? What happens when a nurse speaks up?" It is crucial for you to plan what you will say and how you will approach the needs of all parties to achieve a successful outcome.

Ability to Think Clearly Under Stress

Planning also helps with the second negotiation skill—*the ability to think clearly under stress*. Consider in advance all your options if Plan A does not achieve your designed outcome. If you are prepared with alternatives, you are more likely to stay engaged if you receive backlash. Rackham (1999) even concluded that skilled negotiators do not offer counterproposals as quickly as do average negotiators.

Equally important is a win-win attitude, which avoids a power struggle over opposing solutions. When you are engaged in this type of survival strategy, your ego really wants to say, "Do it my way" (Paterson et al., 2002). But, if you shift the conversation to finding mutually acceptable solutions, you will think more clearly. Being able to self-soothe and reframe the other person's statements will decrease stress and provide support for the next skill, which is practical intelligence.

Ability to Use Common Sense

Common sense, or practical intelligence, is the third skill. Kritek (2002) illustrates this skill with an example of no-nonsense advice you can apply when negotiating in an organization that has a sizable power gap. Because measures of equality change and vary according to organizational culture, you should use common sense in determining when to personally assert and when it is wise to have someone higher up the pecking order intervene (Malhotra & Bazerman, 2007).

Verbal Ability

Verbal ability, the fourth skill, combines assertiveness with listening (Babcock & Laschever, 2007). It emphasizes focusing on the needs of others rather than on preplanned solutions and speaks to the importance of listening to what others need to resolve the conflict. Perhaps, the chief of surgery needs more cooperation from the anesthesiologist to start the cases on time or perhaps more cooperation from the team in room turnover. Rackham (1999) found that skilled negotiators tended to provide a verbal indication of forthcoming behavior. For example, instead of asking a question, they might say, "Can I ask you a question?" They thereby gave a warning that a question was coming.

Content Knowledge

Planning skills can also help with the fifth skill, which is acquiring *content knowledge*. Rackham (1999) found that successful negotiators gave more than three times as much attention to areas of common agreement than to areas of conflict. To do this, however, requires an understanding of the issues. If you are negotiating with the department of surgery, an update by the nursing director of surgical services could provide a framework of crucial questions. Just as nurses always want to know how much the patient knows before they begin patient education, executives need some understanding of the clinical issues before confronting a patient safety clinical matter.

Personal Integrity

But all these skills will not help if you lack the sixth skill, which is *personal integrity*. Integrity is having and consistently holding firm to moral principles and standards. No one will negotiate with any individual in a forthright manner if they believe the individual is dishonest. People with integrity are honest, consistent, open about motives, and treat people with respect and fairness. All physicians are expected to practice "time out" in the surgical suite; any exception undermines the trust patients would like to have in the organization. Maintaining your integrity requires moral courage. There are many ways you can shortchange your integrity, including "simplistic trust, careless neglect, lack of discrimination, laziness and cowardice" (Kritek, 2002, p. 220). You may know the right answer, but you may be more comfortable settling for what is realistic, particularly if someone is trying to discredit you. However, you should always strive for the moral choice when negotiating.

Ability to Perceive and Use Power

The final skill is the ability to perceive and use power. Power is usually defined as the possession of control or influence over others, but another definition is the ability and willingness to exert actions that will result in a desired outcome (Thompson, 2007). As Kritek (2002) points out, our world is fixated on dominance power, but many other forms of power exist.

Power is on of the three key variables you need to juggle in any negotiation (Cohen, 2006). The other two are information and time. Information includes content information, as well as information about your fellow negotiators. The pressure of time can sometimes result in giving in to the demands of someone else, rather than examining options that would satisfy all stakeholders. Therefore, you must always give yourself enough time, or take enough time, to plan and think through what is really needed to resolve the issue. For example, the lack of "time out" may be the tip of the iceberg. What you really want is much bigger, perhaps more interdisciplinary collaboration.

Cohen (2006) describes fourteen different sources of power. Three have already been discussed (i.e., power of knowledge of other person's needs; power of risk taking; and power of legitimacy, such as policy of "time out"). This section discusses the seven most important sources of power for healthcare provider negotiations. Exhibit 5.2 lists all fourteen sources of power.

All healthcare professionals have the power to gain expertise. An executive who takes the time to ask the clinical opinion of the chief nursing or chief medical office, he or she is exercising the power of expertise. "In general the only kind of expertise required for most negotiations is the ability to ask intelligent questions and know whether you are getting accurate answers" (Cohen, 2006, p. 68).

The power of reward and punishment is based on the perception that going along with your solution will help me and not going along with you will hurt me in some way. The reality of this situation is irrelevant. In win-win negotiations,

5.2 The Sources of Power

1. Power of Competition
2. Power of Legitimacy
3. Power of Risk Taking
4. Power of Commitment
5. Power of Expertise
6. Power of Knowledge of Needs
7. Power of Investment
8. Power of Rewarding or Punishing
9. Power of Identification
10. Power of Morality
11. Power of Precedent
12. Power of Persistence
13. Power of Persuasive Capacity
14. Power of Attitude

Cohen, H. (2006). *Negotiate this!: By caring, but not T-H-A-T much.* New York: Business Plus Publishers.

you should only reduce the stress of others in a *quid pro quo* way. Rewards and coercion come in many forms; it is important to make them meaningful to the person with whom you are negotiating.

The power of identification exists in all personal and business communications. You give more credence to a person you respect—a person who has consistently demonstrated cooperation, fairness, or perhaps expertise. When you trust or *identify* with another person, you give that person power. Therefore, you gain power when you choose empathy over pulling rank. This also works in reverse—people will refuse to be identified with people they dislike.

The power of persistence and the power of precedent are closely allied. Most individuals are not persistent enough in negotiations. When the chair of surgery balks at your request for consistent "time out," maintain a resolute attitude. The power of precedent is often the result of the unwavering actions of others, so that any attempt to change a pattern is met with resistance. However, the power of precedent can also be a rallying call for change. Riding the national movement to patient safety is clearly an example of the power of using precedent.

The power of morality is actually the underlying premise of this book. Although our personal moral frameworks may vary based on our culture, religion, and family origin, our moral obligations to our patients bear a remarkable similarity across professions. Patient safety is a moral obligation that has wielded extraordinary power in healthcare institutions across our country.

The final source of power in this discussion is the power of "attitude." The attitude to cultivate in negotiation is one that will increase risk taking, reduce stress, and foster a "can do" approach. Teach yourself to say in every negotiation, "If everything goes wrong, will my life end?" If the answer is no, then do your best to have a win-win outcome.

5.3   Five Steps for Working Out an Agreement

1. Preparation
2. Communicate and listen to needs and interests of others
3. Define objective criteria
4. Search for mutually acceptable solutions
5. Finalize the agreement

Process of Negotiation

How do successful negotiators prepare? How do they behave during negotiations? Generally, they follow five steps listed in Exhibit 5.3.

Preparation

This preparation means doing your homework. Remember that knowledge is power. The more you know about the other party, her needs, and/or the needs of the organization, the better you will be able to negotiate effectively. If you negotiate without this preparation, you will be more likely to respond emotionally. Preparation and research must take place before you enter into the actual negotiation.

Prenegotiation preparation includes three crucial elements:

1. Know Yourself
   - What are my specific needs and interests?
   - What concessions and compromises am I prepared to offer?
     - what I must have
     - what I would like to have
     - what it would be great to have
   - What will I do if we cannot reach agreement?
     - never obligated to accept the deal
     - remember that the person who relies least on a specific outcome is in a better negotiating position.
2. Know your fellow negotiators
   - What are the three facts you must know to better understand the person or group you're dealing with? Investigate to uncover their needs and predict their moves.
   - What are their interests and goals?
   - What alternatives do they have?
   - Who are the key players, and what is their track record?
3. Know Strategy
   - What are the possibilities?
   - What are my alternatives?

- Do I have a deadline or specific time frame?
- Define your response choices
- Practice your opening
- Visualize ultimate success

Communicate and Listen

Never enter a negotiation if you are not clear about your specific needs and interests. In addition to determining your first and second choice outcomes, give equal thought to the minimum you can accept. For example, if you are negotiating with your manager about how to handle the incompetence of a peer, you need to be careful about the level of accountability you take on, especially if this is not the first time you have reported a problem. Unfortunately, many managers expect staff members to deal with problem employees. If you are staff, you need to enter the negotiation knowing the minimum behavior you are willing to accept. Remember *Crucial Conversations* says, "If you ever have the same conversation twice, you are having the wrong conversation" (Patterson et al., 2002).

Remember to define the problem in terms of needs or interests, not solutions. Find out why the person wants the solution he or she initially proposed and seek to understand the advantages that solution has for that person. For example, a physician may suggest admitting the patient through the ER, rather than through the admissions office. His or her motivation is quick access to x-ray and lab studies.

If the conversation becomes heated, stop yourself so that you can reorient the conversation to serve its original purpose. Remember that your goal is a solution to the question of patient admission. If you lose the mutual respect of your colleagues by cutting them off, overstating your facts, or speaking in absolutes, they will begin to find the conversation uncomfortable, stop negotiating, and switch to defending their dignity. *Crucial Conversations* uses the mnemonic CRIB to help with such situations: **C**ommit to staying in the conversation until you find a solution that satisfies everyone. **R**ecognize the reason behind a person's position, and ask, "Why do you want that?" **I**nvent a mutual purpose by discovering your areas of agreement. **B**rainstorm new strategies, and do not become stuck with "either/or" choices. This process is almost identical to the one that I advocate.

Define Objective Criteria

Once you have prepared for the negotiations and have identified everyone's needs and interests, you can move to Step 3. This means confirming that both parties have objective criteria by which to determine what is fair and equitable. One criterion could be existing laws, precedents, polices, JCAHO, or nursing standards, although these criteria do not always prevent problems from developing. For example, "time out" in the surgical suite is considered a patient safety policy, yet wrong site surgery was still the number one sentinel event in 2008 (Joint Commission, 2008).

Step three is where both parties share their interests and needs. It is important to concisely paraphrase the needs of others before stating your own. By asking for clarification of the other negotiators' needs, you demonstrate your interest in an equitable solution. Select the solution (or combination of solutions) that will best meet both parties' needs.

Search for Mutually Acceptable Solutions

Searching for mutually acceptable solutions is the fourth step in the negotiation process. Look for common, shared interests and brainstorm to identify acceptable options. To evaluate options, follow these guidelines:

1. Ask what proposed alternatives are favored for the solution.
2. State which alternatives look best to you.
3. See which of these choices coincide.
4. Jointly decide on one or more of the alternatives.

For example, both the chair of surgery and the executive share a desire to have a safe surgical environment and a desire to avoid patient injury and malpractice suits. Therefore, "time out" and "on-time" starts may initially seem to be conflicting goals, but the latter would actually prevent the backing up of cases into the afternoon, which is when most lapses in judgment occur.

Finalize the Agreement

The fifth step is finalizing the agreement. This entails determining who will do what and by when. Clarify the action steps by which the agreed-upon solution will be implemented. Leave nothing to chance. Make sure all the details are worked out and that all parties understand exactly what is expected of them. This might involve clear statements and education about policy, acknowledgement of who has authority to institute consequences if policy is not followed, and what the first and second offense consequences would be.

Conclusion

Assertiveness and negotiation skills are necessary for the expression component of moral courage. They give voice to your concerns and allow you to deal with a multitude of negative responses to your assertion. Negotiation fosters a workable and yet moral compromise for the patients and families we serve. Moral courage requires these skills, but the true test of moral courage comes when you need to engage in the most difficult of all conversations. How to deliver bad news is the subject of Chapter 6.

Key Points to Remember

1. To deal with emotional upsets, you need to recognize the person or event that triggered your reaction.
2. First you must *identify* what you are telling yourself about the situation or person. *Listen* to your self-talk and *change* it to helpful, supportive talk.

3. Assertive behavior is an honest, direct, and appropriate expression of one's thoughts, feelings, and opinions.

4. Assertiveness focuses on solving a problem, which often requires that another person change his or her behavior.

5. A simple formula to organize your response—"When you do X, I feel Y, because of Z, and what I'd like instead is [request behavior change]."

6. *Pause* before responding to a defensive response, as this gives you time to self-soothe and avoid responding in kind.

7. Antagonistic and argumentative responses may appear as angry, but they are often fueled by fear. It is important to create a safe environment for your conversation so the dialog can be open.

8. The best strategy for responding to tears is to state, "I can see you are upset. I'd like to continue to solve the problem. Are you willing to do that?"

9. If a person chooses withdrawal, remain silent. Reflect on what his or her body language is saying. Then reassert your desire to solve the problem.

10. The technique of *negative inquiry* is used to clarify or make vague criticisms more specific.

11. In the technique of *negative assertion,* you agree with the truth in the criticism and disagree with the part that is not true.

12. Effective boundary setting means saying no to what you do not want to do and yes to what you do want.

13. Negotiation involves two or more parties with common and conflicting interests, who come together to put forth and discuss explicit proposals for the purpose of reaching agreement.

14. Utilize the seven traits of successful negotiators.

15. Three key variables to manage in any negotiation are time, power, and information.

16. Practice the five steps in the negotiation process.

References

Aquilar, F., & Galluccio, M. (2007). *Psychological processes in international negotiations: Theoretical and practical perspectives.* London: Springer.

Babcock, L., & Laschever, S. (2007). *Women don't ask: The high cost of avoiding negotiation—and positive strategies for change.* New York: Bantam Books.

Benun, I. (2006). *Stop pushing me around: A workplace guide for the timid, shy, and less.* Franklin Lakes, NJ: Career Press.

Bishop, S. (2006). *Develop your assertiveness* (2nd ed.). London: Kogan Page.

Clark, C. C. (2003). *Holistic assertiveness skills for nurses: Empower yourself (and others!).* New York: Springer Publishing.

Cohen, H. (2006). *Negotiate this!: By caring, but not T-H-A-T much.* New York: Business Plus.

Cohen, H. (1982). *You can negotiate anything.* New York: Bantam Books.

Dryden, W. (2005). *Assertiveness step by step (Overcoming common problems).* London: Sheldon Press.

Fisher, R., Ury, W., & Patton, B. (1997). *Getting to yes: Negotiating agreement without giving in.* London: Arrow Business Books.

Fred Pryor Seminars. (2006). *Assertiveness skills for managers & supervisors* (Audio CD). Overland Park, KS: Fred Pryor Seminars.

Joint Commission. (September 30, 2008). *Sentinel event statistics.* Retrieved December 19, 2008, from http://www.jointcommission.org/NR/rdonlyres/241CD6F3-6EF0-4E9C-90AD-7FEAE5EDCEA5/0/SE_Stats9_08.pdf

Karrass, G.L. (2003). *Effective negotiating workbook and discussion guide.* Beverly Hills, CA: Karrass.

Kritek, P.B. (2002). *Negotiating at an uneven table: Developing moral courage in resolving our conflicts.* San Francisco: Jossey-Bass.

Leebov, W. (2003). *Assertiveness skills for professionals in health care.* Lincoln, NE: Authors Choice Press.

Lewicki, R.J., Barry, B., & Saunders, D.M. (2006). *Essentials of negotiation* (4th ed.). McGraw-Hill Higher Education.

Lewicki, R.J., & Hiam, A. (2006). *Mastering business negotiation: A working guide to making deals and resolving conflict.* San Francisco: Jossey-Bass.

Malhotra, D., & Bazerman, M. (2007). *Negotiation genius: How to overcome obstacles and achieve brilliant results at the bargaining table and beyond.* New York: Bantam.

Maxfield, D., Grenny, J., Patterson, K., McMillan, R., & Switzler, A. (2005). *Dialogue heals: The seven crucial conversations for the healthcare professional.* Provo, UT: VitalSmarts.

Mayer, R. (2006). *How to win any negotiation: Without raising your voice, losing your cool, or coming to blows.* Franklin Lakes, NJ: Career Press.

McClure, J. S. (2007). *Civilized assertiveness for women: Communication with backbone . . . not bite.* Denver, CO: Albion Street Press.

Patterson, K., Grenny, J., McMillian, R., & Switzler, A. (2002). *Crucial conversations: Tools for when the stakes are high.* New York: McGraw-Hill.

Pfeiffer, R. H. (2003). *Real solution assertiveness workbook* (2nd ed.). New York: Growth Publishing.

Rackham, N. (1999). The behavior of successful negotiators. In Lewicki, R.J., Saunders, D.M., & Minton, J.W. (Eds.), *Negotiation: Readings, exercises, and cases* (3rd ed.) (p. 348). Boston: Irwin/McGraw-Hill.

Raiffa, H. (2005). *The art and science of negotiation.* Boston: Belknap Press.

Raiffa, H., Richardson, J., & Metcalfe, D. (2007). *Negotiation analysis: The science and art of collaborative decision making.* Boston: Belknap Press.

Shell, G.R. (2006). *Bargaining for advantage: Negotiation strategies for reasonable people* (2nd ed.). New York: Penguin.

Small, B. (2006). *What about me, what do I want? Becoming assertive.* New Bern, NC: Trafford Publishing.

Thompson, L. (2007). *The truth about negotiations.* Upper Saddle River, NJ: FT Press.

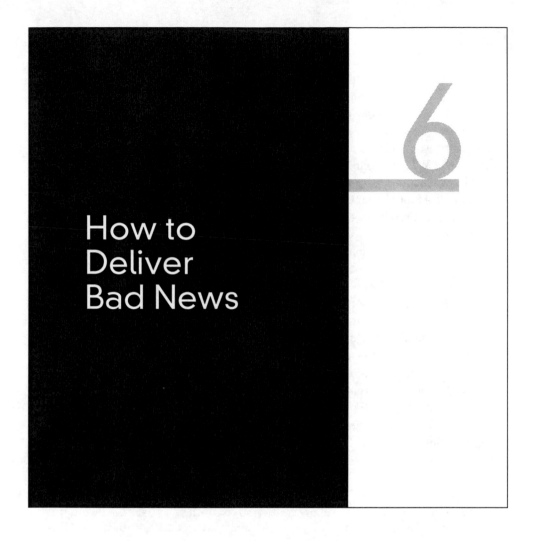

6

How to Deliver Bad News

We need people in our lives with whom we can be as open as possible. To have real conversation with people may seem like such a simple, obvious suggestion, but it involves courage and risk.

> —Thomas Moore, internationally renowned theologian, author, and former Catholic monk

Case 6.1

Mr. Kline had been a patient of mine for more than 20 years. We met when he first moved to my community and wanted "someone to check his heart every once in a while." Because his grandparents and parents had died from heart disease, his goal was to prevent developing the shortness-of-breath his father had experienced. He was in good health, had a cholesterol level of 190, walked three miles into town and back each day to work, and ate a healthy diet. He was happily married to a delightful woman, who was the local librarian, and had two grown kids who lived across the country. He bragged about their success and wished he could see his grandchildren more than three times a year.

On his 70th birthday he came in for his regularly scheduled physical exam, but he did not start with his usual fishing stories or news of his grandchildren. Rather, he wanted to discuss the swelling in his legs, about which he was clearly concerned. We talked and laughed. I put him on a dose of Lasix to "fix the swelling," and he went on his merry way. Three months later, I got a call from the local ER wanting to admit him for congestive heart failure.

Unfortunately, this was the first of six trips to the hospital over the next three years. The admissions directly correlated with his vacations and visits to his grandchildren. He did admit that he was not as rigid about his diet and medications at those times, but he bounced back from each admission.

During one visit with him in the hospital, his was experiencing shortness of breath that did not diminish; he was also distant and very quiet. In short, he was a very different man from his usual jovial self. After about 10 minutes of superficial conversation, he said to me, "You lied. You said that I would outlive my parents because I lived a healthy lifestyle, but here I am with the same symptoms at the same age my father died. Why did you lie to me?"

At that moment, I realized that I had avoided talking with him about changes in his blood pressure, the results of his lab studies, and his symptoms. I had denied his declining condition. How could I have done this? I was, after all, an experienced clinician? In truth, I had been afraid to break the bad news. His condition now was beginning to look like what he had described in his father and grandfather.

Breaking bad news to Mr. Kline or to any patient with seriously declining health is one of the most important and crucial conversations a practitioner will have. In this case, this primary care physician realized that he had avoided the conversation, even though the data were before him. To this day, he remembers the conversation with Mr. Kline as the turning point in his commitment to frank conversations with patients.

How to break bad news to patients and/or their families has been covered extensively in the literature (Buckman, 1992; Baile, Buckman, Lenzi, et al., 2000). Several methods have been developed for teaching these approaches to physicians and nurses. The documented short-term changes in behavior is heartening (Baile, Lenzi, Parker, et al., 2002; Mager & Andrykowski, 2002; Salander, 2002). The perspectives of people who receive bad news show that how you say it does really make a difference (Mager & Andrykowski, 2002; Mast, Kindlmann, & Langewitz, 2005). In 1992, Dr. Robert Buckman published a six-step model for delivering bad news; it is a model I will use to illustrate how to deliver bad news to a patient, manager, and other healthcare providers.

Bad news has been defined in several ways. Some articles indirectly define bad news with such words as "life-threatening diagnosis or death," "treatment failure," "poor prognosis," or "unfavorable medical information." Buckman (1992) defines it as "any information which drastically and negatively alters a patient's view of his or her future" (p. 15). This definition suggests that the seriousness of the bad news depends on what the patient already understands or expects for the future. Bor, Miller, Goldman, and Scher (1993) expanded the definition to include situations in which there is a feeling of no hope, a threat to a person's mental or physical well-being, a risk of upsetting an established lifestyle, and a message is given that leads the patient to understand that life will hold fewer choices. How you convey the meaning of "bad" plays a key role in the emotional response of the receiver. Mr. Kline's criticism of his physician was that he had not been alerted to the seriousness of the threat to his well-being. But, in actuality, the physician had also failed to convey to Mr. Kline that his overall health had been deteriorating—more was involved than just this one incident.

Primary care practitioners communicate bad news because they are required to do so legally. But once the physician delivers the news and leaves, other healthcare professional providers, who are often at the patient's bedside for longer periods of time, are left to provide support to the patient and family members. They need to help the recipients of the bad news understand the meaning of this new information. The ability of the healthcare professional to be part of this painful experience, to reassure and to encourage, is the essence of the primacy of care (Farrell, 1999). Thus, it is imperative that all healthcare professionals know how to deliver bad news in compassionate way.

Breaking "bad news" is a complex communication task, even for the most experienced person. Over the course of a busy career, clinicians may deliver unfavorable medical information thousands of time. The same holds true for an executive, who has to deliver "bad news" about finances or a sentinel event to the board, confront disruptive physicians, or fire/lay-off employees. These crucial conversations are stressful, but they can be made a little easier when you apply well-established communication principles.

Do people want the truth? Would you want to know if your current performance at work would result in your being fired this year? If the likelihood of your dying was 80% this year, would you want to know? From a 1982 survey of 1,251 Americans, 96% wanted to be told if they had cancer, and 85% wished to be receive a realistic estimate of how long they would live when their condition was serious (Morris & Abram, 1982). This support for disclosure has continued, although patient expectations have not always been met (Baile et al., 2002). Providing information on the status of your disease or your job supports the ethical principle of autonomy. So, although we do not want to violate the ethical principle of truth telling (veracity), we want to be sensitive about how disclose information.

Whether you graduated from a medical or business school, you probably did not receive formal training in breaking "bad news" (Baile et al., 2000; Fallowhill & Jenkins, 2004). Published reports have offered little evidence on the best educational strategy for teaching this skill (Rosenbaum, Ferguson, & Lobas, 2004). However, they do indicate that the most effective interventions explain the basic steps for delivering bad news effectively and provide opportunities for learners to discuss concerns, practice, and receive feedback on their skills. As a result of research interventions, using standardized patients, pediatric intensive care clinicians, pediatric emergency room physicians, and medical oncology fellows have improved their informing and counseling skills (Back, Arnold, Baile, Fryer-Edwards, et al., 2007; Greenberg, Ochsenschlager, O'Donnell, Mastruserio, & Cohen, 1999; Vaidya, Greenberg, Patel, Strauss, & Pollack, 1999).

Until recently, limited research was available from the patient's perspective (Kirk, Kirk, & Kristijanson, 2004; Mast et al., 2005); however, there are three classic styles of breaking bad news to patients: (1) disease centered, (2) emotion centered, and (3) patient centered (Mast et al., 2005). In the disease-centered model, the clinician bluntly presents the facts. In the emotion-centered approach, the clinician demonstrates empathy. Finally, in the patient-centered approach, the clinician conveys the information according to the patient's needs, confirms that the patient understands the information, and demonstrates empathy. In the study by Mast and his colleagues, 159 students from the University of Zurich preferred the patient-centered approach. It was more sensitive than the disease-centered approach, provided a greater sense of hope, and conveyed the maximum amount of information.

Kirk et al.'s (2004) study focused on how the clinician's timing and attitude in delivering bad news affected patients and their families. In this study, all of the 72 participants registered in palliative care wanted information about their illnesses and asked that it be totally shared with relatives. Patients and their families identified six important areas in the process of communication (p. 1345):

1. *Playing it straight*—the extent to which healthcare providers are honest and direct in conveying information.
2. *Making it clear*—the extent to which healthcare providers convey information in ways that the patient/family understands.
3. *Showing you care*—the extent to which verbal and nonverbal messages conveyed by healthcare providers are given in a compassionate and empathetic manner.
4. *Giving time*—the extent to which healthcare providers offer the patient and family enough time during the information discussion.
5. *Pacing the information*—the extent to which the healthcare provider gives information in the amounts and at the rate that patients and families can assimilate.
6. *Staying the course*—the extent to which messages given by healthcare providers indicate that they will not abandon the patient/family as the illness progresses.

This raises the question, "Do patient needs differ depending on their diagnosis?" A 2008 study of 11 focus groups says yes, when comparing patients with COPD (chronic obstructive pulmonary disease), cancer, and AIDS (Cutis, Wenrich, Carline, et al., 2008). In this qualitative study, patients, family members, and healthcare professionals gave their perspectives on the physician's skills in providing end-of-life care. The similarities in the patients' perspectives included the importance of emotional support, communication, accessibility, and continuity.

Differences among these patients' perspectives, however, can also speak to the need for the clinician to adjust his or her focus to meet each patient's needs. This can be challenging in the time-stressed environment of health care. For example, the AIDS patient was specifically concerned about pain management, while the cancer patient was more concerned about maintaining a positive outlook despite a terminal diagnosis. Patients with COPD wanted to be better educated about their disease and asked for information in five content areas: diagnosis and disease process, treatment, prognosis, what dying would be like, and advance care planning. All of these requests necessitate professional knowledge, but they also require that the clinician have the ability to deliver unfavorable information in a compassionate and effective way. Unfortunately, this is not what the physician did for Mr. Kline in the case presented at the beginning of this chapter.

How to Deliver Bad News

Effectively and compassionately breaking "bad news" is a complicated communication task in any environment, be it a healthcare facility or business setting. Telling patients and their families the truth about a diagnosis and prognosis—and what to expect along the way—requires the moral courage to tell the truth and the skill to do it compassionately. Employers can use the same skills when they counsel employees about the consequences of failing to meet required job expectations.

This communication process has verbal and nonverbal components, including effective listening, the ability to be present and respond to the emotional reaction of the patient and family members (or employee), and the skill to engage these individuals in the decision-making process. In addition, the clinician must be able to mix in an appropriate amount of hope, no matter how grave the patient's condition. For a terminally ill patient, hope may consist of hospice support that will provide the best possible quality of life during his or her the remaining months. Similarly, a manager who is delivering a written warning to an employee could express hope that the employee will decide to meet the expectations stated. A six-step protocol has been established to facilitate the use of communication and counseling principles.

The mnemonic for the six-steps is SPIKES, as seen in Exhibit 6.1 (Baile et al., 2000; Buckman, 1992), which offers suggestions of statements or questions for each step. In addition, Table 6.2 provides a comparison between delivering bad news to a patient and delivering bad news to an employee.

Step 1. S: Setting Up the Interview

Step one is setting up the interview. The physical setting should be as private as possible, and the possibility of interruptions minimized (e.g., keep your pager on silent and accept no phone calls). Unless absolutely unavoidable, the interview

---

6.1 The Six Steps of SPIKES

1. S—Setting up the Interview
2. P—Assessing the Patient's Perception
3. I—Obtaining the Patient's Invitation
4. K—Giving Knowledge and Information to the Patient
5. E—Assessing the Patient's Emotions with Empathetic Responses
6. S—Strategy and Summary

Baile, W.F., Buckman, R., Lenzi, R., Glober, G., Beale, E.A., & Kudelka, A. P. (2000). SPIKES—A six-step protocol for delivering bad news: Application to the patient with cancer. *The Oncologist, 5*, 302–311.

should be conducted in person, not over the telephone. Sit down, with a distance of 20 to 36 inches between the participants, but not at the foot of the bed. Be able to establish direct-line eyeball-to-eyeball contact. Remove all barriers between you and the other person, such as a desk or bedside tables or clutter. Touching can be a complex issue, and your decision should be based on your relationship to patient, the cultural context, and the clinician's ease with touching. If you decide to touch a patient, be sensitive to the patient's response. (In a management-employee situation, of course, the rule is not to touch.) If requested by the patient, involve family members and significant others.

Step 2. P: Assessing the Patient's Perspective

Step two is assessing the patient's perception. In both steps two and three, the best advice is "before you tell, ask." You need to determine how much the individual knows. To achieve this, use open-ended questions, such as "What have you been told about your medical situation?," "Do you understand why we need to do the MRI?," or "Do you know why I have called you into my office today?" These open-ended questions cannot be answered with a simple yes or no; they require that the patient provide an explanatory answer. Based on these responses, you can correct misunderstandings, identify patients who are in denial about their true condition, and answer questions.

Step 3. I: Obtaining the Patient's Invitation

The real issue here is what *level of detail* does the person or patient really want about the situation. You might ask, "How would you like me to give you the results of the tests?," "Would you like me to give you the full details of your condition, or would you like me to give them to someone else?," "How much detail do you want about why we are suspending you?" or "Do you just want to know the next steps?" Most people will opt for full disclosure, but some need to receive bad news in smaller doses over time.

Step 4. K: Giving Knowledge and Information to the Patient

Step four is sharing your knowledge and information with the patient. Start by warning the individual that "bad news" is coming by opening with such phrases as, "I am sorry to have to tell you this . . ." or "I have 'bad news' to tell you. . . ." Follow this with facts that presented in plain language; avoid the use of medical jargon (Medspeak). Convey the information in small chunks, checking at regular intervals that the patient understands the situation. This is particularly important when conveying serious news. You might say, "The test we did revealed that your cancer has spread to your liver. Do you understand what this means?" Or "The written warning I gave you last week for your lateness has had no effect on your willingness to be on time. Do you know what the next step is in this disciplinary process?"

It is important to repeat important points, because the human brain has a way of screening out information in serious situations. It is often helpful to have written documentation (e.g., X-rays, documented absences) to support your position.

Step 5. E: Assessing the Patient's Emotions With Empathetic Responses

The patient's emotional reaction to the "bad news" might include silence, crying, or anger. These reflect the shock and grief patients may experience. If the response is silence, wait a full minute and then ask, "What are you feeling or thinking right now?" Use empathetic statements, such as "I can see how upsetting this is for you"; exploratory questions, such as "Could you tell me what you are afraid of?"; or validating questions, such as "Your reaction is normal, given the bad news I have given you."

Step 6. S: Strategy and Summary

Depending on the severity of the bad news, the individual might be feeling bewildered, downhearted, or anxious. In addition to empathizing with the patient, you must fulfill your professional responsibilities by summarizing the discussion and describing the next steps that are required to follow through on the diagnosis. Show that you understand the individual's problem and differentiate the fixable from the unfixable. This should lead to a plan that includes actions that address the uncertainties of the problem (e.g., "If the dyspnea does not get better, then we will . . . ," or "If the change of your hours to eliminate lateness does not work, then we will . . ."). In this step it is crucial to identify and reinforce the individual's coping strategies. You want to support the resourcefulness of the patient. What supports do they have to minimize their feeling of loneliness and isolation in facing the diagnosis? Can you recommend any additional supports, such as social services or employee assistance counseling (EAP)?

Sample Dialogs

Exhibit 6.2 offers examples of "bad news" dialogs in both healthcare and business settings. The amount of time required to complete each step will be determined by the individual receiving the news, as each person responds differently to adversity. So, the receiver's response will provide a microcosm of the person's pattern of behavior when reacting to stress. For example, if a person usually copes with stress successfully by withdrawing, he or she is likely to repeat the pattern here. Although experience and maturity might affect the receiver's response, a patient's response to news of a life-threatening illness will likely be very intense. The phrases you use in such circumstances should be based on your assessment of what is best for this person at this time.

Several versions of six steps of SPIKES have been published since Buckman first outlined them. In all the versions, however, steps move from (1) preparation to (2) disclosure to (3) response to the reaction to the disclosure. These steps have been incorporated into medical training and evaluation based on outcomes with simulated patients (Eggly et al., 2008). Eggly and his coworkers analyzed 25 randomly selected videorecorded interactions between oncologists and patients in outpatient cancer clinics. Their findings suggest that three of the assumptions in the SPIKES model had been so oversimplified that they were distorted in the real clinical setting.

6.2 Delivering Bad News

	Patient: Clinician	Manager: Employee
S	"I am pulling the curtain to provide some privacy for our discussion. I would like to sit and have a conversation about your x-ray results with you and your husband."	"Please come to my office so we can sit down and discuss this situation in private."
P	"What is your understanding as to why we did the x-ray?"	"Why do you think I have asked to meet with you today?"
I	"You said that you wanted me to just give you the information straight; is that still your desire?"	"Do you know what the organizational policy is concerning repeated lateness, when a written warning has been given?"
K	"I have bad news. The x-ray shows a reoccurrence of a tumor in your right lung."	"I have bad news. Since you already have received a written warning, I must now give you a three-day suspension."
E	"I can tell you were not expecting this result."	"This is difficult for me to do because you are such a good clinician. This must be upsetting."
S	"The next step is a biopsy, and then the possibility of surgery."	"What strategies do you have in mind to correct this problem?"

The first assumption is that physicians can plan a "bad news" interaction, even though different patients respond differently to the same information. In many cases, the patient's reaction is hard to predict. For example, when a physician suggests that a patient participate in a clinical trial, the patient can see this either as giving hope or as an option of last resort. The physician must be able to adjust the planned dialog to suit the patient's reaction or have alternative dialogs in mind before beginning the discussion. Despite these findings, researchers have continued to suggest that guidelines for giving information should apply to all interactions (Cole & Bird, 2000). I even believe that preparations that include a rehearsal can make a difference in the outcome.

The second assumption is that bad news interactions should focus on one central piece of information. However, the results of the Eggly et al. study show that 24 of the 25 videotape interactions covered an average of 3.2 bad news topics. When this much "bad news" is presented at one time, the patient will most likely be overwhelmed. To cope with this reaction, remember to speak clearly in plain English and be sure to confirm the patient's understanding after each piece of information is presented.

The third assumption is that bad news interactions take place primarily in a physician-patient dyad. Yet, one analysis showed that companions asked 62%

of the questions, while patients asked only 38% of the questions. This result speaks to the need to involve all parties and to ask everyone, not just the patient, the questions outlined in SPIKES.

Are there differences in how patients want to receive bad news based on cultural background (Fujimon et al., 2007)? In Japan, 529 Japanese outpatient cancer patients participated in a study using multiple measures to assess anxiety, mental adjustment, and patient preference. Most items rated as important in U.S. published guidelines were considered equally important in Japan, but two differences emerged. The Japanese norm of formality and privacy was likely the explanation of these differences. The Japanese preferred to be alone and not to be touched when receiving bad news.

Conclusion

For the practitioner, I believe the SPIKES model is effective in delivering bad news. It is particularly helpful for beginning practitioners faced with difficult end-of-life discussions. As with all models, some variation may be necessary, depending on patient and family needs, disease categories, and cultural variations, but these require further study.

Key Points to Remember

1. The perspectives of people who receive bad news shows that how you say it really does make a difference.
2. The patient-centered approach, which is the preferred approach, means conveying the information according to the patient's needs, checking for understanding, and demonstrating empathy.
3. How the patient and his or her family experience the bad news depends on the timing, delivery, and the attitude of the clinician.
4. The clinician must be able to mix in an appropriate amount of hope, particularly if the illness is severe.
5. The six steps to follow in delivering "bad news" has the mnemonic SPIKES.
6. Use English, not medical jargon ("Medspeak").
7. Understand the patient's/family's emotional response.
8. Involve all the people the patient requests for the "bad news" dialog.
9. The SPIKES mnemonic can be used to deliver "bad news" in all business environments, not just healthcare settings.

References

Back, A.L., Arnold, R.M., Baile, W.F., Fryer-Edwards, K.A., Alexander, S.A., Barley, G.E., et al. (2007). Efficacy of communication skills training for giving bad news and discussing transitions to palliative care. *Archives of Internal Medicine, 167,* 453–460.

Baile, W.F., Buckman, R., Lenzi, R., Glober, G., Beale, E.A., & Kudelka, A. P. (2000). SPIKES—A six-step protocol for delivering bad news: Application to the patient with cancer. *The Oncologist, 5,* 302–311.

Baile, W.F., Lenzi, R., Parker, P.A., Buckman, R., & Cohen, L. (2002). Oncologists' attitudes toward the practice of giving bad news: An exploratory study. *Journal of Clinical Oncology, 20*(8), 2189–2196.

Bor, R., Miller, R., Goldman, E., & Scher, I. (1993). The meaning of bad news in HIV disease. *Counseling Psychology Quarterly, 6,* 69–90.

Buckman, R. (1992). *How to break bad news.* Baltimore: Johns Hopkins University Press.

Cole, S.A., & Bird, J. (2000). *The medical interview: The three-function approach* (2nd ed.). St. Louis, MO: Mosby, Inc.

Curtis, J.R., Wenrich, M.D., Carline, J.D., Shannon, S.E., Ambrozy, D.M. & Ramsey, P.G. (2002). Patients' perspectives on physician's skill in end-of-life care: Differences between patients with COPD, cancer and AIDS. *Chest, 122,* 356–362.

Eggly, S., Penner, L., Albrecht, T.L., Cline, R.J., Foster, T., Naughton, M., et al. (2006). Discussing bad news in the outpatient oncology clinics: Rethinking current communication guidelines. *Journal of Clinical Oncology, 24*(4), 716–719.

Fallowhill, L., & Jenkins, V. (2004). Communicating sad, bad and difficult news in medicine. *Lancet, 363,* 312–319.

Farrell, M. (1999). The challenge of breaking bad news. *Intensive and Critical Care Nursing, 15,* 101–110.

Fujimon, M., Parker, P.A., Akechi, T., Sakano, Y., Baile, W.F., & Uchitomi, Y. (2007). Japanese cancer patients' communication style preferences when receiving bad news. *Psychooncology, 16,* 617–625.

Greenberg, L.W., Ochsenschlager, D., O'Donnell, R., Mastruserio, J., & Cohen, G.J. (1999). Communicating bad news: A pediatric department's evaluation of a simulated intervention. *American Academy of Pediatrics, 103*(6), 1210–1217.

Kirk, P., Kirk, I., & Kristjanson, L.J. (2004). What do patients receiving palliative care for cancer and their families want to be told? A Canadian and Australian qualitative study. *British Medical Journal, 328,* 1343–1350.

Mager, W.M., & Andrykowski, M.A. (2002). Communication in the "bad news" cancer consultation: Patient perceptions and psychological adjustment. *Psychooncology, 11,* 35–46.

Mast, M.S., Kindlmann, A., & Langewitz, W. (2005). Recipients' perspectives on breaking bad news: How you put it really makes a difference. *Patient Education and Counseling, 58,* 244–251.

Morris, B., & Abram, C. (1982). *Making healthcare decisions. The ethical and legal implications of informed consent in the practitioner-patient relationship* (p. 119). Washington, DC: United States Superintendent of Documents.

Rosenbaum, M.E., Ferguson, K.J., & Lobas, J.G. (2004). Teaching medical students and residents skills for delivering bad news: A review of strategies. *Academic Medicine, 79*(2), 107–117.

Salander, P. (2002). Bad news from the patient's perspective: An analysis of written narratives of newly diagnosed cancer patients. *Social Science Medicine, 55,* 721–732.

Vaidya, V.U., Greenberg, L. W., Patel, K.M., Strauss, L.H., & Pollack, M.M. (1999). Teaching physicians how to break bad news. *Archives of Pediatric and Adolescent Medicine, 153*(4), 419–422.

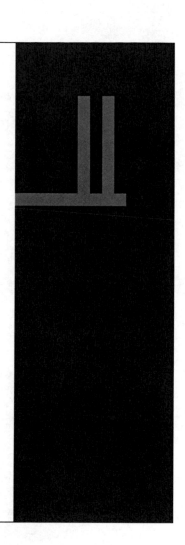

Personal Opportunities for Moral Courage

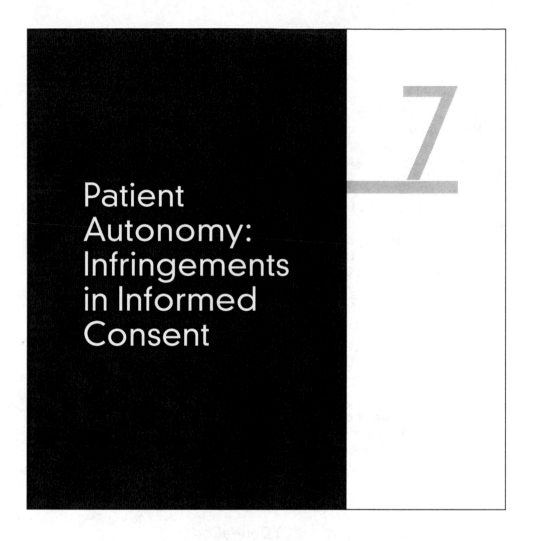

Patient Autonomy: Infringements in Informed Consent

7

To be nobody but yourself—in a world which is doing its best, night and day, to make you like everybody else—means to fight the hardest battle which any human being can fight, and never stop fighting.

—e e cummings, known for his highly idiosyncratic means of poetic expression

Every human being of adult years and sound mind has a right to determine what shall be done with his own body.

—Justice Benjamin Cardozo, U.S. Supreme Court Justice

This chapter on autonomy and informed consent begins with two quotations, the first of which I've carried in my wallet for more than 30 years. It speaks to the moral courage necessary to be your own person and to determine your own destiny. The second I've used in PowerPoint slides on informed consent only since 2002, but the date of the quotation is 1914. The right to self-determination is an issue of such magnitude that it is a central underpinning of any democratic society. On a smaller scale, it is also a significant patient right in any safe healthcare system. This chapter uses a new case study to illustrate the seven steps in the informed consent process. In discussing the implementation of these steps, I will also examine when and why moral courage may be needed.

Patient autonomy is one of the most basic rights in the U.S. healthcare system. This right of patients to self-determination, to determine what will and will not be done to their own bodies, is arguably the most fundamental of moral principles. Because poor health can affect a person's ability to reason and make choices, it is considered a moral imperative to promote good health.

Could there be a valid argument for transitory intrusion on the patient's autonomy if it promotes the patient's health? Perhaps once, but no longer. The medical community long used this argument as a justification for paternalism—for the expectation that the patient would defer to the physician's judgment. However, unquestioning deference to the medical establishment is no longer prevalent, as it was in the mid-twentieth century. Indeed, most patients expect choices, are more aware of their rights, and wish to participate in medical decision-making. Today, patients expect to be informed and viewed as partners in decision making.

The United States is at the extreme end of the continuum in support of patient autonomy (Schneider, 1998). In other countries, a more communal, or family-based, approach is the norm, as can be seen in some first and second-generation Asian, Hispanic, and, at times, African American families. But, many healthcare professionals consider family involvement in decision making a violation of the right of patient autonomy. Patients can, of course, accept support from, or even defer to, others. The key for healthcare professionals is to determine how the patient wants to be involved in treatment decisions and whom else the patient wants to include in the process.

The Healthcare Professional's Obligation to Support Autonomy

Autonomy is the philosophical basis for informed consent. All codes of ethics that apply to healthcare professionals address the obligation to provide accurate information to patients so that they make autonomous decisions. The AMA Code of Medical Ethics states, "A physician shall . . . make relevant information available to patients" (American Medical Association, 2001). The Physician Assistant (PA) Code states, "Provide adequate information comprehensible to a competent patient or patient surrogate. PAs should be committed to the concept of shared decision making, which involves assisting patients in making decisions that account for medical, situational, and personal factors" (American Academy of Physician Assistants, 2007).

The American Nursing Association (ANA) Code (2001) states more specifically to what this information should include:

> *Patients have a moral and legal right to determine what will be done with their own person; to be given accurate, complete, and understandable information in a manner that facilitates an informed judgment; to be assisted with weighing the benefits, burdens, and available options in their treatment, including the choice*

of no treatment; to accept, refuse, or terminate treatment without deceit, undue influence, duress, coercion, or penalty; and to be given necessary support throughout the decision making and treatment process (p. 8).

This Code also focuses on the importance of including the family in the decision-making process. Surrogate decision making is necessary when the patient lacks the capacity to make a decision, although such decisions should be based on the formerly stated wishes and recognized values of the patient. Further discussion of the problems in surrogate decision making will be covered in Chapter 8.

Informed Consent Process

Fletcher, Spencer, and Lombardo (2005) outline seven steps in the informed consent process (see Exhibit 7.1). Insufficient or excessive emphasis on any one of the steps could distort the entire process. For example, patients should be informed of all treatment options and the burdens of those options without an overemphasis that favors the physician's recommendation. Each of the seven steps presents specific concerns that could threaten autonomy. These concerns and the role of moral courage in resolving them are the focus of the case study that forms the basis of our discussion.

Case 7.1

Mrs. Able is a spry and mentally competent 90-year-old widow, who has been living on her own for five years. During a trip to the emergency room, she is diagnosed with gastrointestinal bleeding. The surgeon recommends surgery to stop the bleeding, which will otherwise cause death, but Mrs. Able refuses. Although she understands the diagnosis and the surgeon's proposed treatment, she refuses the surgery and agrees to palliative care because she is convinced that her

"time has come." She discusses her decision with her niece, and both of them confirm it with the surgeon. The surgeon, however, is confused and considers seeking
a psychiatric consult. After all, this is an active and independent women, who seems
to be choosing to die.

Step 1. Determining a Patient's Capacity

Capacity is the ability to understand information relevant to making a particular decision. It requires an appreciation of the possible consequences of each
decision, including choosing not to make a decision (Fletcher, Spencer, & Lombardo, 2005). Whether a patient is capable of making a specific decision is not
always a "yes or no" question; the answer depends on the context of the decision.
To decide whether you will authorize triple-bypass surgery is different from au-
thorizing a lumbar puncture. In the case of Mrs. Able, her capacity is being called
into question because her decision is different from that of the healthcare professional. However, further examination of her thinking reveals her as rational;
she is not basing her decision on distorted perceptions.

Because of the seriousness of the decision, the surgeon's concern is under-
standable. But, it is also true that physicians are less likely to question a patient's
capacity if the patient agrees with their recommendations. As a result, the patient may need a healthcare professional as an advocate when they do not agree
with the physician's recommended treatment.

Step 2. Assuring the Decision Is Voluntary

Once the healthcare professional is confident that the patient is capable, the
professional needs to be certain that the patient is not coerced into changing his
or her mind. The patient's decision must be a voluntary one. Mrs. Able, for example, is not being coerced into having the surgery. She understands what her
decision means and voluntarily accepts comfort measures to ease her dying
process.

Simply put, coercion has no place in informed consent, regardless of its
source, which could include other healthcare professionals, the patient's family,
and significant others. Thus, the healthcare professional needs to watch out for
possible coercion. Consider the following case articulated by a 3–11 staff nurse.

Case 7.2

My patient said to me, "Nurse, I really do not want another amputation. I was able
to manage when just my foot was amputated because of complications from my diabetes. This amputation, however, would be above the knee, and I understand all
the rehab that a prosthesis will require. I am 85 years old and have lived a good life
and am ready to meet my maker, but my daughter just cannot let me go. She was
here last evening, crying and lecturing me about my need to live. Please do not say
anything to her, but I just want to be comfortable and pass on. The nurse finds a

> signed consent form for surgery in the chart. She feels conflicted. Should she honor the requested confidentiality made by the patient or should she raisethe issue with the surgeon at 10 PM to confirm that the patient has truly signed the consent form voluntarily?

In this situation, the nurse's obligation is to help arrange a family meeting with either a social worker or through the ethics committee, as this patient has not freely chosen surgery. At the same time, the patient asked the nurse not to say anything. Is the nurse violating patient confidentiality?

The Code of Ethics for Nurses states "Duties of confidentiality, however are not absolute and may need to be modified in order to protect the patient . . ." (American Nurses Association, 2001, p. 12). This nurse needs to find the courage to speak the truth for the patient and the willingness to provide resources that will help his daughter accept his decision.

Step 3: Disclosing Information

Healthcare professionals have an ethical obligation to provide sufficient information to support the patient in making a decision concerning treatment options. They also must be transparent in supplying this information. This means the health professional is obligated to:

1. State clearly if they are sure or unsure of the diagnosis.
2. Explain why any invasive tests, including blood studies, are necessary, and how these tests will help determine diagnosis, prognosis, treatment, and effects of treatment.
3. Be crystal clear about the benefits and burdens of all recommended treatments.
4. Remember the rule that no test should performed if it will not change the treatment protocol. Healthcare professionals may need to speak out if they see any violation of this rule.

This last obligation grows increasingly important when recommending that a patient participate in a clinical trial. Why? Because clinical trials are usually a treatment of last resort, a treatment recommended when evidence-based practice no longer offers hope. For example, a Phase I trial offers no evidence that it will make any difference in the patient's outcome. In practical terms, this means that the patient's participation is tantamount to donating his or her body to research; the patient needs to understand that this is what they will be doing and that the participation does not offer hope of improved health. Therefore, in terms of a Phase I trial, it would be considered coercion if the healthcare professional said, "We have nothing more to offer you except this Phase I chemotherapy trial." A true disclosure of options would be stated as, "Your options are now limited because the second round of chemotherapy did not slow the growth of your tumor. We can offer you enrollment in a clinical trial that has no proven results as of yet, or we can offer you palliative care that will help keep you comfortable. The first will have some significant side effects that will impact the quality of your life, such as nausea and fatigue. If you choose the palliative care option, clinicians will help you achieve the best quality life you can for your remaining months."

Hope is always offered to the patient, but in the proportion at which it is warranted. Because patients are often desperate at this point, their ability to process information is significantly affected by their anxiety. If the healthcare professional does not present the information properly, it may foster false hope in the patient.

If you know that a patient is not receiving the whole truth about treatment options, it is your ethical obligation to support the patient's right to accurate information, but you must do so without undermining the physician-patient relationship. A comment such as "Mrs. Jones, both your physician and I want what you think is best for you. Your physician has clearly laid out your option for the clinical trial. This will have some effects on the quality of your life that should be mentioned. Would you like to know what they could be?" could open the door to a discussion on palliative care. In many organizations, a referral to a palliative care consultation does not require a physician's order.

Step 4. Making a Recommendation

Almost all patients will eventually ask, "What is your recommendation?" This is an opportunity for the healthcare professional to summarize the choices, benefits, and burdens of each treatment option and to offer their advice about what needs to done next. This is not the same question as "What would you do if you were me?" A reply to this question is irrelevant to the care of this patient and is best refocused with a response such as "What I would do in your circumstances is unknown to me. My job is to help you figure out what you want to do, given who you are and what you value." This is a crucial conversation. Therefore you need to *mirror, paraphrase, and ask questions* that will help the patient determine the outcome most desired.

In the case of Mrs. Able, the patient does not agree with the surgeon's recommendation. When this occurs, a healthcare professional may need to speak out and recommend a second opinion or suggest other options. Moral courage may be necessary if the PA on this surgical service advocates for the patient even though her choice does not conform to her supervising physician's recommendation.

The healthcare professional's recommendation should be based on available scientific evidence and a consideration of the patient's physical, social, psychological, and spiritual needs. This advice needs to consider the patient's goals, whether that be living two more months to greet a first grandchild, using everything in the chemotherapeutic arsenal, or accepting closure and preparing for death.

Step 5. Assurance, Understanding, and Comprehension

The professional's recommendation carries significant authority because of the power differential between the patient and the healthcare professional. Therefore, the healthcare professional needs to help the patient feel safe in discussing the suggested option. Watch carefully for signs of withdrawal or masking. Sometimes, it is best to say, "I suggest you think about the option and discuss this recommendation with your family. We could then reconvene to discuss it further. I want to make sure I have explained this option clearly. Could you please tell me now what you have understood me to say?"

If you have ever received news that could alter the rest of your life, you can understand the importance of slowing down communications so the patient can digest the information. Depending on the severity and intensity of the recommendation, the patient may be in shock and unable to cognitively process the data. If you see that another healthcare professional is not recognizing that a patient is confused or experiencing mental anguish, it is vital that you speak up and stop the conversation. Crucial conversations, in which patients give permission for medical interventions, need to occur in an environment in which the patient feels safe in asking questions.

In the case of Mrs. Able, she demonstrated her understanding of the alternatives and the consequences of her decision. She did discuss her choice with a niece. Both then spoke with the surgeon and reiterated her decision.

Step 6. Finalize the Decision

Dialog ends when the decision is made and an option is chosen. The patient has to decide whom to involve in the decision. Whether the patient chooses to decide by consultation ("I want to hear your opinions and thoughts, but I will decide") or consensus ("I want us to discuss our opinions and ideas until we come up with a decision we can all support"), the healthcare professional needs to provide the patient with breathing space. If the time allotted for the decision is limited, as with a healthcare emergency, then the professional should inform the patient of the time constraints. Years of studies in group dynamics show that problem solving does not really begin until half of the available time has elapsed. Patients and their families must also understand that the dialog cannot continue indefinitely.

Step 7. Authorize the Decision

This is the step during which pen meets paper, as the patient signs the permit and the decision is entered in the physician's orders. If all the other steps have been followed successfully, this final step in the informed consent process is routine. However, no invasive procedure can go forward if this step has not been completed, as many an operating room nurse has discovered when making a final check for the consent form. The only invasive procedure that can be performed on patients without their consent is CPR. It is the only procedure that requires a negative order—one that says the patient does not consent.

Problems With Informed Consent

A series of four articles by Scott et al. (2003) reported findings from a Scottish study on autonomy, privacy, and informed consent on maternal, elderly, and surgical patients. Data was collected by questionnaires completed independently by patients and the professionals who cared for them. The results reveal problems of perception that can arise with informed consent. For example, in a comparative study of midwives and mothers, Scott and her coworkers (2003b) found that the major differences occurred in the information-giving and decision-making steps. On all the information scales, *except* for hospital stay and name and dose of medication, 20 out of 22 items on the autonomy scale were statistically different between mothers and midwives. The midwives perceived themselves as giving more information and involvement to the mothers in determining their care than did the mothers. In the study on the elderly, significant differences were found between patients' and nurses' perceptions (15% versus 54%) concerning information about treatments (Scott et al., 2003c). Other differences concerned the amount of autonomy patients thought they had in making decisions regarding their daily care. The higher the patient's level of education, the more information the nurse provided. Finally, an examination of the perceptions between surgical patients and nurses once again revealed significant differences in the information-giving step of the autonomy subscale. On 8 out of the 11 items, nurses perceived themselves as giving more information than did the patient. The researchers concluded that patients are generally positive about how their autonomy, privacy, and informed consent are sought and protected within the Scottish National Health System, but opportunities for improvement lie in the communication arena of validating, paraphrasing, and assuring comprehension.

Conclusion

Supporting patient autonomy in all decisions is an ethical obligation of healthcare professionals. All seven elements of the informed consent process are important and necessary. The steps need to be performed in the order given, because information is irrelevant if the patient lacks capacity to understand it. At any step, a healthcare professional may need to muster the moral courage to speak out if another healthcare professional is violating the requirement. However, this violation may not originate with the healthcare professional, but with a surrogate decision maker. Therefore, the next chapter includes a considerable discussion about the issue of proxy decision making in advance directives.

Key Points to Remember

1. Patient autonomy—patient's right to self-determination—is one of the most basic rights in the U.S. healthcare system.
2. Autonomy is the philosophical basis for informed consent.
3. Most patients expect choices, are more aware of their rights, and wish to share in medical decision making.
4. The communitarian- or family-based approach to decision making is more common in first- and second-generation Americans of Asian, Hispanic, and, at times, African American descent.
5. Healthcare professionals have an ethical obligation to support the seven steps in the informed consent process.
6. Capacity is the ability to understand information relevant to a particular decision. It requires an appreciation of the possible consequences of each decision, including choosing not to make a decision.
7. The healthcare professional needs to be on the lookout for coercion, not only from other healthcare professionals, but also from the patient's family and significant others.

8. For any invasive test, including blood studies, the patient has a right to know why the test is necessary and how the test will help determine diagnosis, prognosis, treatment, or effects of treatment.
9. Healthcare professionals need to be crystal clear about the benefits and burdens of all recommended treatments.
10. When you see a patient who is not being given the whole truth, your ethical obligation is to support the patient in learning all their treatment options without undermining the physician-patient relationship.
11. The healthcare professional's recommendation is an opportunity to summarize the choices, benefits, and burdens of each and to offer their advice about what needs to done next.
12. The healthcare professional has an obligation to ensure understanding and comprehension of information and recommendations.
13. Though the patient's signature is required on the consent form, the preceding six steps are equally important.
14. A healthcare professional may have to advocate for a patient's decision when it does not agree with the physician's desired treatment.

References

American Medical Association. (2001). *Code of medical ethics.* Chicago: AMA. Retrieved July 1, 2008, from http://www.ama-assn.org/ama/pub/category/2512.html

American Academy of Physician Assistants. (2007). *Guidelines for ethical conduct for physician assistants.* Retrieved June 4, 2008, from http://www.aapa.org/manual/23-EthicalConduct.pdf

American Nurses Association. (2001). *Code of ethics for nurses with interpretative statements.* Silver Spring, MD: American Nurses Publishing. Retrieved July 5, 2008, from http://www.nursingworld.org

Fletcher, J.C., Spencer, E.M., & Lombardo, P.A. (2005). *Fletcher's introduction to clinical ethics* (3rd ed.). Hagerstown, MD: University Publishing Group.

Schneider, C.E. (1998). *The practice of autonomy: Patients, doctors, and medical decisions.* Oxford: Oxford University Press.

Scott, P.A., Valimaki, M., Leino-Kilpi, H., Dassen, T., Gasull, M., Lemonidou, C., & Arndt, M. (2003a). Autonomy, privacy and informed consent 1: Concepts and definitions. *British Journal of Nursing, 12*(1), 43–47.

Scott, P.A., Taylor, A., Valimaki, M., Leino-Kilpi, H., Dassen, T., Gasull, M., Lemonidou, C., & Arndt, M. (2003b). Autonomy, privacy and informed consent 2: Postnatal perspective. *British Journal of Nursing, 12*(2), 117–127.

Scott, P.A., Taylor, A., Valimaki, M., et al. (2003c). Autonomy, privacy and informed consent 3: Elderly care perspective. *British Journal of Nursing, 12*(3), 158–168.

Scott, P.A., Valimaki, M., Leino-Kilpi, H., Dassen, T., Gasull, M., Lemonidou, C., & Arndt, M. (2003d). Autonomy, privacy and informed consent 4: Surgical perspective. *British Journal of Nursing, 12*(5), 311–320.

Tauber, A.I. (2005). *Patient autonomy and the ethics of responsibility.* Cambridge, MA: MIT Press.

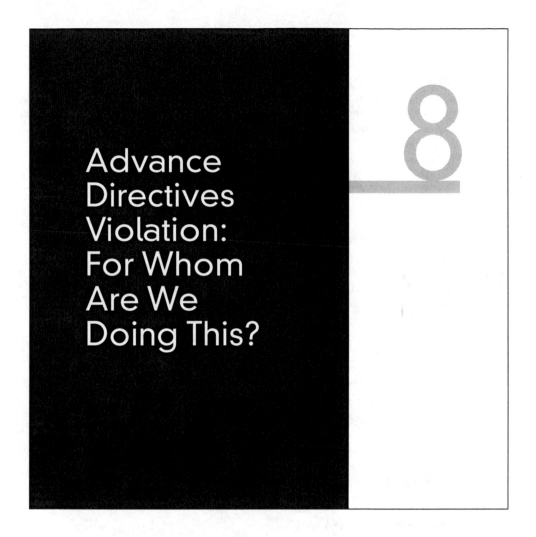

Advance Directives Violation: For Whom Are We Doing This?

8

Death is not the greatest of evils; it is worse to want to die, and not be able to.

—Sophocles, prolific ancient Greek playwright

Americans consider respect for the notion of autonomy as an achievable ideal. The advance directive (AD) was designed to support this ideal by protecting a patient's right to decide not to be kept alive or, on the other hand, to request that all possible technologies be used to prolong life. Although the AD is an ethical and legal document, hospitals across the United States violate it every day. The cases presented in this chapter highlight the disagreements between healthcare professionals and attending physicians and between healthcare professionals and families. The discussion begins with the need for effective and compassionate delivery of the "bad news" and then moves through the specifics of the AD and how ethics committee consultations can help resolve issues. It concludes with applications of the best interests standard. Problems addressed include violation of the AD, lack of a proxy decision maker, and religious objections. Issues surrounding futility are discussed in Chapter 9.

Several highly publicized cases have taught the general public that the lack of written documentation of a patient's wishes can lead to long, drawn out court proceedings about technologically supported life. The Patient Self-Determination Act (PSDA) of 1991 was enacted to support patient autonomy through the AD (Drane, 1991). This law requires hospitals, hospices, and nursing homes to ask if the patient has an advance directive and, if the answer is no, to help the patient fill one out if requested. But, the law does not mandate that the AD be placed on the chart or that the patient's wishes be followed. Busy nurses ask families to bring in the AD or call the nursing home to get a copy, but the lack of follow through is notorious in hospitals. As a result, the autonomous wishes of the patient, even when known, are often ignored or overlooked.

Healthcare professionals need support from their institutions to enforce a policy that every patient either has an AD (including designated proxy decision maker) on his or her chart or a documented conversation in the physician's record of whom to call for proxy surrogate/decision making. To resolve this problem, some hospitals have designated specific people to follow-up on these requirements. The admissions clerk, the nurse admitting the patient, and the resident doing the admission history and physical all have triggers in their on-line documentation that remind them to ask about an AD. Unless the patient hands over the AD right then, a specific follow-up is triggered. If the healthcare facility does not have such a triggering system, a low-tech approach is to designate that a specific person in the hospital, usually a social worker or case manager, be responsible for obtaining an AD. Some facilities require that the responding individual complete a separate form if the patient requests a consultation to discuss the AD. This form becomes part of the patient's permanent record. If the patient creates an AD, the existence of the AD is noted in the physician's record.

Surrogate Decision-Making

Although most people express a desire to execute an AD, only 5 to 25% of patients actually have one in the form of a living will or durable power of attorney (Emanuel, Barry, Stoekle, Ettelson, & Emanuel, 1991; Emanuel, Weinberg, Gonin, Hummel, & Emanuel, 1993). This gap between desire and completion is mainly the result of a reluctance to discuss end-of-life issues. These issues are best discussed in the office of the patient's primary care physician at a time when the patient is stable (Emanuel, 2008; Johnson, Pfeifer & McNutt, 1995; Steinbrook, Lo, Moulton, et al., 1986). Patients believe it is the responsibility of their physicians to initiate such conversations (Edinger & Smucker, 1992; Johnson et al., 1995; Steinbrook et al., 1986), but physicians barely have enough time for routine visits, let alone the multifaceted conversations that an AD requires. So, the issue is often left unaddressed, and the patient's preferences remain unspecified. Then, when the patient is in a critical care unit and/or in the final stage of a terminal illness, the physician is forced to have these discussions with a family member. Studies have projected that surrogates make 75% of the decisions for critically ill hospitalized patients and 44% to 66% of the decisions for nursing home resident (Hiltman, Medich, Chase, Peterson, & Forrow, 1999; Kim, Karlawish, & Caine, 2002). Thus, in large part, the proxy decision maker must substitute his or her judgment ("substituted judgment") for the patient's judgment, with an overarching responsibility to inform the healthcare team what the patient would have wanted and not what the proxy wants for the patient.

Studies of proxy decision making have had inconclusive results. Some find that the surrogate has a better than average chance in predicting the patient's wishes, while others suggest that surrogates are able to predict accurately only in extreme situations (Layde, Beam, Broste, et al., 1995; Sulmasy, Terry, Weisman, et al., 1998). In one study that compared the proxy's choices with random choices, the proxy matched the patient's preferences only 62% of the time (Suhl, Simons, Reedy, & Garrick, 1994).

Engleberg, Patrick, and Curtis (2005) used the Preferences about Dying and Death (PADD) in a hospice population to explore the degree to which a person's end-of-life preferences agreed with observations of others. The PADD is based on published studies, valid measurements, and qualitative interviews with patients who had AIDS, COPD, and cancer. Almost 73% of the population studied had a cancer diagnosis, where the projectory of dying is more defined. The results indicate that family members were able to predict patient preferences in about half of the situations that patients acknowledged as essential in coping with the end of life. Good agreement (>60%) was achieved in 8 of 30 items. All items in which the percentage of concurrence was greater than 55% were regarded as very important to a good death (e.g., pain under control, breathing comfortably, funeral arrangements made, etc.). Greater agreement was seen with patients who had an AD, higher income, and multiple conversations with their surrogates about preferences.

Families overestimated the need for resolving family conflicts, but undervalued the significance of the patient's concerns about being a strain or burden. The bad news is that even in this hospice population, where both patient and family members have made the physical and emotional transition, there is lack of agreement. The good news, however, is that discussions and an AD did help. Clearly, the 31 items in the PADD could be used as an outline for a discussion between family members and patients before an end-of-life decision arises. In addition, when healthcare professionals know what is most important to terminally ill patients, they can facilitate the conversation to cover the most important points. The PADD may just represent a social consensus of the definition of a good death.

The PADD study indicated, not surprisingly, that patients close to death experience an urgency about end-of-life issues that is not present in healthy people. This is why more than one conversation is necessary, and that conversation should focus on life issues rather than on completing the AD. For example, in initial conversations, patients could focus on designating a surrogate and identifying outcomes they find unacceptable, such as a Persistent Vegetative State (PVS). They could be encouraged to discuss preferences with their surrogates using the PADD as a guide.

Case 8.1

Mrs. M. is a 75-year-old widow who has been a patient on your unit about twice a year for the last three years. Her congestive heart failure, chronic obstructive pulmonary disease, and diabetes have significantly impacted the quality of her life since her last admission three months ago. She now needs oxygen 24 hours a day and still has shortness of breath at rest. Her ejection fraction, EKG, and functional status on NYHA assessment all fit the criteria for hospice referral. She is remaining symptomatic despite maximum medical management with vasodilators and diuretics.

She tells you, "This is my final trip. I know I will not make it this time. I have made my peace with my family and God. I am ready to go." You ask if her son, who is her proxy decision maker, knows her wishes. She says "Yes, I filled out the advance directive with him, and he is supposed to bring it to the hospital."

When her son visits that day, you are surprised when you hear him say to her physician, "I cannot find the AD, but my mother wants everything done, including CPR, so no, I do not want to make her a DNAR (do not attempt resuscitation)." You take the son aside outside the room and voice your confusion over what you just heard. He responds defensively. You talk about how difficult it is to let go of loved ones. He cries, but says "I am in charge of my mother's healthcare, and I will do what I know is best."

When a healthcare professional discovers that the patient's preferences and the surrogate's actions differ, he or she has an ethical obligation to stand up and advocate for the patient. You can suggest that the family member discuss the situation with you or the physician or look to a social worker or pastoral counselor to cope with their emotional pain. If these suggestions are rejected, it is time to call for an ethics consultation. The surrogate's "job description" has two major responsibilities: know what the patient wants as a result of in-depth discussions and assertively advocate for those preferences with the healthcare team. When a surrogate, who is not performing his or her obligations properly, also refuses coaching and offers of support, healthcare professionals must begin the process of removing the surrogate from that position. It does not matter if the person is court appointed or a volunteer. It is unethical to violate a patient's right to self-determination. You will need moral courage to stand up to a surrogate, who is not acting in the patient's best interests, but it is your obligation.

Several codes of ethics speak directly to the issue of the responsibility of the healthcare professional in surrogate decision making. The American Nurses Association Code of Ethics for Nurses (2001), for example, provides the following guidance:

> The nurse supports the patient self-determination by participating in discussions with surrogates, providing guidance and referral to other resources as necessary, and identifying and addressing problems in the decision-making process (p. 9).

The American Academy of Physician Assistants Code for Physician Assistants (2007) states, "To the extent possible, honor patient and surrogate preferences, using the most appropriate measures consistent with their choices, including alternative and non-traditional treatments" (p. 6).

In the case of Mrs. M., an ethics consultation may be needed if the healthcare professionals are unsuccessful in convincing the son to honor his mother's wishes. Although the exact operations of an ethics committee consultation will be discussed in Chapter 18, a brief explanation of how the ethics committee can help in this situation might be useful. According to Fox, Myers, and Pearlman (2007), the two primary reasons for ethics consultations are: (1) intervening to protect a patient's rights and (2) resolving real and imagined conflicts. Representatives from the Ethics Committee will take the time to assess the issues from all sides, facilitate a meeting for discussion, and make recommendations for resolution of the problem. This is a time-intensive process; time the busy clinician often does not have. Sometimes, it takes moral courage to call for an ethics consultation and participate in the meeting, but the ethics consultant will support an honest discussion of the issue and provide the support you need to move forward with clarification of the surrogate's ethical responsibilities.

Not all conflicts arise because of disagreements between healthcare professionals and surrogates. An ethics consultation may also be useful when there is conflict between the healthcare professional and physician over the care of the patient. The following case illustrates this problem.

Role of Culture in Advance Directives and Delivering Bad News

Case 8.2

Mr. Weld is a 65-year-old African American who seemed healthy until he arrived in the ER complaining of severe abdominal pain and vomiting for the past 24 hours. An X-ray revealed a massive bowel obstruction. He wanted to wait until his family arrived to discuss treatment options, but the surgeon stated this was an emergency that required an immediate bowel resection. The emergency surgery revealed that the tumor causing the bowel obstruction was cancerous and had already metastasized to the liver.

The nurse practitioner who worked closely with this surgeon was present when the surgeon delivered the bad news to the patient. Afterward, she approached the surgeon with some concerns about the message the surgeon had sent to the patient. She was disturbed because the surgeon had simply told the patient that he found a tumor, but he did not inform the patient that the tumor was cancerous or that it had significant metastasis. The surgeon replied that it was the oncologist's responsibility to deliver the "fatal blow," not his. The nurse practitioner asked what she should say when the patient asked about his condition. The physician said, "Just punt to me, and I will punt to the oncologist who will see him this afternoon." As a result, she avoided the patient all day. She did not want to be in the position of having to respond to questions about his diagnosis, or worse, his prognosis.

Whether you are a PA, advanced practice nurse, nurse, or resident, you are likely to encounter this situation during your medical career. Whether this surgeon acted out of fear or paternalism is hard to determine, but the patient's "right to know" was clearly violated. The surgeon's motivation is not the issue. What is crucial for the nurse practitioner is the ability to ensure that the patient has the necessary information to make informed medical decisions. I believe the nurse practitioner should use the "delivering bad news" model to prepare the patient and his family for the conversation with the oncologist. Therefore, I recommend that "you ask forgiveness and not permission" and share your actions with the surgeon after you meet with the patient and family. This requires moral courage, because the physician has clearly indicated that he believes this communication is not necessary.

Honesty is the key to fostering trust, particularly with cultural groups that already lack faith in the medical system. For example, people with strong religious convictions, who believe in miracles and the power of God (not physicians) to determine when a person dies, are often hesitant to limit medical treatment (Johnson, Elbert-Avila, & Tulsky, 2005). Unfortunately, even with church-initiated programs to encourage the preparation of ADs, use among African Americans remains low. When this nurse practitioner discusses the options with her patient, she needs to keep these cultural leanings in mind and to determine if these issues are relevant for this patient (Barclay, Blackhall, & Tulsky, 2007)

Take this case a step further. What if Mr. Weld had no one to act as his surrogate? He arrived at the emergency room with "no next of kin," has no one to speak for him, and has no idea that his condition is now terminal. If we really are serious about honoring nonmalfeasance, autonomy, and veracity, moral courage is necessary to put in motion the supports this man will need to have a quality end-of-life scenario.

Advance Directives: Successful and Unsuccessful Outcomes

Have advance directives been successful in improving clinical outcomes in end-of-life care? The evidence is inconclusive at best, thereby giving rise to the conclusion that ADs have not been successful in this country (Kolarik, Arnold, Fischer, & Hanusa, 2002). The results of the famous SUPPORT study have also led to further concerns about the effectiveness of the advance care planning intervention. This study concluded that even with the assistance of an APRN, DNAR orders were still written late and had no effect on duration of ICU stays or cost (Teno, Licks, Lynn, et al., 1997). However, findings from more recent studies indicate that ADs do help contain costs, reduce hospitalization time, and ease family stress (Kolarik et al., 2002). In this later review, as well as in one by Singer, Martin, Lavery, et al. (1998), the AD was judged successful from the patient's perspective because it increased communication between the patient and family members. Therefore, while ADs may not change clinical outcomes, they do provide support for important end-of-life conversations.

One criticism has focused on the AD document itself. Treatment-based AD directives are difficult to apply to all situations. An AD that contains the patient's values and goals can be generally applied to diverse clinical scenarios, but may be insufficient for application to difficult end-of-life decisions.

A study by Kolarik et al. (2002) examined two types of ADs as applied to 63 patients. The patients were randomly assigned to either Emanuel's Medical Directive (EMD) or Pearlman's values history (PVH). The EMD form has been well studied, describes six different clinical scenarios (e.g., coma, dementia), and asks the individual to select items from a list of treatments (e.g., CPR, dialysis). The PVH has also been evaluated in a randomized trial. Using Likert scales of importance, PVH asks questions such as, "If you were dying, how important would it be for you to avoid pain and suffering, even if it means that you might not live as long?" Of the initial 278 patients approached to participate in the PVH study after a routine office visit, 25% already had an AD. Of the 143 who refused to participate, 54% said they did not have time for the process.

Both the EMD and the PVH were viewed favorably by researchers. Participants in both groups thought the forms would reduce the emotional burden on the surrogate decision maker and would make it easier for them to talk with their family members. Completed PVH forms showed 100% compliance with the request to designate a surrogate as compared with 80% for completed EMDs, where the request was on the last page instead of the first. Although patients were encouraged to discuss the results with their physicians, only one had the discussion. Researchers concluded that the type of form is not relevant and that the physician's participation is desired, but not required. The name of the surrogate needs to be requested on the front of form.

A more recent approach used a cluster of doctors' orders concerning life-sustaining intervention, such as the Physician Orders for Life-Sustaining Treatment (POLST) form (Cantor, 2000). This approach can optimize discussions with patients and families. It is very helpful if the patient transitions from one setting to another.

Ironically, the more inclusive and complex the document, the more examination it is likely to receive. Why? Because all parties assume that a lawyer was involved in its preparation. In today's litigious society, the risk-averse physician and the risk manager will be more guarded when a form is more detailed.

Advance Directives Reduce the Family Burden of Decision Making

Besides supporting the patient's autonomy, ADs also reduce the strain and burden on families. The Azoulay and Sprung (2005) study found that 83% of surrogates who made medical decisions in intensive care units had symptoms of posttraumatic stress disorder (PTSD). Studies have also shown that the burden of decision making is decreased when the (1) patient's preferences are known from conversations or an AD and (2) the patient's family receives honest medical information from providers (Chambers-Evans & Carnevale, 2005; Tilden, Tolle, Nelson, & Fields, 2001). If healthcare professionals knew what information surrogates needed to make their decisions, they could provide the necessary support to ease this burden. Thus, Vig, Starks, Taylor, Hopley, and Fryer-Edwards (2007) studied 50 designated surrogate decision makers of older, chronically ill veterans. They identified the following factors as those that make surrogate decision making easier.

1. Encourage a surrogate to use existing social networks for support in decision making, including friends and representatives from a religious community who are not emotionally involved with the patient. Normalize the need to talk it out again and again.
2. Recognize a surrogate's courage in following the patient's preferences even though the surrogate will lose a loved one.
3. Help surrogates to understand the medical condition. Include them in decision making and focus on relief of suffering.
4. Have one clinician be the spokesperson clinician, who coordinates the information received from everyone else involved in the case.
5. Answer the surrogate's questions with honest information expressed in plain English. Explain treatment recommendations and provide reassurances that the surrogate is making good decisions for the loved one.
6. Encourage surrogates to use coping strategies they have used in other stressful situations (e.g., hobbies and praying).

This study pointed out that family conflict, the surrogate's own health, competing responsibilities, geographical distance from the patient, financial concerns, and an inability to follow the patient's wishes may all hamper the surrogate's perceived effectiveness. If healthcare professionals recognize these as potential red flags, they should offer the surrogate organizational or community support.

No Proxy Decision Maker

When the patient is incompetent and has no proxy decision maker or AD, the standard switches from "substituted judgment" to "a best-interest standard." The best-interest standard is the guiding principle for decision making in health care and promotes the most good for the patient in making life-saving or life-sustaining treatment decisions. Thus, the decision must include consideration of the individual's quality of life if intervention is made or withheld/withdrawn.

Bailey (2006) offers three essential components for a minimal explanation of quality of life. The *first* is the absence of absorbing and intractable pain and suffering. Pain is distress of the body or mind resulting from injury or illness, while suffering is the endurance of a particular life experience that includes a feeling of being overwhelmed by the negativity of the circumstances. One may suffer without experiencing pain, but if one is in pain, the person is also likely to be suffering. Most people are willing to bear some pain and suffering to remain alive, but only if they know it will eventually stop.

The *second* component is the presence of bodily integrity and relatively normal bodily function. Loss of a limb, severe burns, gaping war wounds—all of these are severe insults to bodily integrity, which refers to the wholeness or soundness of the body. Bodily integrity means that the body is not seriously damaged from injury, disease, or illness. However, some people believe that being a quadriplegic would not meet this definition, while others consider being a paraplegic to be acceptable bodily integrity. Here, quality of life embraces not only the lack of bodily integrity, but also the ability of the person to come to terms with his or her new body and compensate for physical obstacles.

The *third* component is the capacity to live as an autonomous individual. Autonomy, which is the right to self-determination, requires that the individual critically assess, reflect, and act on basic wants and values. Many people in the disabled community have made peace with their dependence on others for support in performing some of the basic functions of life; to them, life is worth living. But what if cognitive function is lost and the individual will never regain consciousness or possess the capacity to make decisions about how to live life? In my opinion, decisions made for patients who are critically ill and incompetent should be based on their future capacity to become autonomous. A patient with severe dementia will never again be autonomous, nor will the patient who suffered extended anoxia in a resuscitation effort. In these cases, I would recommend against prolongation of treatment.

Conclusion

Since 1991, Americans have made minimal progress in completing and using advanced directives. Such directives would be more useful if they emphasized advance care planning, particularly discussions of end-of-life care with physicians, rather than serving merely as a legal document (Lo & Steinbrook, 2004). Many emotional, cultural, and physical barriers exist to the use of ADs. Even more troubling is the violation of patient autonomy when the medical professional fails to honor ADs. We can offer explanations and excuses, but the fact remains that many of these violations occur because the healthcare professional refuses to stand up for the patient's predetermined statement because of fear of litigation. Equally troubling is the refusal of the healthcare professional to withdraw treatment when the only purpose it serves is to prolong dying. Patients and surrogates have a right to request any treatment, but the healthcare professional has an obligation not to provide treatment with insignificant benefit or no possibility of improvement. This applies not only to the patient's underlying clinical condition, but also to the patient's values and goals. Providing treatment that will not alter the outcome is futile and will be discussed in Chapter 9.

Key Points to Remember

1. The advance directive (AD) was designed to protect a patient's right to decide not to be kept alive against one's will or, on the other hand, to request that all possible technologies be used to prolong life.
2. Surrogates made 75% of the decisions for critically ill hospitalized patients and 44% to 66% of the decisions for nursing home residents.
3. When a healthcare professional discovers that the patient's preferences and the surrogate's actions differ, he or she has an ethical obligation to stand up and advocate for the patient.
4. The best-interest standard is the guiding principle in healthcare decision making and centers on what would promote the most good for this patient, whether it be life sustaining or life ending.

References

American Academy of Physician Assistants. (2007). *Guidelines for ethical conduct for physician assistants*. Retrieved June 4, 2008, from http://www.aapa.org/manual/23-EthicalConduct.pdf

American Nurses Association. (2001). *Code of ethics for nurses with interpretative statements*. Silver Spring, MD: American Nurses Publishing. Retrieved July 5, 2008, from http://www.nursingworld.org

Azoulay, E., & Sprung, C.L. (2005). Family physician interactions in the intensive care unit. *Critical Care Medicine, 32*(11), 2323–2328.

Bailey, S. (2006). Decision making in acute care: A practical framework supporting the "best interests" principle. *Nursing Ethics, 13*(3), 284–291.

Barclay, J.S., Blackhall, L.J., & Tulsky, J.A. (2007). Communication strategies and culture issues in the delivery of bad news. *Journal of Palliative Medicine, 10*(4), 958–977.

Cantor, M.D. (2000). Improving advance care planning: Lessons from POLST. Physician orders for life-sustaining treatment. *Journal of the American Geriatrics Society, 48*(10), 1343–1349.

Chambers-Evans, J., & Carnevale, F.A. (2005). Dawning of awareness: The experience of surrogate decision making at the end of life. *Journal of Clinical Ethics, 16*(1), 28–45.

Drane, J.F. (1991). The patient self-determination Act (PSDA) and the incapacitated patient: Policy suggestions for healthcare ethics committees. *HEC Forum, 3*(6), 309–320.

Edinger, W., & Smucker, D.R. (1992). Outpatients attitudes regarding advance directives. *Journal of Family Practice, 35*, 650–653.

Emanuel, E.J., Weinberg, D.S., Gonin, R., Hummel, L.R., & Emanuel, L.L.(1993). How well is the patient self-determination act working: An early assessment. *American Journal of Medicine, 95*, 619–628.

Emanuel, L.L. (2008). Advance directives. *Annual Review of Medicine, 59*, 187–198.

Emanuel, L.L., Barry, M.J., Stoekle, J.E., Ettelson, L.M., & Emanuel, E.J. (1991). Advance directives for medical care—a case for greater use. *New England Journal of Medicine, 324*, 889–895.

Engleberg, R.A., Patrick, D.L., & Curtis, J.R. (2005). Correspondence between patients' preferences and surrogates' understandings for dying and death. *Journal of Pain and Symptom Management, 30*(6), 498–509.

Fox, E., Myers, S., & Pearlman, R.A. (2007). Ethics consultation in United States Hospitals: A national survey. *American Journal of Bioethics, 7*(2), 13–25.

Hiltman, E.F., Medich, C., Chase, S., Peterson, L., & Forrow, L. (1999). Family decision making and end-of-life treatment: The SUPPORT nurse narratives. *Journal of Clinical Ethics, 10*(2), 126–134.

Johnson, S.C., Pfeifer, M.P., & McNutt, R. (1995). The discussion about advance directives: Patient and physician opinions regarding when and how it should be conducted. *Archives of Internal Medicine, 155*, 1025–1030.

Johnson, K.S., Elbert-Avila, K.I., & Tulsky, J.A. (2005). The influence of spiritual beliefs and practices on the treatment preferences of African Americans: A review of the literature. *Journal of the American Geriatrics Society, 53*, 711–719.

Kim, S.Y.H., Karlawish, J.H.T., & Caine, E.D. (2002). Current state of research on decision-making competence of cognitively impaired elderly persons. *American Journal of Geriatric Psychiatry, 10*(2), 151–165.

Kolarik, R.C., Arnold, R.M., Fischer, G.S., & Hanusa, B.H. (2002). Advance care planning: A comparison of values statements and treatment preferences. *Journal of General Internal Medicine, 17*, 618–624.

Layde, P.M., Beam, C.A., Broste, S.K., Connors, A.F., Desbiens, N., Lynn J., et al. (1995). Surrogates' predictions of seriously ill patients' resuscitation preferences. *Archives of Family Medicine, 4*, 518–524.

Lo, B., & Steinbrook, R. (2002). Resuscitating advance directives. *Archives of Internal Medicine, 164*(14), 1501–1506.

Singer, P.A., Martin, D.K., Lavery, J.V., Thiel, E.C., Kelner, M., & Mendelssohn, D.C. (1998). Reconceptualizing advance care planning from the patient's perspective. *Archives of Internal Medicine, 158*, 879–884.

Steinbrook, R., Lo, B., Moulton, J., Saika, G., Hollander, H., & Volberding, P.A. (1986). Preferences of homosexual men with acquired immunodeficiency syndrome for life-sustaining treatment. *New England Journal of Medicine, 314,* 457–460.

Suhl, J., Simons, P., Reedy, T., & Garrick, T. (1994). Myth of substituted judgment. Surrogate decision making regarding life support is unreliable. *Archives of Internal Medicine, 154*(1), 90–96.

Sulmasy, D.P., Terry, P.B., Weisman, C.S., Miller, D.J., Stallings, R.Y., Vettese, M.A., et al. (1998). The accuracy of substituted judgment in patients with terminal diagnosis. *Archives of Internal Medicine, 128*(8), 621–629.

Teno, J.M., Licks, S., Lynn, J., Wenger, N., Connors, A.F., Phillips, R.S., et al. (1997). Do advance directives provide instructions that direct care? SUPPORT investigators. Study to understand prognoses and preferences for outcomes and risks of treatment. *Journal of the American Geriatrics Society, 45,* 508–512.

Tilden, V.P., Tolle, S.W., Nelson, C.A., & Fields, J. (2001). Family decision-making to withdraw life-sustaining treatments from hospitalized patients. *Nursing Research, 50*(2), 105–115.

Vig, E.K., Starks, H., Taylor, J.S., Hopley, E.K., & Fryer-Edwards, K. (2007). Surviving surrogate decision-making: What helps and hampers the experience of making medical decisions for others. *Society of General Internal Medicine, 22,* 1274–1279.

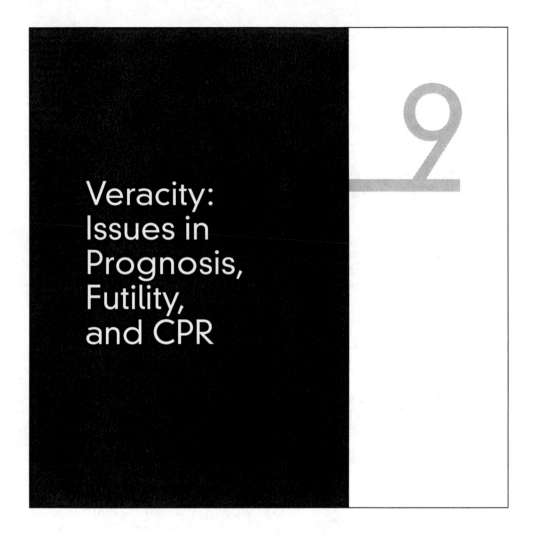

Veracity: Issues in Prognosis, Futility, and CPR

9

The task of medicine is to cure sometimes, to relieve often, and to comfort always.

—Ambroise Paré, a 16th-century French surgeon

Most people who watch the television show *ER* would assume that almost all people who arrive at a hospital ER in critical condition can be saved (Diem, Lantos, & Tulsky, 1996). The patient is stabilized using new technology and then transferred to the operating room or critical care unit, where life is sustained beyond that which would otherwise be possible. People have transferred to technology a sense of the sacred; they hold on to the belief that the magic of technology will intervene to stop death. But, in truth, sometimes no amount of technology can be effective in saving a life. Sometimes, particularly in the technologically driven environments of hospitals, we forget that death is the natural end of life. Technology is only a tool to be used thoughtfully with an evidence-based understanding of its limitations. As a consequence of technology, the difference between *"prolonging life"* and *"prolonging death"* has become progressively in need of further clarification.

Although the death of a patient is likely to be more immediate with the withdrawal of mechanical ventilation than with withdrawal of artificial nutrition or hydration, medications, or dialysis, the ethical, legal, and clinical implications remain the same. In the past, all of these technologies would have been labeled "extraordinary," but today a natural death is becoming more and more unusual.

This chapter focuses on the ethical principle of veracity and the ethical dilemmas involved in futile treatment. Information about cardiopulmonary resuscitation (CPR), do not resuscitation (DNR) status, and the current definition of futility will be based on the most recent research. I will offer suggestions about how to interpret prognostic indicators about a patient's chance of survival and probable functional outcome following surgery. Unfortunately, in futility cases, the staff members who care for the patient and family members also suffer. These effects and ways to cope with them are offered. The chapter ends with a brief look at the use of palliative sedation as an alternative approach to treatment in futility cases.

Importance of Veracity

Veracity is the obligation to tell the truth. In the medical environment, truthfulness is a legal principle requiring that a health professional be honest and give full disclosure to a patient, abstain from misrepresentation or deceit, and report known lapses in standards of care to the proper agencies.

But why is truthfulness especially important in a healthcare professional–patient relationship? The most compelling argument in favor of full disclosure is to ensure that patients receive relevant information about their own medical conditions that respects and enhances their autonomy, that is, their ability to control, make decisions about, and determine the course of their medical treatment (Tuckett, 2004). Autonomy is closely related to dignity, and a patient's dignity is undermined when a healthcare professional lies and misleads by withholding or through selective disclosure of information.

Because a surrogate decision-maker is a patient's only voice in these critical medical situations, the surrogate also deserves to hear the truth—the same truth that the patient would have received. If, for example, a healthcare professional is discussing options with a surrogate concerning a critically ill son and omits selected prognostic indicators or offers options that will not improve the outcome, the professional is concealing or deceiving the surrogate. Further, a healthcare professional needs to use clear language; the use of technical terms or medical jargon, such as "growth" or "neoplasm," can be misleading. The surrogate is entitled to the truth about the diagnosis, prognosis, and probable functional outcomes for the patient. Only then can the family or surrogate even begin to make the difficult decisions about DNR or transitioning from the hope of a cure to palliative care.

Defining the Concept of Futility

The notion of medical futility surfaced in the literature in the 1980s, when patients' families insisted on life-prolonging treatments that healthcare professionals considered to be only death prolonging (Lo & Jonsen, 1980). Since then, the debate about the definition of futility has continued. Healthcare professionals and bioethicists have tried to develop techniques for mediating the conflicts between healthcare professionals and surrogates. Most recently, Texas enacted legislation to assist with decisions about futile cases. According to its provisions, healthcare professionals can decide not to treat a patient if they deem the treatment inappropriate from a medically scientific perspective (Heitman & Gremillion, 2001). Furthermore, this law encourages a shift toward the communitarian value that no one has unlimited claims on community resources by promoting the use of available healthcare resources only for patients with a good chance of survival.

Clinical paradigms about futile care often involve life-sustaining intervention for patients in a persistent vegetative state or resuscitation efforts for people who are terminally ill. Other paradigms include the use of aggressive therapies, such as hemodialysis, chemotherapy, and surgery, for patients with advanced fatal illnesses that have no realistic expectation of cure or even palliation, and the use of less invasive treatments, such as antibiotics or intravenous hydration, to patients in near-moribund conditions. In these circumstances, healthcare professionals and surrogates may be using these interventions as an excuse to avoid difficult and crucial discussions. Some healthcare professionals forget that when an intervention is medically inappropriate, it is justifiable not to offer it.

The concept of futility evolved from the understanding that if an intervention cannot change the underlying pathophysiological parameters of a patient's condition, it is a futile rather than a beneficial intervention. Although the healthcare literature offers many definitions of futility, a consensus has not been reached. It tends to be defined situationally, rather than by an accepted standard. Why? Because what may be considered futile in a community hospital may not be considered futile in an academic medical center. However, after a brief review of the available definitions, I will combine several to form a pragmatic definition for clinicians.

The word futility is derived from Greek, where it means useless, or an effort that is useless because it is undertaken to achieve an unattainable goal. Therefore, any action undertaken to achieve that goal is ineffective, senseless, and pointless.

In 1990, Schneiderman, Jecker, and Jonsen proposed this approach:

When physicians concluded (either through personal experience, experiences shared with colleagues, or considerations of published empirical data) that in the last 100 cases a medical treatment has been useless, they should regard the treatment as futile. If the treatment merely preserves permanent unconsciousness or cannot end dependence on intensive medical care, the treatment should be considered futile (p. 953).

Then, in 1993, Murphy and Finucane listed seven clinical conditions for which treatment should not be continued. The choice of conditions was based on the potential outcomes of these treatments and represented the beginning of studies on prognostic indicators.

More recently, the American Medical Association adopted a quantitative definition of futility based on well-designed studies. Treatment is defined as futile if the patient has no more than a 1% chance of functional survival after treatment (Jonsen, Siegler, & Winslade, 1998). However, some individuals disagree with this definition. There are patients who consider life in a persistent vegetative state (PVS) or tethered 24 hours a day to critical care equipment to be a life still worth living. But for most people, the image of Terri Schiavo in a PVS only increased their need for assurances from loved ones that they would never be left to exist in such a state.

A healthcare professional's assertion that a treatment is medically futile inherently involves a value judgment (Council on Ethical and Judicial Affairs, AMA, 1999). Therefore, to make these value judgments, one needs a workable understanding of futility.

Brody and Halevy (1995) identified four reasons for physicians to justifiably withhold futile treatments:

1. If the proposed treatment does not fulfill medicine's purpose, which is to cure the patient or, at a minimum, to comfort the patient and reduce suffering.
2. If the proposed treatment is known to be ineffective. Otherwise, the physician is guilty of nonadherence to the standards of scientific competence.
3. If the proposed treatment risks loss of public confidence because it is known to be ineffective.
4. If the proposed treatment violates the physicians' first rule of ethics, which is "first do no harm." When physicians inflict procedures on patients that they know provide no benefit, they are violating this oath.

Some authors distinguish between quantitative and qualitative futility (Cantor, Braddock, Derse, et al., 2003). Quantitative futility is based on evidence in the literature, Applied Physiology and Chronic Health Evaluation (APACHE) system parameters, and the extensive knowledge and experience of clinicians involved in the case. Although quantitative determinations of futility may seem objective, they are, in fact, value judgments. A subject still open to debate is whether experienced physicians using state-of-the-art evidence should be allowed to make this value judgment. The qualitative approach is based on the principle that physicians should not to be required to offer treatments to reach objectives that are not worthwhile medical goals. Is it futile to attempt resuscitation on a patient who is in a permanent vegetative state? Advocates of patient autonomy criticize this approach because it replaces the perspective of the patient with that of the physician. In a qualitative futility decision, the rejected treatment is likely to be an effective one, just not for this patient. Physiologic futility is present when a certain treatment cannot achieve a desired effect (e.g., medication cannot raise blood pressure to sustain life). This approach prioritizes the value of physiological homeostasis above other values.

Physicians and ethicists have conducted comprehensive examinations of unwarranted care for almost thirty years. For example, Paris and Schreiber (1996) stated: "When a requested intervention will not succeed in achieving its goal, the action would be ineffective or futile" (p. 565). "Treatments offering no benefit and serving to prolong the dying process should not be employed" (p. 569). Yet, even in medicine, we continue to disregard metaanalysis of futility. Lofmark and Nilstun (2002) stated that we must decide when to overlook inappropriate treatment measures. Despite these and many other recommendations, healthcare professionals continue to overuse technology on dying patients.

It is important to distinguish between futility and rationing (Jecker & Schneidermann, 1992). Futility asks the question, "Will the intervention work?," whereas rationing raises the question, "Is the intervention worth it?" Rationing arguments must always balance the benefits of a diagnostic or therapeutic intervention against its costs, compare the intervention with other competing interventions, and consider the total funds available for healthcare (Burns & Truog, 2007). Futile interventions are entirely lacking in benefit or offer such a minimal benefit that no balancing is necessary. Rationing will be discussed in Section V.

After reviewing the literature, I propose the that futility be defined as "the provision of treatment that would provide insignificant benefit or improvement in the patient's underlying clinical condition and the use of an intervention that would be highly unlikely to result in a meaningful survival for the patient." When reasoning and medical experience indicate that the intervention would either leave the patient in a PVS or permanently dependent on critical care supports, I would consider the intervention futile.

Prognostic Indicators to Predict Futility

When physicians question the futility of care, they give uncertainty as the reason. Prognostic tools, such as the SUPPORT and APACHE systems, can assist decision making (Luce & Rubenfeld, 2002). However, these tools cannot accurately and consistently predict survival or death (Nelson, Danis, & Meier, 2001; Higgins, McGee, Steingrub, Rapoport, Lemeshow, & Teres, 2003). Prognostic indicators of mortality rates range from 5% to 40% in intensive care units (ICUs) across the United States, depending mainly on the severity of a patient's illness at admission (Knaus, Wagner, Zimmerman, & Draper, 1993). Thus, "Mortality prediction models provide very precise and highly accurate estimates of patient mortality when applied to populations; however in the case of the individual patients even the best model remains limited" (Szalados, 2007, pp. 321–322). Several studies have shown that prognostic indicators can be reasonably accurate and significantly influence treatment decisions (Kruse, Thill-Baharozian, & Carlson, 1988; Lloyd, Nietert, & Silvestri, 2004). The Therapeutic Intervention Severity Score relies on the relationship between resource use and mortality to predict outcomes (Cullen, Civetta, Briggs, & Ferrara, 1974).

A 2007 study was designed to analyze the content of physicians' prognostic reports to family members of ICU patients (White, Engelberg, Wenrich, Lo, & Randall, 2007). The researchers autotaped 51 discussions between physicians and family members from four hospitals, which represented a 75% participation rate. At each conference, the physician was asked to rate the degree of conflict within the family about whether treatment should be withdrawn, how strongly the physician felt such treatment should be withdrawn, and the physician's comfort level in discussing the bad news. The in-hospital mortality rate was 80%. All but two conferences focused on whether to withdraw life support or prepare a DNAR order. The conferences lasted from 7 to 74 minutes, with a mean of 32 minutes. Although physicians discussed a patient's chances for short- and long-term survival in only 63% of the conferences, they did discuss the patient's potential functional outcomes in 86% of conferences. The latter is good news. Four factors were associated with the greater number of prognostic statements: (1) longer duration of the conference; (2) increased conflict between the physician and the family about withdrawing treatment; (3) the physician being White; and (4) a family with a higher education level (p. 449). No difference was noted in the physicians' specialty, years of practice, or comfort in breaking news. These results indicate that families with low literacy receive less information about the potential outcome of treatment. As a result, these family members may be more likely to misunderstand the patient's true clinical picture. In relation to veracity and futility, the patient's prognosis for survival was discussed in only 33% of the conferences.

Practitioners have an ethical obligation to decide whether a specific treatment would be useful. They are not obligated to provide care they consider physiologically futile, even if the patient and family insist. It is generally agreed that physicians should not offer or provide treatments that have no chance of benefiting a patient (Schmidt, 2006). This is based on the ethical principles of beneficence and nonmaleficence. Too often, resuscitation or other technological interventions are provided because practitioners want to avoid legal action.

CPR: The Truth

Cooper, Cooper, and Cooper (2006) provide an interesting historical perspective on CPR. The first case of successful human closed-chest defibrillation occurred in 1955, the first portable external defibrillator was developed in 1979, and the first article on an implantable defibrillator appeared in 1981. The last of these developments changed the lives of many people by preventing sudden death.

Although it may be hard to believe, external cardiac massage was not widely taught until 1958. The first CPR guidelines that encouraged practice with mannequins—some of you may remember "Resusei Anne"—were issued in 1966. Although many physicians recommended teaching the technique to the lay public, these initial guidelines disapproved of this policy. Teaching the public was not officially sanctioned until 1974. Finally, in 1991, advanced cardiac life support (ACLS) was sanctioned for use by paramedics. However, the Ontario Prehospital Advanced Life Support (OPALS) Study found no improvement in outpatient survival with the addition of ACLS (Stiell, Mello, Burns, et al., 2004).

Fast forward the discussion to today's statistics. Most rates of survival are recorded based on hospital discharge and range from 1% to 25% for outpatients and 0% to 29% for inpatients (Cooper et al., 2006). A summary of results from four large studies of cardiac arrest survival demonstrates that the probability of survival for all cardiac rhythms increases when the cardiac arrest happened in the hospital (6.4% versus 17.6%). Patients with ventricular fibrillation fare markedly better than patients found in asystole. Today's statistics fail to match the outcomes shown on TV dramas, where 75% of the patients survive in the *ER* (Diem et al., 1996).

These dismal survival statistics are attributed to the higher level of patient acuity and noncardiac causes of arrest. In addition, the cohort of 50 years ago was primarily surgery patients who benefited from intense monitoring. This cohort also did not demonstrate the brain damage we see today, damage that is a frequent cause of death after cardiac arrest (Safar & Kochanek, 2002). Perhaps, these poor outcomes also reflect the performance of CPR on patients who should never have received it. CPR was never meant to be used on patients in multiorgan failure or with terminal illnesses.

The statistics for children who experience in-hospital cardiac arrest also reveal high mortality and morbidity (deMos, van Litsenburg, McCrindle, Bohn, & Parshuram, 2006; Morris, Wernovasky, & Nadkarni, 2004). Studies show that CPR duration of 30 or more minutes yields a survival rate of between 0% and 5%. Alsoufi, Al-Radi, Nazer, et al. (2007) examined the records on survival after extracorporeal cardiopulmonary resuscitation (ECPR) was performed on 80 children who suffered a cardiac arrest. The application of extracorporeal membrane oxygenation (ECMO) resulted in a favorable outcome in 30% (hospital survival with grossly intact neurologic status). Heart transplantation was often needed for a successful ECPR exit strategy. Of the noncardiac pediatric patients, only one survived, yielding an 89% mortality versus 63% mortality for children with cardiac disorders. These findings are consistent with those of a large Philadelphia study, in which children with isolated heart disease were more likely to survive (Morris, Wernovasky, & Nadkarni, 2004).

Could we conclude that such treatment should not be offered to noncardiac patients? Solomon, Sellers, Heller, et al. (2007) would most likely say no. In their study of 781 nurses and physicians, 80% agreed with the statement, "We are saving children who should not be saved," 45% agreed with statement, "I have acted against my conscience," and 50% agreed with the statement, "the treatments I offer are overly burdensome" (p. 872).

Shared Decision Making

However, many healthcare professionals refuse to accept sole responsibility for defining futility and prefer shared decision making. The Studdert, Mello, Burns, et al. (2003) study of 656 patients with prolonged stays in seven ICUs discovered that the major source of conflict in 33% of the cases was disagreements over life-sustaining treatments. Several models to help resolve these disagreements will be offered.

In 2004, both the North American and European critical care societies approved shared decision making as the preferred process by which physicians and family members decide to forgo life-sustaining treatment (White et al., 2007). Eighty-one percent of family members of ICU patients wished to participate actively in treatment decisions (Heyland, Cook, Rocker, et al., 2003), but to participate, they need to understand the patient's clinical condition and prognosis (Charles, Whelan, & Gafni, 1999).

The AMA Council on Ethical and Judicial Affairs (1999) recommended a "process-based" approach to futility determinations at end of life. The approach emphasizes a fair process between parties, rather than an externally imposed definition. The Council offers the following seven-step procedure for resolving disagreements between physicians and patients or their proxies. Four of the steps are targeted at deliberation and resolution that includes all concerned parties, two steps are aimed at developing alternatives in the case of irreconcilable differences, and the final step strives for closure when all alternatives have been exhausted. The steps are:

1. Deliberation and negotiation among patient, proxy, and physician about what comprises futile care for the patient and what treatment options fall within acceptable limits for the physician, family members, and sometimes the health-care institution.
2. Joint decision making should be done at the bedside with the patient or proxy and the physician using outcome data and discussing goals of treatment.
3. Assistance of an ethics consultant and/or a patient representative to facilitate discussion to reach resolution on a definition of the appropriate limits of care.
4. An institutional committee, such as an ethics committee, may be involved if disagreements cannot be resolved.
5. If outcome of the institutional process coincides with the patient's desires, but the physician remains unconvinced, arrangements may be made for transfer to another physician within the facility.
6. If the outcome of the deliberation process coincides with the physician's position, but the patient and/or proxy remains unconvinced, arrangements for transfer to another facility may be sought.
7. If transfer is not possible, because no physician and no institution can be found to follow the patient's and/or proxy's intervention wishes, then the intervention in question need not be provided, although the legal ramifications of this course of action are uncertain.

Advantages to a fair process approach are that arbitration can occur rapidly in the immediate clinical setting with people knowledgeable in medicine. In addition, such arbitration is less expensive in financial and emotional terms than court action. But what if the conflict is intractable?

Procedural Approaches and State Laws

Every U.S. state has enacted legislation to address end-of-life decision making. Up to the time of Texas law, however, no law has effectively dealt with medical futility—an issue that has engendered significant debate in the medical and legal literature, as reflected in many court cases and a formal opinion from the American Medical Association's Council on Ethical and Judicial Affairs. In 1999, Texas became the first state to adopt a law regulating end-of-life decisions by providing a legislatively sanctioned, extrajudicial due process mechanism for resolving medical futility disputes and other end-of-life ethical disagreements (Heitman & Gremillion, 2001; Truog, 2007). After two years of practical experience with this law, data collected at a large tertiary care teaching hospital strongly suggest that the law represents a first step toward practical resolution of this controversial area of modern health care. As such, the law may be of interest to practitioners, patients, and legislators elsewhere (Fine & Mayo, 2003).

Policymakers in many states are now looking to develop the purely process-based approaches that are outlined in the Texas Advance Directives Act (TADA) (Heitman & Gremillion, 2001). With this legislation, Texas also became the only state to provide a formalized review process to resolve the conflict when the situation reaches step seven in the review process. Patients or their representatives are notified 48 hours in advance of a review committee meeting. If the ethics or medical review committee agrees with the physician's judgment, the physician and facility are not obligated to provide treatment after the tenth day that follows notification of the patient or patient's representative. This 10-day waiting period can be extended if transfer to another physician or facility is likely.

In the initial study of the process at Baylor University in 2003, 91.5% of the time the committee agreed with the clinicians that further treatment was futile. In a larger study reported in 2007, the rate was 70% (Fine & Mayo, 2003; Smith, Gremillion, Slomka, & Warneke, 2007). This 2007 study examined the Texas medical appropriateness reviews during the first five years since enactment of the legislation (1999–2004) by sending a survey to the 409 members of the Texas Hospital Association. A response rate of 42.2% indicated that only 30% used the policies to review actual cases. Of the 256 cases, the review committee disagreed with physicians in 78. In 44% of these cases, the patients died within a 10-day period, suggesting that medical inappropriateness determinations were accurate. In the remaining 71 cases, the patient or patient representative agreed to discontinue treatment. Thirty patients were transferred and only eight of these improved. One could argue that this data indicates that the TADA process worked. But what of the eight patients (.04%) who improved in the 10 days? We do not know the level of clinical expertise on these review committees at the three non-specialty teaching hospitals, but this statistic does speak to the importance of the ten-day waiting period. Written comments on the survey indicated that some did not review cases because patients were projected to die within the 10-day period or were reluctant to use a process prone to becoming adversarial.

Ethical Decision-Making Models

Iserson, Saunders, and Mathieu (1995, p. 803) developed an ethical decision making model for emergency settings to be used when the patient's wishes are not known. The authors suggest three steps. First ask the question, "Is this the type of ethics problem for which you have already worked out a rule, or is this at least similar enough so that an existing rule could reasonably be extended to cover it?" If no rule is applicable, the next step is to ask, "Is there an option that will buy time for deliberation without excessive risk to the patient?" If you have no rule to cover the situation and no option to buy time for deliberation, then the third step suggests you evaluate your proposed solution using these three rules:

1. *Impartiality*—"Would you be willing to have this action performed if you were the patient?"
2. *Universality*—"Would you be willing to use the same solution in similar cases?"
3. *Interpersonal justifiability*—"Would you be willing to defend the decision to others, to share the decision in public?"

All of these lead you to the question, "Which action would I be willing to defend on the front page of the *New York Times*?"

9.1　Jonsen Model for Ethical Decision Making

Medical Indications	Quality of Life
Patient Preferences	Contextual Features

Jonsen, A.R., Siegler, M., & Winslade, W.J. (1998). *Clinical ethics* (4th ed.). New York: McGraw-Hill.

The second model for ethical decision-making, developed by Jonsen, Siegler, and Winslade (1998), was designed to answer the question, "What medical interventions should be made in this case at this time?" The decision-making model considers four factors: medical indications, patient preferences, quality of life, and contextual factors (see Exhibit 9.1).

We will use this model with a case example with clear-cut medical indications.

Case 9.1

Mr. Thomas is in severe respiratory failure and needs intubation and ventilation. The patient's preferences are known because he has an AD. The patient's approach to quality-of-life issues was simply expressed by his wife, "He no longer wants to live because he is unable to leave the house and is severely short of breath even sitting in his easy chair."

In this case, the medical indications, patient preferences, and quality-of-life factors were clearly defined. Contextual factors included family wishes, laws, and hospital policies that could impact this circumstance. In this case, the interventions were palliative in nature—doses of morphine and lorazepam to ease his struggling. He died quietly two hours later with his wife by his side.

Some participants in the futility debate suggest the use of other words, such as "clinically nonbeneficial interventions," to clarify intent (Schmidt, 2006). Others focus strictly on providing comfort to individuals whose underlying pathophysiology indicates that all further interventions are futile. But regardless of what we call it, we also have to recognize the effects of futile cases on frontline healthcare professionals.

Effect of Futility on Healthcare Professionals

Burns and Truog (2007) suggest that when their "principled negotiation" approach fails, healthcare professionals should find ways to support each other while honoring the family's wishes for futile care. The authors also state that surrogates should never be allowed to make decisions that are harmful to patients.

But these authors are physicians who do not spend 8 to 12 hours a day caring for these patients and interacting with their families, so perhaps it is more appropriate to ask nurses and other healthcare professionals what they need to ensure continuity of care for their patients. Otherwise, if we accept Burns and Truog's suggestion at face value, we could inadvertently reduce healthcare professionals to mutant acceptance of the family's wishes and the consequent patient suffering. According to Soelle (1975, p. 680), it means that further discussion is not possible, so healthcare professionals cease serving as agents. Most of the literature has focused on the moral distress of nurses, but experience has taught me that they are not the only frontline healthcare professionals who are significantly affected by such decisions.

Peter and Liaschenko (2004) address the perils created by proximity in the nurse-patient relationship. A satisfying nurse-patient relationship, one in which nurses know they did their best and patients benefited from their care, is a major reward of nursing. The very nature of nurses' work results in close proximity to the physical, emotional, and, at times, spiritual being of the patient. The nurse listens to the patient's story to understand what this particular patient needs.

This proximity encourages nurses, as moral agents, to act on behalf of those for whom they feel responsible. Because nurses feel this moral responsibility acutely, they find moral violations very distressing. Perhaps it is less burdensome to give orders than to carry them out or live so close to the consequences of futile interventions, but if you are the one who "bears witness" to the unnecessary suffering of a patient, you face the moral complexity of feeling responsible for that patient.

The moral distress could perhaps be alleviated by temporary breaks from patient care, but nurses can less easily escape proximity from the patient. This is simply not a realistic option in critical care units. Instead, the staff rotates the suffering among themselves by changing patient assignments. Lost is continuity of care, but gained is one more day as a bedside nurse.

Attention needs to be given to the human impact on nurses caring for patients whose treatment is futile. Moral distress is a real phenomena that causes suffering and, for some nurses, results in an exodus from bedside nursing (Corley & Minick, 2002). Nurses have consistently identified futile care as a major stressor in the ICU. They are also aware that the continued emphasis on the use of technology to sustain life denies patients the benefits of palliative care that are found when the focus shifts from cure to comfort.

Meltzer and Huckabay (2004) evaluated the relationship between nurse burnout and nurse perception of futile care in 60 critical care nurses. The frequency of futile care situations had a significant relationship to a nurse's emotional exhaustion. Beckstrand and Kirchhoff (2005) reported the results of a national random sample of 844 critical care nurses. They identified the most common obstacles to good end-of-life care (see Exhibit 9.2). Nurses have a ring-side seat in the futility debate, as they listen to disagreements about the direction of dying patients' care, witness prolonged patient suffering, watch physicians behave evasively, and hear family members override the patient's AD, often because they fail to accept the reality of the diagnosis.

Ferrell (2006) studied the effect of moral distress on nurses by examining 108 nurse narratives. The nurses were asked to (1) describe a distressing clinical experience in which you witnessed the administration of care that you describe as futile and (2) to describe how this experience impacted you as a nurse.

9.2 Common Obstacles to Good End-of-Life Care

1. Disagreement about the direction of dying patients' care
2. Actions that prolong patient suffering
3. Physicians who were evasive and avoided conversations with families
4. Family lack of understanding about the care of patient
5. Family nonacceptance of a poor prognosis
6. Overriding a patient's advance directive

Beckstrand, R.L., & Kirchhoff, K.T. (2005). Providing end-of-life care to patients: Critical care nurses' perceived obstacles and supportive behaviors. *American Journal of Critical Care, 14*(5), 395–403.

Many of these stories were not recent, but the nurses recalled situations that caused moral distress in vivid detail. In 71% of the narratives, the nurses indicated that futile care usually occurred because of a conflict between a surrogate decision maker and a healthcare professional. The conflict of "aggressive care denying palliative care" was by far the primary source of disagreement. As might be assumed from the Peter and Liashenko (2004) study, the nurses did not perceive themselves as passive observers, but as forcefully involved in the conflict.

Therefore, I cannot agree with Burns and Truog's approach to resolving intractable conflicts between family members and physicians by honoring the family's request for futile care. The American Nurses Association Code of Ethics (2001) does not support acceptance of action. The following is taken from provision five:

> *Moral respect accords moral worth and dignity to all human beings irrespective of . . . life situation. Such respect extends to oneself as well. . . . Nurses have a duty to remain consistent with both their personal and professional values and to accept compromise only to the degree that it remains an integrity-preserving compromise. An integrity-preserving compromise does not jeopardize the dignity or well-being of the nurse or others. (pp. 18–19)*

Nurses and other healthcare professionals need the organization to step in and take action, action that shows these front-line healthcare professionals that they are supported. When ethics committee mediations do not work, the physician is the one responsible for doing whatever is necessary to end medically inappropriate and unbeneficial care. Otherwise, the healthcare professional of the future might choose conscientious objection.

Conscientious objection is identified as a right in the ANA Code of Ethics (2001).

> *When nurses are placed in situations of compromise that exceed acceptable moral limits or involve violations of the moral standards of the profession, whether in direct patient care or in any other forms of nursing practice, they may express their conscientious objection to participation. Where a particular treatment, intervention, activity, or practice is morally objectionable to the nurse, whether intrinsically so or because it is inappropriate for the specific patient,*

or where it may jeopardize both patients and nursing practice, the nurse is jus-
tified in refusing to participate on moral grounds (p. 20).

Catlin et al. (2008) formulated the following defining statement for their pilot
study:

For the nurse, consciousness objection may occur when the nurse interprets that
the care that has been assigned for a patient is harmful or causes suffering.
The nurse does not wish to provide this form of care and feels sincerely and has
felt for some time that this is a question of conscience. The nurse objects to the
care orders, is willing to assist in other forms of care, and is not wishing to
abandon the patient (pp. 104–105).

In this pilot study, the researchers asked 66 neonatal and 13 pediatric intensive
care experienced nurses about their understanding of conscientious objection.
The nurses objected most strongly to situations in which aggressive interventions did not change outcomes, interventions for 22- to 24-week gestational age
newborns or newborns with conditions incompatible with life and with parents
who would not agree to shift from treatment to palliative care. Forty-five percent of the nurses had objected to such futile care, while 56% had not. The primary barriers to expressing an objection was physician's orders for futile care
(44%), administrative polices and legal consequences (42%), and undue influence
from parents (19%). These results clearly point to the need for practice guidelines from national organizations and administrative protocols that support the
moral courage of these healthcare professionals.

Palliative Sedation as an Alternative

The doctrine of double effect embraces the concept that it is morally acceptable
to cause an otherwise unacceptable result if the result was not the intended consequence of the legitimate act. For example, the intent is the relief of intractable
pain, but the unintended effect could be sufficient respiratory depression to
cause death. The justifiable distinction between high dose analgesia, or palliative sedation, and euthanasia is a fine line that distinguishes the risk of providing comfort at end of life from behavior consistently recognized as lethal. "The
natural death and living will statutes uniformly state that withdrawal of life support in a patient who is terminally ill, per the patient's instructions, is not considered suicide or assisted suicide" (Szalados, 2007, p. 320). The established legal
structure regards this as the patient's right to a natural death.

Euthanasia is defined as "the act or practice of ending the life of an individual suffering from a terminal illness or an incurable condition, as by lethal injection or the suspension of extraordinary medical treatment." The intentional
taking of a patient's life by another, whether it be an act of mercy or not, is considered homicide in every U.S. state. This differs from the issue of futility, in which
the termination of life-supporting treatment is based not on the intent to kill,
but on the desire to honor the patient's autonomy and relieve suffering.

Another critical distinction could be made between inaction (withholding
treatment) and intervention (withdrawing treatment). Fortunately, the courts

have rejected such a distinction. Instead, they have focused on the patient's right to self-determination and bodily integrity. The fear was that differentiating withholding from withdrawing could create a disincentive to trial-of-life support technology.

Conclusion

To honor a patient's autonomy, we have to tell the truth (veracity). To help surrogates make decisions in the final stages of life for their loved ones, we need to be certain they understand the scientific truth about the patient's chances of survival with technological interventions. For many, the decision is a confusing array of options. However, when they are told the truth in a direct and compassionate way, most families will come to terms with the reality. Meetings with individuals who are knowledgeable about the patient's pathophysiology, the patient's desires, and the family's fears can usually help surrogates work through the process of letting go. In cases where surrogates do not understand or refuse to accept the truth about the futility of the interventions, healthcare professionals need state protection as they attempt to honor the dignity of the patient. Research has shown that it is not only the patient who suffers. Healthcare professionals in close proximity to patients receiving futile care also suffer. We need to establish effective organizational polices and state laws that minimize this suffering by developing procedures to resolve futile cases.

Key Points to Remember

1. As a consequence of technology, the difference between *"prolonging life"* and *"prolonging death"* has become progressively in need of clarification.
2. Truthfulness is a legal principle requiring that a health professional be honest and give full disclosure to a patient, abstain from misrepresentation or deceit, and report known lapses in the standards of care to the proper agencies.
3. Futility is "the provision of treatment that would provide insignificant benefit or improvement in the patient's underlying clinical condition and the use of an intervention that would be highly unlikely to result in a meaningful survival for the patient."
4. Follow the seven-step procedure for resolving disagreements between physicians and their patients or their proxies about what constitutes futile treatment.
5. Every U.S. state has enacted legislation to address end-of-life decision making.
6. Attention needs to be given to the human impact on nurses caring for patients whose treatment is futile. Moral distress is a real phenomenon that causes suffering.
7. Nurses and other healthcare professionals need the organization to step in and take action, action that shows these front-line healthcare professionals that they are supported.
8. The doctrine of double effect embraces the concept that it is morally acceptable to cause an otherwise unacceptable result if the result was not the intended consequence of the legitimate act.

References

Alsoufi, B., Al-Radi, O.O., Nazer, R.I., Gruenwald, C., Foreman, C., et al. (2007). Survival outcomes after extracorporeal cardiopulmonary resuscitation in pediatric patients with refractory cardiac arrest. *Journal of Thoracic and Cardiovascular Surgery, 134,* 952–959.

American Nurses Association. (2001). *Code of ethics for nurses with interpretative statements.* Silver Spring, MD: American Nurses Publishing. Retrieved July 5, 2008, from http://www .nursingworld.org

Beckstrand, R.L., & Kirchhoff, K.T. (2005). Providing end-of-life care to patients: Critical care nurses' perceived obstacles and supportive behaviors. *American Journal of Critical Care, 14*(5), 395–403.

Brody, B.A., & Halevy, A. (1995). Is futility a futile concept? *Journal of Medicine and Philosophy, 20,* 123–144.

Burns, J.P., & Truog, R.D. (2007). Futility: A concept in evolution. *Chest, 132*(6), 1987–1993.

Cantor, M.D., Braddock, C.H., Derse, A.R., Edwards, D.M., Logue, G.L., Nelson, W., et al. (2003). Do-not-resuscitate orders and medical futility. *Archives of Internal Medicine, 163,* 2689–2694.

Catlin, A., Volat, D., Hadley, M.A, Bassir, R., Armigo, C., Valle, E., et al. (2008). Conscientious objection: A potential neonatal nursing response to care orders that cause suffering at the end of life? Study of a concept. *Neonatal Network, 27*(2), 101–108.

Charles, C., Whelan, T., & Gafni, A. (1999). What do we mean by partnership in making decisions about treatment? *British Medical Journal, 319,* 780–782.

Cooper, J.A., Cooper, J.D., & Cooper, J.M. (2006). Cardiopulmonary resuscitation: History, current practice and future direction. *Circulation, 114,* 2839–2849.

Corley, M.C., & Minick, P. (2002). Moral distress or moral comfort. *Bioethics Forum, 18*(1/2), 7–14.

Council on Ethical and Judicial Affairs, AMA. (1999). Medical futility in end-of-life care. *JAMA, 281*(10), 937–941.

Cullen, D.J., Civetta, J.M., Briggs, B.A., & Ferrara, L.C. (1974). Therapeutic intervention scoring system: A method for quantitative comparison of patient care. *Critical Care Medicine, 2,* 57–60.

deMos, N., van Litsenburg, R.R., McCrindle, B., Bohn, D.J., & Parshuram, C.S. (2006). Pediatric in-intensive-care-unit cardiac arrest: Incidence, survival, and predictive factors. *Critical Care Medicine, 34,* 1209–1215.

Diem, S.J., Lantos, J.D., & Tulsky, J.A. (1996). Cardiopulmonary resuscitation on television: Miracles and misinformation. *New England Journal of Medicine, 334,* 1578–1582.

Ferrell, B.R. (2006). Understanding the moral distress of nurses witnessing medically futile care. *Oncology Nursing Forum, 33*(5), 922–930.

Fine, R.L., & Mayo, T.W. (2003). Resolution of futility by due process: Early experience with the Texas advance directives law. *Annals of Internal Medicine, 138*(9), 743–746.

Heitman, E., & Gremillion, G. (2001). Ethics committees under Texas law: Effects of Texas Advance Directives Act. *HEC Forum, 13,* 98–102.

Heyland, D.K., Cook, D.J., Rocker, G.M., O'Callaghan, C.J., Dodek, P.M., & Cook, D.J. (2003). Decision-making in the ICU: Perspectives of the substitute decision-maker. *Intensive Care Medicine, 29,* 75–82.

Higgins, T.L., McGee, W.T., Steingrub, J.S., Rapoport, J., Lemeshow, S., & Teres, D. (2003). Early indicators of prolonged ICU stay. *Critical Care Medicine, 31*(1), 45–53.

Iserson, K.V., Saunders, A.B., & Mathieu, D. (1995). *Ethics in emergency medicine* (2nd ed.). Tucson: Galen Press.

Jecker, N.S., & Schneidermann, L.J. (1992). Futility and rationing. *American Journal of Medicine, 92,* 180–196.

Jonsen, A.R., Siegler, M., & Winslade, W.J. (1998). *Clinical ethics* (4th ed.). New York: McGraw-Hill.

Knaus, W.A., Wagner, D.P., Zimmerman, J.E., & Draper, E.A. (1993). Variations in mortality and length of stay in intensive care units. *Annals of Internal Medicine, 118*(10), 753–761.

Kruse, J.A., Thill-Baharozian, M.C., & Carlson, R.W. (1988). Comparison of clinical assessment with APACHE II for predicting mortality risk in patients admitted to a medical intensive care unit. *JAMA, 260,* 1739–1742.

Lloyd, C.B., Nietert, P.J., & Silvestri, G.A. (2004). Intensive care decision making in the seriously ill and elderly. *Critical Care Medicine, 32,* 649–654.

Lo, B., & Jonsen, A.B. (1980). Clinical decisions to limit treatment. *Annals of Internal Medicine, 93,* 764–768.

Lofmark, R., & Nilstun, T. (2002). Conditions and consequences of medical futility—From literature review to a clinical model. *Journal of Medical Ethics, 28,* 115–119.

Luce, J.M., & Rubenfeld, G.D. (2002). Can health care costs be reduced by limiting intensive care at the end of life? *Respiratory Critical Care Medicine, 165,* 750–754.

Meltzer, L.S., & Huckabay, L.M. (2004). Critical care nurses' perceptions of futile care and its effect on burnout. *American Journal of Critical Care, 13,* 202–208.

Morris, M.C., Wernovsky, G., & Nadkarni, V.M. (2004). Survival outcomes after extracorporeal cardiopulmonary resuscitation instituted during active chest compressions following refractory in-hospital pediatric arrest. *Pediatric Critical Care Medicine, 5,* 440–446.

Murphy, D.J. & Finucane, T.E. (1993). New do-not-resuscitate polices: A first step in cost control. *Archives of Internal Medicine, 153,* 1642–1648.

Nelson, J.E., Danis, J.E., Meier, D.E., Oei, E.J., Nierman, D.M., Senzel, R.S., et al. (2001). Self-reported symptoms of critically ill cancer patients. *Critical Care Medicine, 29*(2), 277–282.

Paris, J. & Schreiber, M.D. (1996). Physicians' refusal to provide life-prolonging medical interventions. *Clinics in Perinatology, 23,* 563–571.

Peter, E., & Liaschenko, J. (2004). Perils of proximity: A spatiotemporal analysis of moral distress and moral ambiguity. *Nursing Inquiry, 11*(45), 218–225.

Pope, B.B., Rodzen, L., & Spross, G. (2008). Raising the SBAR: How better communication improves patient outcomes. *Nursing, 38*(3), 41–43.

Safar, P.J., & Kochanek, P.M. (2002). Therapeutic hypothermia after cardiac arrest. *New England Journal of Medicine, 346,* 612–613.

Schmidt, T.A. (2006). Moral moments at the end of life. *Emergency Medical Clinics of North America, 24,* 797–808.

Schneiderman, L.J., Jecker, N.S., & Jonsen, A.R. (1990). Medical futility: Its meaning and ethical implications. *Annals of Internal Medicine, 112,* 949–954.

Smith, M.L., Gremillion, G., Slomka, K., & Warneke, C.L. (2007). Texas hospitals' experience with Texas advance directive act. *Critical Care Medicine, 35*(5), 1271–1276.

Soelle, D. (1975). *Suffering.* Philadelphia: Fortress Press.

Solomon, M., Sellers, D.E., Heller, K.S., Dokken, D.L., Levetown, M., Rushton, C., et al. (2005). New and lingering controversies in pediatric end of life. *Pediatrics, 116,* 872–883.

Stiell, I.G., Wells, G.A., Field, B., Spaite, D.W., Nesbitt, L.P., DeMaio, V.J., et al. (2004). Advanced cardiac life support in out-of-hospital cardiac arrest. *New England Journal of Medicine, 351,* 647–656.

Studdert, D.M., Mello, M.M., Burns, J.P., Puopolo, A.L. Galper, B.Z., Trug, R.D., & Brennan, T.A. (2003). Conflict in the care of patients with prolonged stay in the ICU: Types, sources, and predictors. *Intensive Care Medicine, 29*(9), 1489–1497.

Szalados, J.E. (2007). Discontinuation of mechanical ventilation at end-of-life: The ethical and legal boundaries of physician conduct in termination of life support. *Critical Care Clinics, 23,* 317–337.

Truog, R.D. (2007) Tackling medical futility in Texas. *New England Journal Medicine, 357,* 1–3.

Tuckett, A.G. (2004). Truth telling in clinical practice and the arguments for and against: A review of the literature. *Nursing Ethics, 11*(5), 500–513.

White, D.B., Engelberg, R.A., Wenrich, M.D., Lo, B., & Randall, C.J. (2007). Prognostication during physician-family discussions about limiting life support in intensive care units. *Critical Care Medicine, 35*(2), 442–448.

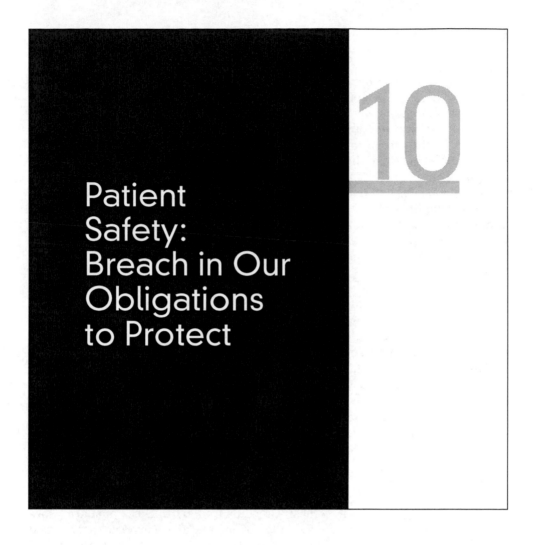

Patient Safety: Breach in Our Obligations to Protect

Safeguards are often irksome, but sometimes convenient, and if one needs them at all, one is apt to need them badly.

—Henry Adams, a mid-nineteenth-century author

The imperative for patient safety began with the Institute of Medicine's (IOM) 1999 landmark report, "To Err is Human," that shocked everyone with the statistic that as many as 98,000 people die annually as a result of medical errors (Kohn, Corrigan, & Donaldson, 2000). This report listed medical errors as the eighth most common cause of death—outpacing traffic accidents, breast cancer, and HIV/AIDS. The cost of this unanticipated loss of life is estimated at $9 billion dollars annually. It is equivalent to one jumbo jet full of passengers crashing every day (Watcher, 2004). This is not just a U.S. problem. Vincent, Neale, and Woloshynowych (2001), in the first epidemiological study of British patients, found that 10.8% of patients had experienced a medical error. The published international rates on unintentional harm in hospitals range from 2.9% to 16% (Kohn, Corrigan, & Donaldson, 2000). Since 1999, other U.S. research supports the gravity of the problem (Blendon, DesRoches, Brodie, et al., 2002; Healey, Shackford, Osler, et al., 2002; Starfield, 2000).

Just as we can no longer pretend that medical error is not a serious problem, we need to stop pretending that healthcare professionals will always perform perfectly. Healthcare professionals and researchers in other fields have shown us where we can make the most difference in saving lives and preventing the complications, as well as the pain and suffering that result from these errors. Healthcare professionals need to start using lessons from other industries to create a commitment to a culture of safety that includes improved teamwork, communication among team members, and redundancy in safety measures. It is time to integrate the National Patient Safety Goals into the very fabric of our practice, so that no safety measures are considered optional (Joint Commission, 2008a).

Safety goals have been articulated since the 2001 Institute of Medicine's report, *Crossing the Quality Chasm*. However, they are still not followed or consistently enforced. It is time for all healthcare professionals to take their ethical obligation of "do no harm" seriously and to muster the moral courage necessary to speak out when they see or hear violations. This chapter focuses on how the individual can maintain his or her ethical obligations in relation to these safety goals. We will also discuss how to confront individuals who are not following polices designed to protect patients. We are not perfect, but we can show the public that we take their safety seriously by personally adhering to the National Patient Safety Goals and holding our colleagues equally accountable.

Defining Our Terms

Defined narrowly, patient safety means freedom from harm. Since "no harm" does not mean "safe," a more common definition of error is "an occurrence that harmed or could have harmed a patient." The IOM (2000) defines error as a "the failure of a planned action to be completed as intended or the use of a wrong plan to achieve an aim" (Kohn, Corrigan, & Donaldson, 2000). The intended outcome is not achieved. Errors are mistakes, inaccuracies, or oversights. They include both omissions (failing to do something) and commissions (doing the wrong thing or not doing what was expected or needed) (Banja, 2004).

Reliability is inherent in these definitions and is defined as delivering best-practice care to patients in a timely manner to achieve the best possible outcomes (Valentin & Bion, 2007). Reliability is the number of errors expressed as a proportion of the total opportunity for error—percent per million. For example, the most reliable medical processes are blood transfusion and anesthesia, which have an error level of 10^{-5} (1–9 deaths per 100,000).

Systems Approach Versus Individual Blame

The principle classification of causes of error is system and human factors. The error is seen as the consequence of the interplay between the two (Chang, Schyve, Croteau, et al., 2005). Error analysis must therefore be based on both factors—the human operators and the systems in which they work.

This IOM report identified safety as "primarily a systems problem" (Leape, Berwick, & Bates, 2002, p. 504). First, systems theory holds that individuals make mistakes because of faulty design in processes. Therefore, healthcare professionals have been challenged to examine the policies, protocols, and procedures that guide current practice. Second, systems theory holds that individuals should not be punished for errors. This has resulted in the reporting of "near misses" and more openness with "lessons learned." Catching the initial error is crucial, because it may lead to a cascade of events that results in continuing deterioration of a patient's condition.

A strong case could be made for holding healthcare managers and executives just as responsible for errors as the frontline clinicians (Sharpe, 2003). After all, they have significant control over the decision making that affects patient welfare. They are responsible for creating the vision for a culture of safety that will be discussed in Chapter 17.

However, this systems approach does not eliminate the individual responsibility of the healthcare professional. When a healthcare professional makes an error, that person has a responsibility to report the mistake, participate in investigating the causal systems failures, and reveal the error to the attending physician and patient. The systems approach actually empowers healthcare professionals to contribute to systems improvement, but my focus in this chapter is the individual's personal responsibility.

My approach is based on the need for all healthcare professionals, regardless of their position in the organizational hierarchy, to be patient safety leaders. This type of leadership requires the moral courage to insist that everyone on the healthcare team always takes the extra steps and time needed to ensure the safest action. Surgery cannot start until the "time out" has occurred to reidentify the correct site. The sterile procedure can not be started at bedside until the contaminated gloves are changed. The patient's meds need to be reconciled each time the patient is transitioned, regardless of whether there are 5 or 25 medications. Commitment to safety is the responsibility of each person in the healthcare environment.

Let us begin with the most prominent problem the Joint Commission has identified in achieving patient safety goals. Despite amplified efforts to prevent wrong site, wrong procedure, and wrong person surgeries, recent data from the Joint Commission revealed that wrong site surgeries are the number one reported sentinel event (Sentinel event statistics, 2008). The Joint Commission's implementation expectation for use of a universal protocol for prevention is detailed and clear (Joint Commission, 2008b). If the error is not picked up in preoperative verification, then the "time out" immediately before starting the procedure could stop the error.

Speaking Out for Patient Safety: Lessons Learned

Findings from a survey of nurses about safety revealed that more than one in three nurses found it difficult to speak up when they found a problem with a patient's care (Pronovost, Wu, & Seaton, 2004). On July 9, 2008, the Joint Commission issued an alert entitled "Behaviors that undermine a culture of safety" (The Joint Commission, 2008d). This document specifically addresses the effects of intimidating and disruptive behaviors on creating preventable adverse events. To protect our patients, all healthcare professionals must be able to challenge erroneous care processes. Let us examine what some researchers have found to be helpful in giving a voice to healthcare professionals.

The Association of Operating Room Nurses (AORN) Foundation, in conjunction with grants from Kimberly-Clark Health Care and Safer Healthcare, launched demonstrations at five sites to determine how human factors training could impact the 12 key areas of patient safety identified by Agency for Healthcare Quality Research (AHRQ, 2007). IOM, in its 1999 report, recommended the use of Crew Resource Management (CRM), an approach has been in place in the aviation industry for 30 years. The programs share some common elements:

- Teamwork
- Communication
- Decision making
- Situational awareness (thinking ahead and planning for contingencies)
- Education about limitations of human performance and the stressors that precipitate the commission of errors, including fatigue, emergencies, and work overload (Pizzi, Goldfarb, & Nash, 2007).

The demonstration sites used a CRM version of training adapted to healthcare settings. The results of the training clearly indicated that several procedures could decrease the risks of speaking up. The teams learned that the failure to voice concerns was responsible for many preventable errors. Team briefing and debriefing checklists encouraged open communication and respect in the perioperative setting (see Exhibits 10.1 and 10.2) (Marshall & Manus, 2007).

The briefing time is 90 seconds—just a few minutes taken from the surgical time that can increase patient safety. As seen in both checklists, communication about the patient is encouraged before, as well as after, the "time out." In one hospital, a question was added to the end of briefing—"What is the destination of the patient after surgery?" Because some patients in this 1,700-bed facility go directly

---

10.1 Team Briefing Checklist

Yes	No	Elements Performed (check yes or no)
☐	☐	Announce team briefing
☐	☐	Introduce all personnel/team members
☐	☐	Share critical information about patient and procedure
☐	☐	Encourage team input and continued communication
☐	☐	Conduct Time Out
☐	☐	Review contingency plans as needed
☐	☐	Ask for questions or comments from the team

Reprinted with permission from Marshall, D.A., & Manus, D.A. (2007). A team training program using human factors to enhance patient safety. *AORN Journal, 86*(6), 994–1011.

10.2	Team Debriefing Checklist

Yes	No	Elements Performed (check yes or no)
☐	☐	Announce team debriefing
☐	☐	Discuss what went well and not well during surgery
☐	☐	Ask what and how the team could improve the next time
☐	☐	Assign follow-up roles and responsibilities
☐	☐	Ask for any last minute questions

Reprinted with permission from Marshall, D.A., & Manus, D.A. (2007). A team training program using human factors to enhance patient safety. *AORN Journal, 86*(6), 994–1011.

to the intensive care unit (ICU), this simple question stopped double transfers (e.g., transfers to the postanesthesia unit followed by a second transfer to the ICU).

The debriefing should focus on quality improvement. Its implementation has improved efficiency and patient safety. To increase an individual's comfort in speaking up, one team instituted the phrase, "I have a question." When any member voices this, all procedures that can be safely halted are, and the surgeon is required to pay attention. All of these tools could be refigured for ICU team rounds, shift reports, and other handoffs.

"SBAR" was seen as the most effective simulation in this training. Fortunately, it is a helpful model to promote concise communications from healthcare professionals to physicians. Both the Joint Commission and the Institute for Healthcare Improvement are recommending that this method of communication be standardized as the best practice (Pope, Rodzen, & Spross, 2008). The SBAR acronym stands for:

Situation
Background
Assessment and
Recommendation

An example of SBAR can be seen in Exhibit 10.3. This standardized process provides a structure so healthcare professionals know what data to collect and organize before calling physicians. By following this procedure, they do not rely on their memories for information. In turn, the physician knows what to expect during the communication. This communication model fits the physician's cognitive style of information processing and has significantly reduced frustrating late night calls to physicians from healthcare professionals. Instead, the SBAR format makes it easier to call when necessary, regardless of the hour. SBAR and the briefing and debriefing all work to help us realize Goal #2 of the National Patient Safety Goals—to improve effectiveness of communication among healthcare professionals.

There are also simple practices, such as hand washing, that reduce nosocomial infections (Gerberding, 2002). Yet compliance with this practice is pathetically

10.3   An Example of SBAR Communication

Dr. Mabley, this is Mary Harrison, RN, calling from Lansdale Hospital about your patient, Laura Palm.

Here is the situation: Mrs. Palm is having increased dyspnea and is complaining of chest pain.

The background information is that she had extensive varicose vein stripping two days ago. About 20 minutes ago, she began to complain of chest pain. Her pulse is 122 and blood pressure is 130 over 74. Her respirations are 24, and she is restless.

My assessment of the situation is that she may be having an MI or pulmonary embolism.

I recommend that you see her immediately and that we start her on O_2 at once.

low for nurses (Larson, Aiello, & Cimiotti, 2004). Rather than blaming nurses or any other healthcare professional, a systems approach to problem solving directs us to look at the structural layout of hand hygiene resources that limit the practice of consistent hand washing. Suresh and Cahill (2007) recently found that the following situations hindered the hand-washing process: poor visibility of hand-washing devices; difficulty with device access; and wide separation of resources needed to complete hand washing.

In addition, Hugonnet, Chevolet, and Pittet (2007) found a relationship between staffing levels and infection. When there is a nurse-patient ratio of more than 2.2 instead of a median of 1.9/24 hours, 26.7% of all infections are prevented. Inadequate staffing and poor structural layout of hand hygiene resources speaks to system problems in reducing infection.

However, neither explanation is an excuse for the personal accountability of healthcare professionals to wash their hands before touching any patient. It does, however, speak to the responsibility of healthcare professionals to participate on a QI team to determine how to improve the poor process design and to advocate for the staffing necessary to prevent infections.

Nurses report that that the majority of errors are caused by job overload. Therefore, nurse staffing plays a major role in preventing errors (American Nurses Association, 2000). The fatigue from this overload affects critical thinking and may cause nurses to "cut corners" in an effort to complete tasks. Furthermore, the connection between the number and mix of competent nurses must be considered in light of patient census and acuity.

Another example is National Patient Safety Goal #9, which is to reduce the risk of patient harm resulting from falls. In one year, almost 14,000 people aged 65 and older died from injuries related to falls, and 1.8 million people in the same age group were treated in emergency departments for nonfatal injuries (Centers for Disease Control, 2007). This research found that 20% to 30% of these older adults suffered moderate-to-severe injuries, such as hip fractures and traumatic brain injury. For people over the age of 85, the rate increases four to five times.

Nurses need to complete a fall risk evaluation for each patient on admission and then as often as policy dictates (Gustafson, 2007). Many organizations now place wristbands on patients who are at high risk for falls. To prevent falls, healthcare professionals need to get into the habit of rechecking patients before leaving the room to assure that the call bell is within reach, the bed is locked in the low position, all clutter is removed from the patient's path, the night light is on, and nonslip footwear and adaptive equipment, such as walkers and bedside commodes, are within reach. This one-minute check could save a patient from a devastating fall. Recommendations also include making rounds every hour to assess positioning and pain and to assist with toileting needs.

Other members of the healthcare team can be very helpful. Physical therapists and occupational therapists could be consulted for gait and balance assessment. Sometimes sitters are needed to provide protection for confused and disoriented patients. Since most falls occur during shift changes, it is important to use nurses' aides during this time to check on and assist patients.

Opportunities for Improvement in Patient Safety in Intensive Care

The complexity of processes in the ICU, including the acuity of illness, the volume of work, and the intensity of interventions, increases opportunities for error. However, the monitored environment and levels of documentation should increase the ability to confirm errors. Valentin and Bion (2007) conducted a multinational study of sentinel events in ICUs and found 38.8 events per 100 days in five categories (medications, catheters and drains, equipment, airway, and alarms). The authors also explored the cause of errors and made recommendations for changes to prevent their occurrence (see Exhibit 10.4). Many of these recommendations have to do with timely communication among and action by members of the team. Others have to do with the use of evidence-based protocols to reduce infection and rapid response teams to catch problems early.

For example, the sixth step in abolishing catheter-related bloodstream infections includes empowering the nurse to stop unsafe practices (Pronovost, Needham, & Berenhotz, 2006). In this case, the nurse would need the moral courage to speak up to protect the patient if any of the previous five steps had not been followed. A number of articles about stopping unsafe practices point to the importance of teamwork, optimal communication, mutual respect, and effective interdisciplinary collaboration. The role of leadership in fostering these components of a culture of safety will be discussed in-depth in Chapter 17.

Dorman and Pronovost (2002) added other recommendations to this list based on nine studies. Inadequate nurse staffing in the ICU (in which one nurse needs to care for more than one or two patients) increased the risk for pulmonary complications. Daily rounds by ICU physicians was a powerful predictor of risk-adjusted patient mortality and morbidity. All nine studies found a significant reduction in mortality rates with intensivist physician staffing. Using a case study example of a multipronged medication error, the authors clearly point out the problem when production—and not safety—is the focus. The time pressures created by a production focus can also lead to "work-arounds."

10.4 Recommendations for Improvement in Patient Safety in the ICU

Nurse staffing at 2.2/24hrs. (Hugonnet et al., 2007);

Intensivists decrease mortality and morbidity

Newly admitted patients seen immediately by physician. 1.6% increase in mortality for each hour of delay (Engoren, 2005).

Unless absolutely necessary do not transfer patient during afternoon or evening. Increased risk of death (Tobin and Santamaria, 2006)

Early goal-directed care in severe sepsis and septic shock. Each hour of delay is a mean decrease in survival of 7.6% (Kumar, Roberts, Wood et al., 2006)

Audit current practice against benchmarks (gap analysis) is simple effective error detection tool

No working beyond working hours, especially in 12 hour shifts for nurse or physicians (Scott, Rogers, Hwang, & Zhang, 2006; Landrigan, Rothschild, Cronin et al., 2004)

Rapid medical response teams available 24 hours a day

Six-step intervention to abolish catheter-related bloodstream infections (Pronovost et al., 2006)

Standardization of hand-offs (Catchpole, de Leval, McEwan et al., 2007)

Culture of safety is top priority for leadership (McCauley & Irwin, 2006)

Valentin, A., & Bion, J. (2007). How safe is my intensive care unit? An overview of error causation and prevention. *Current Opinion in Critical Care, 13*, 697–702.

Work-Arounds and Patient Safety

Robert Frost, one of America's favorite poets, wrote: "Don't ever take a fence down until you know why it was put up." Work-arounds are defined as "clever methods for getting done what the system does not let you do easily" (Ash, Berg, & Doiera, 2004; Ash, Gorman, Lavelle, et al., 2003, p.195). Frequently, work-arounds bypass safety elements and medical technology (e.g., safety alarms and Pyxis). An example of a technology work-around can be seen in barcode medication administration. The system is designed to reduce medication administration errors, but some nurses ignore the system. They keep copies of patient wristbands in a central location, thereby allowing numerous meds to be given at one time. A work-around may be the result of extensive informal testing. While it deviates from the prescribed plan, the process is not necessarily of lower quality. Many times, work-arounds, also called short-cuts, are used because the required procedure is seen as an unnecessary demand on a nurse's time (Patterson, Rogers, Chapman, & Render, 2006). A poor process can lead to blocks in workflow.

National Patient Safety Goal # 8 (to accurately and completely reconcile medications across a continuum of care) might be easily accomplished in a hospital with a computerized system. Stop flags can also be instituted, so that patient transfer is blocked until reconciliation is completed. However, in a hospital where patients are taking more than ten medications, the process is onerous. In noncomputerized systems, the chance for error is significant, and the time required often puts medication reconciliation low on the priority list.

Work-arounds may be practical problem-solving behaviors in organizations, but they do not address the underlying problems. As a result, they can exacerbate operational failures by continuing to repeat bad procedures. While these procedures may not cause harm, they increase the risk of harm. Repeated procedures become routine procedures. Ultimately, they are accepted as the normal way to address a problem. For example, the medication ordering process for admissions may be seen as cumbersome by physicians. The work-around is verbal orders, but this is not the safest process.

To prevent work-arounds from becoming normative within an organizational culture, healthcare professional providers must speak out about the possible harm these shortcuts are creating for patients. Without these voices, work-arounds become set in unit or organizational culture.

Conclusion

Patient safety is everyone's responsibility, although blame is not the way to meet the 2009 National Patient Safety Goals. To remedy the problems, a systems approach is needed, as are procedures that block the creative work-arounds that healthcare professionals develop. There are numerous evidence-based solutions to reduce risk of infections, prevent errors in surgery and falls, improve communication, and administer medications safely. For example, SBAR and team debriefing checklists can improve team member communication. They provide a format that makes it easier for healthcare professionals to speak up if they detect a potential or realized problem. We need to use the Patient Safety Solutions that have been developed. They are defined as "any system design or intervention that has demonstrated the ability to prevent or mitigate patient harm stemming from the processes of health care" (Joint Commission, 2008c).

Key Points to Remember

1. Healthcare professionals need to start using lessons from other industries to create a commitment to a culture of safety that includes improved teamwork, communication among team members, and redundancy in safety measures.
2. Patient safety means freedom from error.
3. To protect our patients, all healthcare professionals must be able to challenge erroneous care processes. Failure to speak up is responsible for many preventable errors.
4. SBAR (situation, background, assessment, and recommendation) is a helpful model to promote concise communications from healthcare professionals to physicians.
5. Frequently, work-arounds bypass safety elements and medical technology. To prevent work-arounds from becoming normative within an organizational culture, healthcare professional providers must speak out about the possible harm these shortcuts are creating for patients.

References

Agency for Healthcare Research and Quality (AHRQ). (2007). *Hospital survey on patient safety culture*. Retrieved March 6, 2008, from http://ahrq.gov/qual/haspculture

American Nurses Association. (2000). *New ANA study provides more proof of link between RN staffing and quality patient care*. Retrieved September 30, 2007, from http://nursingworld .org/MainMenuCategories/ThePracticeofProfessionalNursing/PatientSafetyQuality/ RNStaffingandQualityPatientCare.aspx

Ash, J.S., Berg, M., & Coiera, E. (2004). Some unintended consequences of information technology in health care: The nature of patient information system-related errors. *Journal of American Medical Informatics, 46,* 104–112.

Ash, J.S., Gorman, P.N., Lavelle, M., Payne, T.H., Massaro, T.A., Frantz, G.L. et al. (2003). A cross-site qualitative study of physician order entry. *Journal of American Medical Informatics, 10,* 188–200.

Banja, J.D. (2004). Persisting problems in disclosing medical error. *Harvard Health Policy Review, 5*(1), 14–20.

Blendon, J., DesRoches, M., Brodie, M., Benson, J.M., Rosen, A.B., Schneider, E., et al., (2002). Views of practicing physicians and the public on medical errors. *New England Journal of Medicine, 347*(24), 1933–1940.

Catchpole, K.R., de Leval, M.R., McEwan, A. et al. (2007). Patient handover from surgery to intensive care: Using Formula 1 pit-stop and aviation models to improve safety and quality. *Paediatric Anaesthology, 17,* 470–478.

Centers for Disease Control and Prevention Injury Center. Retrieved March 6, 2008, from http://www.cdc.gov/ncipc/wisqars

Chang, A., Schyve, P.M., Croteau, R.J., O'Leary, D.S., & Loeb, J.M. (2005). The JCAHO patient safety event taxonomy: A standardized terminology and classification schema for near misses and adverse events. *International Journal of Quality Healthcare, 17,* 95–105.

Dorman, T., & Pronovost, P. (2002). Intensive care unit errors: Detection and reporting to improve outcomes. *Current Opinion in Anaesthesiology, 15,* 147–151.

Engoren, M. (2005). The effect of prompt physician visits on intensive care unit mortality and cost. *Critical Care Medicine, 33,* 727–732.

Gerberding, J.L. (2002). Hospital-onset infections: A patient safety issue. *Annals of Internal Medicine, 137,* 665–670.

Gustafson, S.E. (2007). Assess for fall risk, intervene—and bump up patient safety. *Nursing 2007, 12,* 24–25.

Healey, M.A., Shackford, S.R., Osler, T.M., Rogens, F.B., & Burns, R. (2002). Complications in surgical patients. *Archives of Surgery, 137,* 611–618.

Hugonnet, S., Chevrolet, J.C., & Pittet, D. (2007). The effect of workload on infection risk in critically ill patients. *Critical Care Medicine, 35,* 76–81.

Institute of Medicine. (2001). *Crossing the quality chasm: A new health system for the 21st century*. Washington, DC: National Academies Press.

The Joint Commission. (2008a). *2009 National Patient Safety Goals*. Retrieved July 11, 2008, from http://www.jointcommission.org/PatientSafety/NationalPatientSafetyGoals/

The Joint Commission. (2008b). *Implementation expectations for the universal protocol for preventing wrong site, wrong procedure and wrong person surgery*. Retrieved July 11, 2008, from http://www.jointcommission.org/NR/rdonlyres/4CF3955D-CD1F-4230-86C5-D04485 CAFBEA/0/IG_final.pdf

The Joint Commission. (2008c). *Patient Safety Solutions*. Retrieved July 11, 2009, from http:// www.jointcommission.org/PatientSafety/Solutions/

The Joint Commission. (2008d). *Behaviors that undermine a culture of safety*. 40. Retrieved March 6, 2009, from http://www.jointcommission.org/SentinelEvents/SentinelEventAlert/ sea_40.htm

Kohn, K.T., Corrigan, J.M., & Donaldson, M.S. (2000). (Eds.) *To err is human: Building a safer health system*. Washington, DC: National Academies Press.

Kumar, A., Roberts, D., Wood, K.E., Light, B., Parrillo, J.E., Sharma, S., et al. (2006). Duration of hypotension before initiation of effective antimicrobial therapy is the critical determinant of survival in human septic shock. *Critical Care Medicine, 34,* 1589–1596.

Landrigan, C.P., Rothschild, J.M., Cronin, J.W., Kaushal, R., Burdick, E., Katz, J.T., et al. (2004). Effect of reducing interns' work hours on serious medical errors in intensive care units. *New England Journal of Medicine, 351*(18), 1838–1848.

Larson, E.L., Aiello, A.E., & Cimiotti, J.P. (2004). Assessing nurses' hand hygiene practices by direct observation or self-report. *Journal of Nursing Measurement, 12*(1), 77–85.

Leape, L.L., Berwick, D.M., & Bates, D.W. (2002). What practices will most improve safety? Evidence-based medicine meets patient safety. *Journal of the American Medical Association, 288,* 501–507.

Marshall, D.A., & Manus, D.A. (2007). A team training program using human factors to enhance patient safety. *AORN Journal, 86*(6), 994–1011.

McCauley, K., & Irwin, R.S. (2006). Changing the work environment in ICUs to achieve patient-focused care: The time has come. *Chest, 130,* 1571–1578.

Patterson, E.S., Rogers, M.L., Chapman, R.J., & Render, M. (2006). Compliance with intended use of bar code medication administration in acute and long-term care: An observational study. *Human Factors, 48,* 15–22.

Pizzi, L., Goldfarb, N.I., & Nash, D.B. (2001). Crew resource management and its application in medicine. In *Making health care safer: A critical analysis of patient safety practices.* Rockville, MD; AHRQ (Publication # 01-E058). Retrieved March 6, 2008, from http://www.ahrq .gov/clinic/ptsafety/

Pope, B.B., Rodzen, L., & Spross, G. (2008). Raising the SBAR: How better communication improves patient outcomes. *Nursing 2009, 38*(3), 41–43.

Pronovost, P.J., Wu, A.W., & Seaton, J.B. (2004). Acute decomposition after removing central line: Practical approaches for increasing safety in intensive care unit. *Annals of Internal Medicine, 140,* 1025–1033.

Pronovost, P., Needham, D., Berenholtz, S., Sinopoli, D., Chu, H., Cosgrove, S., et al. (2006). An intervention to decrease catheter-related bloodstream infections in the ICU. *New England Journal of Medicine, 355,* 2725–2732.

Scott, L.D., Rogers, A.E., Hwang, W.T., & Zhang, Y. (2006). Effects of critical care nurses' work hours on vigilance and patient safety. *American Journal of Critical Care, 15,* 30–37.

Sentinel event statistics as of March 31, 2008. The Joint Commission. Retrieved July 11, 2008, from http://www.jointcommission.org/NR/rdonlyres/241CD6F3-6EF0-4E9C-90AD-7FEAE 5EDCEA5/0/SE_Stats_03_08.pdf

Sharpe, V.A. (2003). Promoting patient safety: An ethical basis for policy deliberation. *Hastings Center Report, 33*(5), S3–18.

Starfield, B. (2000). Is US health really the best in the world? *JAMA, 284,* 483–485.

Suresh, G., & Cahill, J. (2007). How "user friendly" is the hospital for practicing hand hygiene? An ergonomic evaluation. *Joint Commission Journal on Quality & Patient Safety, 33*(3), 171–179.

Tobin, A.E., & Santamaria, J.D. (2006). After-hours discharges from intensive care are associated with increased mortality. *Medical Journal of Australia, 184,* 334–337.

Valentin, A., & Bion, J. (2007). How safe is my intensive care unit? An overview of error causation and prevention. *Current Opinion in Critical Care, 13,* 697–702.

Vincent, C., Neale, G., & Woloshynowych, M. (2001). Adverse events in British hospitals: Preliminary retrospective review. *British Medical Journal, 322,* 517–519.

Wachter, R.M. (2004). "The end of the beginning: patient safety five years after: To Err is Human." *Health Affairs.* (suppl Web exclusives) *6,* W4-534–545.

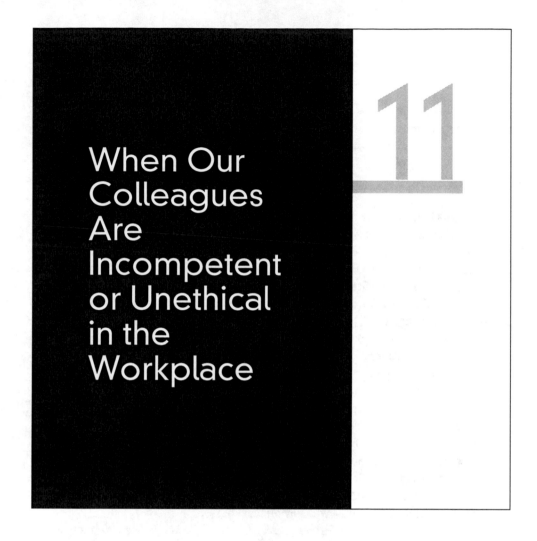

When Our Colleagues Are Incompetent or Unethical in the Workplace

11

Step Four: Make a searching and fearless moral inventory of ourselves.
—Alcoholics Anonymous

I have had the honor of hearing about a dozen Step Four stories from members of Alcoholics Anonymous. Each required the teller to demonstrate a high degree of moral courage in relating the raw truth of his or her life. This chapter does not require that you engage in that level of soul searching, but it will hopefully challenge you to reconsider how you look at colleagues who are impaired, either because of drugs/alcohol abuse and/or a mental illness. My hope is that you will no longer pretend "all is well," but that you will instead speak up when you realize that a colleague is suffering with impairment. Many of you know someone who is impaired, but rather than confront the situation, you label the person difficult or overemotional.

Codes of ethics explicitly state that healthcare professionals are responsible for reporting chemically dependent and mentally ill individuals when their performance is impaired. Most codes also address the importance of confronting any person whose behavior is threatening the well-being of patients and other members of the healthcare team. This chapter examines how to identify and confront colleagues whose performance threatens patient safety, regardless of the reason. It will also discuss how to confront unethical behaviors, such as lying and lateral violence. You will also read Sarah's story.

Case 11.1 Sarah's Story

Sarah was born and raised on a farm in Minnesota, as the youngest in a family of ten. As she says "by the time my mother had me, she was exhausted, so she just let me do what I wanted. My father worked us so hard that I really did not have time to get into much trouble until I was ten. One day, a friend and I set off fireworks, but the barn caught on fire. To this day, my father has no idea how this happened. Because I valued my life, I never said a word. It was the first step in my sensation seeking. At the age of 12, I discovered beer, and at 14, I found vodka. My father had always been a heavy drinker, but he drank bourbon, and I could not stand the smell. I was pretty much a loner and did not make friends easily, but there were three of us who hung out together. We would do mischievous things, but nothing that broke the law, except for our underage drinking. I decided to join the Army and see the world as a corpsman, because I thought it would be great to get away and exciting to see places I had never seen. During those five years, I was a heavy drinker, discovered sex, and was brutally raped. I decided I needed to grow up and wanted to become a professional nurse, because I had discovered that I liked medicine. Back then, schools did not engage in drug testing, so I was admitted and somehow made it through with good grades. My weekends with my 'drinking buddies' were a blur, and now I know I was having blackouts.

In my third year as a nurse, I discovered Demerol. It was innocent enough. No one was around to watch me waste it, so I decided to give myself the injection. Remember, this was pre-AIDS. Well, I fell in love from the first moment. I transferred to the critical care unit, where I had access to all the Demerol I wanted. As my tolerance grew, I needed more and more. So here I am, getting blitzed on the weekend and shooting up Demerol during the week, but I had no idea I was an alcoholic or an addict. Denial is truly amazing.

I got caught when I fell asleep in the ladies room booth with a needle in my vein. I had many signs of addiction outside of work and, in retrospect, I had signs at work, but I was very good at maintaining excellent care for my patients. I was given the option to go into rehab or lose my license. I figured I would do what they asked and, when I got out, I would be more careful and just stick to alcohol. I remember nothing of rehab because I was detoxifying the entire 30 days. It was really rough and the rules drove me crazy. Then I had to go to AA meetings three days a week, a peer assistance meeting on Fridays, get a sponsor, and, the part I really hated, see this psychologist. I did it all, and gradually woke to the fact that I was one sick person. My sponsor was relentless, and the psychologist asked me all kinds of dumb questions about my family. But I was learning things about myself that helped me understand 'why did I drink and drug.'

I will never forget the first day I returned to work. People stared at me, no one asked me to lunch, and I watched people give Demerol to patients knowing I would never be able to even touch it again. I never did touch it again, but I did relapse with alcohol for a week. This occurred when the strain of work, school, and my dying mother got to me. My sponsor read me the riot act, and I had to go to 90 AA meetings in 90 days. That was torture at first, but then I finally got it—these people really did care about me. Gradually, the people at work warmed up to me again. Some really reached out and told me they admired how brave I was. Most days, I was one step away from a drink, but gradually the therapy insights, the support from AA meetings, and my sponsor's 'take no prisoners' attitude got me through it all. I never knew I had such low self-esteem, but step-by-step that psychologist guided me through the AA steps, and I unloaded years of self-loathing. Finally, I saw the person she said she saw the first day she met me. I really gave her a run for her money, but she hung in there—she was caring, direct, and very helpful.

I have been clean and sober for 20 years. The strangest thing is that I work in a cardiac cath lab and give narcotics every day, but never have the urge. I have new ways to manage my stress, and my excitement seeking now involves helping people of all colors and ages. It is so exciting to see a child learn to read."

When Practice Is Impaired by Alcohol and/or Drugs

The American Medical Association (AMA) defines impairment as "any physical, mental or behavioral disorder that interferes with the ability to engage safely in professional activities" (Taub, Morin, Goldrich, & Ray, 2006). The American Nurses Association (ANA) Code supports this definition, as it also recognizes that a variety of conditions may hamper healthcare professionals in practicing with reasonable skills and safety. The ANA Code also speaks directly to the issue of patient protection by requiring "appropriate action regarding any instances of incompetent, unethical, illegal, or impaired practice by any member of the health care team . . ." (ANA, 2001, p. 14).

The statistics on impaired healthcare professionals raise safety issues that affect patients. Since 1984, the ANA has estimated that 6% to 8% of nurses have a drug and/or alcohol abuse problem (ANA, 1984). Sullivan, Bissel, and Williams (1988) recorded a similar incidence rate, which is comparable to the incidence of drug/alcohol problems in the general population. Because two-thirds of nursing state board actions stem from impaired functioning and alternative-to-discipline programs are not reporting statistics to the state board of nursing (SBN), the actual percent of drug/alcohol problems is hard to calculate (Sullivan, 1987a). The debate continues as to whether the rate is actually higher among nurses than in the general public.

Physicians develop chemical dependence problems at the rate of 10% to 15% (Joranson, Ryan, Gibson, & Dall, 2000). McGovern, Angre, and Leon (2000) assessed 108 physicians who were attending a treatment program. They found that the physicians' drugs of choice were alcohol (61.4%) and prescription opiates (26.3%). Family physicians and internists were the largest groups of physicians affected. They were followed by psychiatrists, obstetricians/gynecologists, and emergency medicine physicians. In an Australian study, 42.1% of male doctors and 52.9% of female doctors admitted to writing prescriptions for themselves in the past year (Joranson et al., 2000). Findings from these studies heighten the need for healthcare professionals to speak up when they see patient safety risks and the potential for medical error based on impairment.

All codes of ethics for healthcare professional include statements about the professional's obligation to confront colleagues whose performances show signs of impairment. The examples below come from the nursing, physician, and physician assistant codes of ethics. But even when done appropriately, this reporting may present substantial risks to the healthcare professional (e.g., retaliation).

For nurses, the requirement to hold individuals accountable for incompetent, unethical, illegal, and impaired practice is found in Provision 3.6, Addressing impaired practice, of the Code (ANA Code, pp. 15–16). It clearly states that the nurse is responsible for taking action when any member of the healthcare system puts the best interests of a patient in jeopardy. The focus of this crucial conversation should be on the possible harmful effects on the patient. If you meet with a lack of accountability for the action, then the problem needs to be reported to the appropriate person in the organizational hierarchy or to an appropriate external authority, such as the State Board of Nursing or other regulatory board.

The nurse detecting the impairment has an obligation to protect the patient and to ensure that the impaired individual receives needed care. If the organization has no guiding policies or if they are inappropriate (i.e., they deny legal access to due legal process or demand resignation), the nurse should ask for guidance from an employee assistance program (EAP), state peer assistance program, or professional organization. This Code supports the return to work for an impaired individual who has sought assistance.

The AMA *Code of Medical Ethics* (2001) states that "A physician shall uphold the standards of professionalism, be honest in all professional interactions, and strive to report physicians deficient in character or competence, or engaging in fraud or deception, to appropriate entities." This Code recognizes that some type of intervention may be required in the case of a physician who is impaired, incompetent, or behaving unethically. The requirement is grounded in the physician's responsibility to self-regulate (professionalism) (Taub et al., 2006).

The American Association of Physician Assistants (AAPA) *Guidelines for Ethical Conduct for the PA Profession* (2007) instructs PAs to report illegal or unethical conduct by healthcare professionals to the appropriate authorities. In the AAPA guidelines, "impaired" means being unable to practice medicine with reasonable skill and safety because of physical or mental illness, loss of motor skills, or excessive use or abuse of drugs and alcohol. The code charges PAs with being able to recognize impairment in all healthcare professionals and to seek the resources necessary to encourage impaired professionals to get treatment.

Risk Factors

If we could identify some of the risk factors, could we help prevent or intervene earlier in cases of chemical dependency? There is no one risk factor. Rather, the interplay of multiple factors put an individual at risk of chemical dependence. Exhibit 11.1 compares risk factors from five studies. In Donovan's (1986) study,

11.1	Comparison of Risk Factors for the Development of Chemical Dependence in Nursing				
Authors	Donovan (1986)	Sullivan (1987a)	Trinkoff et al. (2000)	Burns (1991)	West (2002)
Risk factors/ contributors	Heredity		Greater substance abuse with more depressive symptoms	Sensation seeking	Sensation seeking
	Family history of alcoholism	Family history of alcoholism			Family history of alcoholism
	Gender	Experienced sexual abuse	Increased role strain	Hassles	
	Psychological deficits	Academically and professionally successful	Social network contained significantly more drug users	Peers involved with drugs?	Knew more impaired nurses
	Antisocial personality	Extensive medical histories	High access to substances	High scores on alcohol risk survey	High score on alcohol risk survey
	Ego weakness			Low self-esteem	
	Socio-cultural factors		Religiosity decreased		

seven risk factors are identified. Sullivan (1987b) discovered five characteristics in substance-impaired nurses. Burns (1991) found that high scores on the alcohol risk survey and low self-esteem were the dominant predictor variables for substance abuse. Trinkoff, Zhou, Storr, and Soeken (2000) found five factors that were likely to predict nurse's substance use. West (2002) studied differences among 100 substance-impaired and 100 nonimpaired nurses using three questionnaires. Role strain was measured through job demands, and depressive symptoms were assessed. West further reported that after interventions with substance impaired nurses, substance abuse decreased, although it was not completely absent.

Sarah's story shows many of these predictors, including a history of alcoholism (father), peer group pressure (drinking buddies), sexual abuse (brutal rape), low self-esteem, and easy access to substances (ICU nurse). Sarah most likely would have also scored high on the alcohol risk survey. Before we examine the intervention process, let us also look at the mental and physical illnesses that cause incompetence in the workplace.

Success of Peer Assistance

The United States has no unified policy or approach for the treatment of chemical dependence in healthcare professionals, so wide variation in treatment exists. Physicians have the most highly developed network of addiction providers and peer assistance programs that are available independent of licensing boards.

The treatment model for nurses varies significantly from state to state. Some use a medical model, others use a deterrence model, and some use both. The SBN could use a deterrence model and place the nurse on probation or suspension, impose practice restrictions, or revoke the nurse's license to practice. Some state boards have developed an alternative model that protects the public, but also focuses on the treatment and rehabilitation of impaired nurses.

Haack and Yocum (2002) studied 100 nurses from a discipline deterrence model and 119 from an alternative model in four regions of the United States over a six-month period. With attrition, the final number of nurses studied was 65 in the discipline and 82 in the alternative model group. There was no statistically significant difference in the relapse rate between the two groups. Less than 15% of the nurses in both groups experienced a relapse, with alcohol and crack cocaine being the most common problems. With today's nursing shortage, the most important statistic was that 74% of nurses in the alternative model group were employed, whereas only 52% of the discipline deterrence model were employed. Without employment, they likely lacked the health insurance needed to pay for their recovery. The alternative model provides a more humane and rehabilitative model for the problem of chemical dependence.

Sarah's story indicates the importance of providing the needed resources to stop the chronic illness of addiction with an intervention, treat the illness, and then provide the needed supports for the individual to maintain recovery. This professional was not lost to the illness of addiction because other healthcare professionals would not support her denial. From the list of signs and symptoms of addiction in Exhibit 11.2, Sarah had long coffee breaks, requested change to a less supervised shift, presented with changes in physical/emotional condition during a shift, and had an increased use of narcotics recorded for patients. For most people, these actions would not be enough to trigger questioning of her professional capacity.

Recognizing the importance of physician health, a 2000 Joint Commission on Accreditation of Healthcare Organizations (JCAHO) mandate required all hospital medical staff to have physician wellness committees or to work with already established physician health programs in each state. More specifically, it insists that medical personnel implement a process to identify and manage matters of individual physician health that is separate from the medical staff disciplinary function. The responsibilities of this committee include educating medical staff about illness and impairment and referring impaired physicians to appropriate resources for diagnosis and treatment. Perhaps it would be most useful to duplicate this model for all healthcare professionals.

Mental and Physical Illness

Depression and anxiety are the two most common psychiatric disorders. The World Health Organization has acknowledged that depression is the principal cause of disability in the world after cardiovascular disease (Michaud, Murray, & Bloom, 2001). U.S. National Comorbidity Survey estimates reveal that 17.1% of the population suffers from major depressive episodes at some point in their lifetimes, 10.3% in the last twelve months (Kessler, McGonagle, Zhao, et al., 1994). The probability of a depressive disorder increases 1.5 to 3.5 times if the patient has a chronic illness, chronic pain, significant recent stress, or undiagnosed symptoms and signs (Kroenke, Jackson, & Chamberlin, 1997). According to Kessler and Wang (2008), some anxiety disorders (phobias, separation anxiety disorder) and impulse-control disorders have the earliest age of onset distributions. Other anxiety disorders (panic disorder, generalized anxiety disorder, post-traumatic stress disorder), mood disorders, and substance disorders typically have later ages of onset. The signs and symptoms of depression or anxiety can cause significant interpersonal difficulty and concentration problems, leaving the healthcare professional open to making mistakes and being isolated from other team members. Research also suggests that most women who suffer from depression do not seek treatment (Mann, 2005).

My experience, after having treated more than 100 healthcare professionals for addiction, shows that most were using the drugs to either medicate their undiagnosed depression and/or anxiety or were using the drugs to cope with physical pain, often from a work injury. Early on, I learned to probe for possible sexual abuse in their history, because three patients who had relapsed finally shared for the first time the sexual abuse they experienced at the hands of brothers and uncles. All of these nurses and physicians were trying to continue to work, but they needed the help of legal and illegal drugs to cope. Through the use of 12-step AA/NA program, peer assistance groups, and counseling, they learned other ways to manage their emotions.

Sarah's case was typical—a history of undiagnosed depression in the family and the attitude that psychotherapy was only for "really crazy" people. This attitude leaves most people to struggle with their mental illness alone, rather than receiving the skills that cognitive-behavioral therapy (CBT) can offer. Sarah's low self-esteem was covered up with bravado, but underneath she was in deep pain from family rejection, the brutal rape, and her codependent relationship with her substance-abusing partner. Although she did not have depression or anxiety, she did have a deep fear of intimacy and fear of failure.

Today these fears, as well as depression and anxiety, are very treatable with CBT. When possible, therapists like to avoid giving recovering individuals any mind-altering substance, but sometimes depression or anxiety is so severe that medication is necessary in addition to the CBT.

Cognitive dysfunction can occur with any disease, but it is slightly more likely in progressive multiple sclerosis (MS). Cognitive changes are common in people with MS—approximately 50% of afflicted people will develop cognition problems (National MS Society). Certain functions, such as memory, information processing, attention and concentration, planning and prioritizing, and word finding, may be more affected than others. Clearly, some of these problems could lead to

11.2 Checklist for Detecting Potential Chemical Dependence in an Employee

1. Absenteeism
   - ___ a. Frequent, unscheduled short-term absences
   - ___ b. Higher absenteeism rate than other employees for colds, flu, gastritis, etc.
   - ___ c. Absences after payday or days off
   - ___ d. Inconsistent or increasingly improbable excuses for absences
   - ___ e. Absences for traffic or home accident injuries
2. "On-The-Job" Absenteeism
   - ___ a. Long coffee breaks
   - ___ b. Physical illness on the job (frequent trips to Occupational Health)
   - ___ c. Excess time for charting/record keeping
   - ___ d. "Locked door syndrome"—excessively long use of restroom
3. Difficulty in Concentration
   - ___ a. Assignment takes more time (despite skill/experience)
   - ___ b. Difficulty in assigning priorities in clinical caseload
   - ___ c. Medication errors (wrong medication, wrong dose, administration to wrong patient)
   - ___ d. Omitted, illogical, incomplete, or illegible charting
   - ___ e. Deteriorating handwriting during shift
   - ___ f. Errors in transcribing orders and/or taking verbal orders
   - ___ g. Overlooking signs of a patient's deteriorating condition
4. Inconsistent Work Patterns
   - ___ a. Alternate periods of high and low efficiency
   - ___ b. Becoming or has become less dependable
   - ___ c. Doing minimal or substandard work in comparison with peers
   - ___ d. Frequent requests for help with patient assignments
5. Physical/Emotional Problems
   - ___ a. Changes in physical/emotional condition during shift
   - ___ b. Marked nervousness on the job
   - ___ c. Excessive sweating
   - ___ d. Tremors of hands
   - ___ e. Lack of attention to personal cleanliness or grooming
   - ___ f. Reports to duty despite physical or emotional contraindication
6. Decreasing Job Efficiency
   - ___ a. Omits treatments
   - ___ b. Makes bad decisions or shows poor judgment
   - ___ c. Lacks usual initiative or enthusiasm
   - ___ d. Requests change to less supervised shift
7. Poor Relationships on the Job
   - ___ a. Wide swings in mood from isolation to angry outbursts
   - ___ b. Uncooperative with coworkers
   - ___ c. Avoids contact with nurse-leader or supervisor
   - ___ d. Complaints by patients of irritability, physical roughness, or verbal abuse

11.2 *Continued*

8. Medication-Centered Problems
____ a. Frequently around medication chart or closet
____ b. Increased use of prn psychoactive medications or narcotics recorded for patients
____ c. Increase in wastage/breakage of controlled substances
____ d. Missing drugs, unaccounted drugs
____ e. Seeks out on-duty physicians for personal complaints of pain, backache, migraines, etc.
____ f. No dates/times on narcotic sign outs
____ g. Complaints by patients about decreased pain relief
9. Personal Life Interferes With Job
____ a. Frequent or excessively long phone calls
____ b. "Visitors" or unexplained errands during work shift

mistakes that cause patient errors. Fatigue and cognitive fog are the major reasons why many people with MS eventually leave the workforce.

Both type 1 and type 2 diabetes mellitus have also been linked with reduced performance because of cognitive dysfunction. The precise pathophysiology of cognitive dysfunction in diabetes is not understood, but it is likely that hyperglycemia, vascular disease, hypoglycemia, and insulin resistance play significant roles (Kodl & Seaquist, 2008). Type 2 diabetes is associated with poor cognitive performance in middle-aged men and women (Kumari & Marmot, 2005). Obviously, not all individuals with diabetes will show loss of cognitive function, but as we understand these changes better, the individual may be able to compensate in some way.

Both physical and mental illness can bring with it a variety of cognitive changes that can lead to incompetent practice that result in errors of judgment. To protect patients, managers have a responsibility to counsel any individual whose performance is unacceptable, regardless of the cause. This can be done in a compassionate and firm way, just as it would be done for individuals suffering from an addiction. All are diseases that can interfere with practice. Some of the interventions that led to Sarah's success in recovery could also be applied to patients with physical and mental illnesses.

Courage to Care: Intervention

Our role is not to foster denial in our colleagues who are suffering from untreated illness or chemical dependency. It is our moral obligation to be knowledgeable so we are able to identify the problem, help people face up to their problems, know how to refer them for treatment, and support them when they return to the workplace. This section focuses on how to confront the impaired individual. The signs and symptoms have already been presented in Exhibit 11.2.

Remember that the purpose of confronting inappropriate or unethical behavior is not to punish the healthcare professional, but to protect the patient. It
is important to focus on the troubling behaviors and facts, not on hearsay. It is
usually best to concentrate on the individual's well-being by using a phrase such
as, "You are usually so organized and clear in your documentation and I have
noticed in the last two weeks that I am having trouble reading and following your
notes. Is something wrong?" The response could be the first step toward rehabilitation or a defensive denial. You may find out that the change has a legitimate
explanation, such as a new medication for rheumatoid arthritis that is clouding
judgment and pain that is making legible handwriting difficult.

However, if you get a denial and are still concerned, then it is time to contact the next person in line in the organizational hierarchy. If this person does not
intervene, then it is your ethical obligation to go one step higher and/or contact
the regulatory body for that profession. Reports can be anonymous. However, if
you file a report with your name, you are protected from reprisals if the report
is written in good faith.

When the signs of addiction are obvious and the person in question denies
it, sometimes the confronting person will say this person is lying. The truth is
that the person is lying to himself or herself. One's false view of oneself causes
duplicity. The best way to confront lying, regardless of the cause, is to point out
the inconsistency between behavior and reality. For example, "Sarah, you say you
have not signed out any more narcotics than any other nurse, but look at these
sign out sheets on which your name is highlighted. You are three times as likely
as any other staff member to have signed out a narcotic, even though your nurse's
notes do not indicate significant pain for any of these patients. How do you account for this inconsistency?"

Dunn (2005) gives an excellent overview of the of the manager's role in the
intervention. It is not acceptable for managers to stand by idly and watch a professional self-destruct. Dunn points out the myth that an addicted person must
reach "rock bottom" before considering treatment options, but that does not
change the fact that it is very rare for a chemically addicted person to suddenly
gain insight into the severity of his or her problem without outside help. One
person may not be able to break through the powerful defense mechanisms of
denial, rationalization, minimization, and projection. Therefore, the manager will
likely have several other people in the room for the conversation/confrontation.
The goal is to obtain the willingness of the healthcare professional to accept help
and get a fitness-to-practice evaluation.

If this evaluation shows a chemical dependency and/or mental illness, then
the goal becomes referral for treatment, hopefully in an alternative program
rather than a discipline/deterrence program. If the healthcare professional refuses evaluation or treatment, then the manager has no alternative but to report
the individual to the regulatory body.

After successful treatment, the healthcare professional returns to work. Returning to work and facing one's colleagues often requires significant courage
because of the stigma associated with addiction and/or mental illness. Exhibit
11.3 describes the recommended employment conditions for people in recovery
returning to work and suggestions for ways that coworkers can prepare and be
supportive.

11.3	Responsibilities of Recovering Healthcare Professionals and Helpful Support from Colleagues

Responsibilities of Recovering Healthcare Professionals and Suggested Working Conditions

1. If possible, not in clinical setting with exposure to drug of choice
2. Practice in less stressful clinical setting
3. Not personally distributing any type of controlled substance in first six months; under direct supervision for next six months.
4. Limited work hours, part-time or full time with restrictions of no overtime and no night shift
5. Work in structured setting under direct supervision, but never alone
6. Submit to random, supervised drug and alcohol screening
7. Monitored attendance at self-help recovery group and counseling sessions
8. Delineated consequences of relapse or violation of agreement
9. Performance feedback and appraisals indicate satisfactory performance

Helpful Support From Colleagues for Recovering HCP

1. Be welcoming and supportive of their courage to return, not judgmental
2. If confidentiality is not an issue, a debriefing for the staff prior to return to discuss feelings, concerns and to understand nurses present limitations
3. If confidentiality is not issue, ask how they are doing with recovery process and if there is any way you can help

Dealing With the Unethical Conduct of Horizontal Violence

You may recognize many alternative names for horizontal violence, such as lateral violence, horizontal hostility, workplace incivility, and bullying. In nursing, this violence applies to nurses who covertly or overtly direct their dissatisfaction toward each other, toward themselves, and toward those less powerful than themselves (Griffin, 2004). We use the term violence because there is a victim. The most vulnerable are newly licensed nurses, newly hired nurses, the hospital float pool, and traveling nurses. Griffin names many forms of horizontal violence, including nonverbal innuendo, verbal affront, undermining activities, withholding information, sabotage, infighting, scapegoating, backstabbing, failure to respect privacy, and broken confidences.

The theoretical basis for horizontal violence lies in the fact that nurses are dominated by the medical profession in the hierarchical structure of many healthcare organizations. This excludes them from the power structure that drives change. For many nurses aged 50 years and older, there are also some gender and role socialization issues. As a result, they tend to exhibit the characteristics of an "oppressed population" (see Figure 11.1).

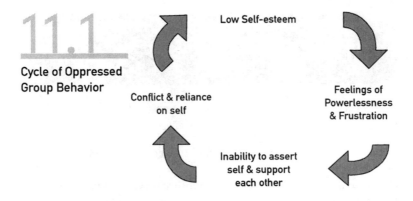

11.1

**Cycle of Oppressed
Group Behavior**

Low Self-esteem

Conflict & reliance
on self

Feelings of
Powerlessness
& Frustration

Inability to assert
self & support
each other

The ramifications of horizontal violence are significant for both the individual nurse and the healthcare organization. Such behaviors can impact patient satisfaction, as they see the lack of cooperation and support among members of the nursing staff. The following is a partial list of the consequences:

1. Low morale
2. Diminished teamwork
3. Increased stress
4. High turnover rates
5. Increased labor costs
6. Difficulty in recruiting new staff
7. Decreased quality of patient care

The ANA Code (2001) demands respect and compassion in *all* relationships. Disrespect breaches the nursing profession's Code of Ethics, which states:

> *The principle of respect for persons extends to all individuals with whom the nurse interacts . . . In each of these roles, the nurse treats colleagues, employees, assistants, and students with respect and compassion. This standard of conduct precludes any and all prejudicial actions, any form of harassment or threatening behavior, or disregard for the effect of one's actions on others (p. 9).*

To stop this violation of unethical conduct, we need to raise awareness about the unacceptability of the behavior (Rowe & Sherlock, 2005). Healthcare organizations need to adopt nonnegotiable professional behavior standards. Using the skills learned in Chapter 5, healthcare professionals can address these behaviors as they occur. By using cognitive rehearsal, healthcare professionals can recognize behavior when it occurs, plan ahead for ways to respond, actually practice what they will say, and then respond in a professional manner when the behavior occurs. Moral courage is still a necessary ingredient, but by practicing the response, the situation will be easier to tackle. Effective preceptor and mentoring programs can also provide training and role modeling to help vulnerable new nurses. Management can support the change to a collaboration norm by having a "zero tolerance policy." This culture change in attitude needs support with skill building if long-term change in civility is to occur (Bartholomew, 2006).

Conclusion

Incompetent and unethical practices by healthcare professionals always need to be addressed in a firm, yet compassionate, way. Whether the problem is addiction, mental or physical illness, or lateral violence, managers and executives have the responsibility to protect patients and to identify and intervene with employees. Discomfort and fear of causing discomfort are frequent obstacles to holding individuals accountable for their performances. However, the ethical obligation to do so and training in the skills of moral courage make such confrontations less upsetting.

Key Points to Remember

1. Codes of ethics explicitly state that healthcare professionals are responsible for reporting chemically dependent and mentally ill individuals when their performance is impaired.
2. The healthcare professional detecting the impairment has an obligation to protect the patient and to ensure that the impaired individual receives needed care.
3. Depression and anxiety are the two most common psychiatric disorders.
4. The purpose of confronting inappropriate or unethical behavior is not to punish the healthcare professional, but to protect the patient.
5. The theoretical basis for horizontal violence lies in the fact that nurses are more likely to attack each other because they experience a lack of power in making changes in the hierarchical structure of many healthcare organizations.

References

American Academy of Physician Assistants. (2007). *Guidelines for ethical conduct for physician assistants.* Retrieved June 4, 2008, from http://www.aapa.org/manual/23-EthicalConduct.pdf

American Medical Association. (2001). *Code of medical ethics.* Chicago, IL: AMA. Retrieved July 1, 2008, from http://www.ama-assn.org/ama/pub/category/2512.html

American Nurses Association. (2001). *Code for ethics for nurses with interpretative statements.* Silver Spring, MD: American Nurses Publishing. Retrieved July 5, 2008, from http://www.nursingworld.org

American Nurses Association. (1984). *Addictions and psychological dysfunctions in nursing: The profession's response to the problem.* Kansas City, MO: ANA.

Bartholomew, K. (2006). *Ending nurse-to-nurse hostility.* Marblehead, MA: HCPro.

Burns, L.J. (1991). *An investigation of risk factors for substance abuse among nurses* (Doctoral dissertation, University of Pennsylvania). UMI Dissertation Services.

Donovan, J. (1986). An etiologic model of alcoholism. *American Journal of Psychiatry, 143,* 1–11.

Dunn, D. (2005). Substance abuse among nurses—Intercession and intervention. *AORN Journal, 82*(5), 775–799.

Griffin, M. (2004). Teaching cognitive rehearsal as a shield for lateral violence: An intervention for newly licensed nurses. *Journal of Continuing Education in Nursing, 35*(6), 257–263.

Haack, M.R., & Yocum, C.J. (2002). State policies and nurses with substance abuse disorders. *Journal of Nursing Scholarship, 34*(1), 89–94.

Joint Commission on Accreditation of Healthcare Organizations. (2000). Medical staff revisions reflect current practices in the field. *Joint Commission Perspectives, 20*(6).

Joranson, D., Ryan, K., Gilson, A., & Dahl, J. (2000). Trends in medical use and abuse of opioid analgesics. *JAMA, 283,* 1710–1714.

Kessler, R.C., McGonagle, K.A., Zhao, S., Nelson, C.B., Hughes, M., Eshlemann, S., et al. (1994). Lifetime and 12-month prevalence of DSM-III psychiatric disorders in United States: Results from National Comorbidity Survey. *Archives of General Psychiatry, 51,* 8–19.

Kessler, R.C., & Wang, P.S. (2008). The descriptive epidemiology of commonly occurring mental disorders in the United States. *Annual Review of Public Health, 29,* 115–129.

Kodl, C.T., & Seaquist, E.R. (2008). Cognitive dysfunction and diabetes mellitus. *Endocrine Reviews, 29*(4), 494–511.

Kroenke, K., Jackson, J.L., & Chamberlin, J. (1997). Depressive and anxiety disorders in patients presenting with physical complaints: Clinical predictors and outcome. *American Journal of Medicine, 103*(5), 339–347.

Kumari, M., & Marmot, M. (2005). Diabetes and cognitive function in a middle-aged cohort: Findings from the Whitehall II study. *Neurology, 65,* 1597–1603.

Mann, J.J. (2005). The medical management of depression. *New England Journal of Medicine, 353,* 1819–1834.

McGovern, M., Angre, D., & Leon, S. (2000). Characteristics of physicians presenting for assessment in a behavioural health center. *Journal of Addiction Diseases, 19,* 59–73.

Michaud, C.M., Murray, C.J., & Bloom, B.R. (2001). Burden of disease: Implications for future research. *JAMA, 285,* 535–539.

National MS Society. Retrieved August 4, 2008, from http://www.nationalmssociety.org/about-multiple-sclerosis/symptoms/cognitive-function/index.aspx

Rowe, M.M., & Sherlock, H. (2005). Stress and verbal abuse in nursing: Do burned out nurses eat their young? *Journal of Nursing Management, 13,* 242–248.

Sullivan, E.J. (1987a). A descriptive study of nurses recovering from chemical dependency. *Archives of Psychiatric Nursing, 1*(3), 194–200.

Sullivan, E.J. (1987b). Comparison of chemically dependent and nondependent nurses on familial, personal and professional characteristics. *Journal of Studies of Alcohol, 48,* 563–568.

Sullivan, E.J., Bissel, L., & Williams, L. (1988). *Chemical dependency in nursing: The deadly diversion.* Menlo Park, CA: Addison-Wesley.

Taub, S., Morin, K., Goldrich, M.S., & Ray, P. for Council on Ethical and Judicial Affairs of the American Medical Association. (2006). Physician health and wellness. *Occupational Medicine, 56*(2), 77–82.

Trinkoff, A.M., Zhou, Q., Storr, C.L., & Soeken, K.L. (2000). Workplace access, negative proscriptions, job strain, and substance use in registered nurses. *Nursing Research, 49*(2), 83–90.

West, M.M. (2002). Early risk indicators of substance abuse among nurses. *Journal of Nursing Scholarship, 34*(2), 187–193.

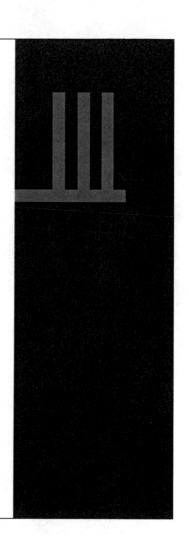

Organizational
Development
of Moral
Courage

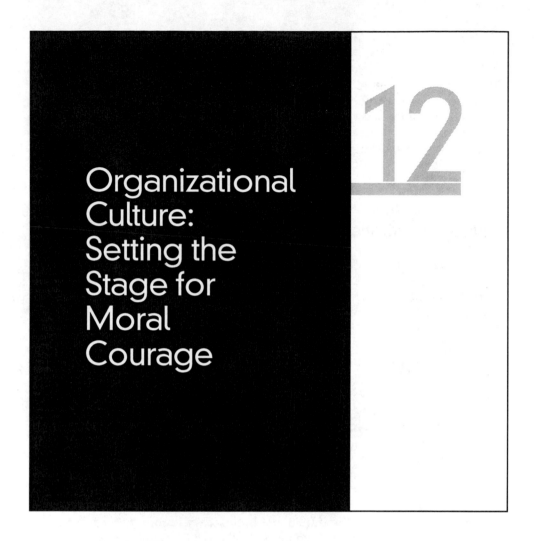

Organizational Culture: Setting the Stage for Moral Courage

> Organizational culture is the key to organizational excellence . . . and the function of leadership is the creation and management of culture.
> —Edgar Schein, prolific writer and consultant on organizational development

The phrase organizational culture refers to the personality of the organization, which is principally created by the repeated actions of senior leadership acting on their beliefs and values. Their behaviors determine what is morally acceptable. You can tell the culture of an organization by looking at the arrangement of offices, what employees brag about, and how people are treated. This is the way you develop an impression about someone's personality.

The role of executive leadership in creating a moral culture is delineated in the Code of Ethics from the American College of Healthcare Executives (ACHE)

(2007). After a brief definition of organizational culture, and this Code, a tool is offered for the assessment of your organizational culture—the Organizational Courage Assessment. An ethical culture goes beyond mere corporate compliance and prevents the need for whistleblowing. This chapter focuses on the key components of organizational culture that are necessary to create a social order that not only supports "do no harm," but also sets the stage for "one of the best places to work" awards.

Defining Organizational Culture

Organizational culture is a set of beliefs and values which, over time, are validated by the organization and transformed into shared underlying assumptions about the world. They are manifested in myths, stories, rituals, a special language, and ideology. Culture includes beliefs (that is, opinions about how things are) and values (that is, how things ought to be). Culture creates a sense of belonging for the people in the organization and organizational loyalty. Because culture guides organizational behavior, it has the potential to do great good or do harm.

Samuel (2006) defines culture as the way people function together to achieve desired business outcomes. He sees it as the single most important factor in an organization's ability to achieve desired results. It represents the framework of the organization, but it is also the collective mindset of the people. The culture is held together "by the way we do things around here." These patterns of behavior or habits direct the behavior of members in predictable ways. It directs how decisions are made and at what level, how poor performance is managed, and how effective the up-down communication is in accomplishing outcomes. The culture is the sum total of its functional habits (continuously providing feedback on performance) and dysfunctional habits (conflict avoidance).

What is necessary to create a moral culture that supports accountability, patient safety, and quality patient care? Rest (1984) conceptualizes moral behavior as having four elements: (1) moral sensitivity to the effects of actions on the well-being of others, (2) moral reasoning to discover the most ethically justifiable resolution, (3) motivation to place morality above other considerations, and (4) perseverance and practical strategy for implementing the moral decision. *Moral sensitivity* is the level of concern about ethical dilemmas that exist in the organization. *Moral reasoning* is the individual's critical thinking and principle approach to protecting the mission, values, patients, and staff. *Moral commitment* is the person's promise to uphold professional and ethical standards. In a moral culture, the executives and managers always make the patient the highest priority.

American College of Healthcare Executives Code of Ethics

The American College of Healthcare Executives Code of Ethics (2007) serves as the conduct guide for the profession of healthcare management. It includes responsibilities to patients, employees, organization, and community. According to this Code:

> *The fundamental objectives of the healthcare management profession are to enhance overall quality of life, dignity and well-being of every individual needing healthcare services; and to create a more equitable, accessible, effective and efficient healthcare system. Healthcare executives have an obligation to act in ways that will merit the trust, confidence and respect of healthcare professionals and the general public. Therefore, healthcare executives should lead lives that embody an exemplary system of values and ethics (pp. 1–2).*

The Code sees executives as moral advocates who are responsible for supporting the rights of patients (e.g., honoring advance directives and access to emergency care) and anticipating the possible outcomes of their decisions. The values mentioned in the code—honesty, integrity, respect, fairness, and good faith are very similar to Kidder's (2005) international values of honesty, responsibility, respect, compassion, and fairness. Executives are to "demonstrate zero tolerance for any abuse of power that compromises patients and others served" (p. 3). Zero tolerance means that no disruptive physician would be tolerated and any delivery of bad news to a patient would be truthful about prognosis and compassionate.

In Section IV of the Code, covering responsibilities to employees, the executive is required to "provide a work environment that encourages a free expression of ethical concerns and provides mechanisms for discussing and addressing such concerns" (p. 4). If this goal is achieved, there would be no need for whistleblowing, as all ethical concerns would be resolved within the healthcare organization.

Organizational Courage Assessment

The Organizational Courage Assessment (Kilmann, O'Hara, & Strauss, 2004) is another assessment instrument that lists 20 possible acts of courage. You are first asked to evaluate whether you have observed these acts or if they are not necessary because personnel are already addressing the issues appropriately. Second, you are asked to assess how afraid people would be of negative consequences if they acted in such a manner. An example of a question for the first section is, "Have you observed people speaking out against illegal or unethical actions"; for the second section, an example is, "How afraid would people be of speaking out against illegal or unethical actions?" This assessment then describes four types of organizations:

1. courageous organizations

2. quantum organizations

3. fearful organizations

4. bureaucratic organizations

The difference between courageous organizations and quantum organizations is that the quantum organizational culture is already supportive. As a result, courage is not required to overcome fear. In bureaucratic organizations, individuals are resigned to doing the expected and few acts of courage are seen. Both fearful and bureaucratic organizations require organizational transformation. Without an organizational intervention to change processes, structures, and practices blocking empowerment of employees to do the right thing, the organization will never be able to support an ethical climate.

Baptist Health Care was an organization in which a transformational intervention changed the organizational culture (Stubblefield, 2005). The story started in 1995, when the organization received patient satisfaction ratings at only the 18th percentile and an employee survey that ranked top management eight deviations below the industry norm. In 2005, this same organization received the coveted Malcolm Baldrige National Quality Award. This ten year turn-around changed the culture of Baptist. The actions management took and the lessons learned from other winners of this award will be scattered throughout Sections III and IV. A few examples of what they did include are: placing a greater emphasis on quality; taking cost out of the process, and improving efficiency; encouraging transparency in all information from the executive office; determining what to measure and managing what was measured; adopting best practices from within the healthcare field; and looking to other industries for examples. Lessons from Disney, Quint Studer, and Jim Collins will also be used to illustrate the human resources and leadership development strategies necessary to set the stage for moral courage (Collins, 2001; Lee, 2004; Studer, 2008).

Organizational Ethical Codes of Conduct

The value of these codes is a topic for debate. Codes are statements of organizational norms against which an actual or proposed action is evaluated, standards to which an action must conform, or values/principles we are asked to follow. On the positive side, codes of conduct can make behavioral expectations clear by establishing consistent standards and showing an accountable image to the community. If enforced, the code could strengthen ethical conduct, deter moral misconduct, and reduce organizational risk of liability (Schwartz, 2002). Such guidelines reduce an organization's criminal liability for misconduct if an ethics program is in place.

However, research has found no correlation between these programs and a decline in illegal conduct. Most are too vague to be useful in guiding individuals in resolving day-to-day ethical dilemmas. Some are too long and focus more on legal issues of compliance than on ethical resolution of problems. As of today, no significant relationship exists between codes and actual conduct. Organizational ethical standards need to be integrated into the ethical climate. If not enforced, they are merely shelf decoration.

Compliance Programs

The amendment to the U.S. Sentencing Commission Guidelines (2004) said that organizations must not only be conscientiousness in identifying criminal conduct, but that they must promote an organizational culture that encourages ethical conduct and a commitment to compliance with the law. Incentives and sanctions are used to support compliance, as is ethics training for top personnel. Health-care organizations need to give the compliance officer the authority and resources to evaluate the ethics programs. Too often, this is delegated to a mid-level manager, and program evaluations are minimal. In some organizations, the compliance officer is now working hand in hand with organizational ethics committee. More on how such a committee can support an ethical culture is discussed in Chapter 17.

The University of Medicine and Dentistry of New Jersey created a code of conduct, entitled "Maintaining an Ethical and Compliant Environment: A Guide to University Hospital's Compliance Program and Code of Conduct" (2006). But like most codes I have examined, 90% focuses on compliance. An example of a code of conduct that is practical and utilizes organizational values can be seen in the "Code of Mutual Respect," designed by a group of physicians and nurses at Summit Healthcare in Pennsylvania (See Exhibit 12.1).

Creating a Moral Organizational Climate

Does an organization's commitment to an ethical culture make a difference? Trevino and Weaver (2003) found the following:

Employees who view their organization as supporting fair and ethical conduct and its leadership as caring about ethical issues observe less unethical behavior and perform better along a range of dimensions; they are more willing to share information and knowledge and "go the extra mile" in meeting job requirements.

When employers show concern for employees, employees show concern for customers. When employees experience justice, they feel respected and their loyalty increases. This leads to the retention of ethical employees, which, in turn, leads to a culture in which ethical conduct is the norm.

Zimbardo (2006) discusses organizational designs for the support of evil and strategies to support a virtuous environment. He says "evil is intentionally behaving or causing others to act in ways that demean, dehumanize, harm, destroy or kill innocent people" (p. 129). He suggests it is not only the blind obedience to authority seen in Milgram (1974) studies, in which 67% of research participants went all the way to the highest shock level of 450 volts to help another person learn appropriate behaviors. By changing one variable, such as the introduction of peer modeling (obedience to authority or rebellion against authority), he demonstrates the importance of situational differences and peer pressure. If you want people to act ethically, you need to provide role models who refuse to engage in evil. The rescuers of the Holocaust survivors discussed in Chapter 1 come to

12.1 Summit Health's Code of Mutual Respect

At Summit Health we believe in open respectful communication with our patients and within the health care team. We demonstrate this belief through conduct that reflects our core values of integrity, compassion, excellence, and service.

Integrity

- I treat all members of the health care team with dignity and compassion.
- I remain appropriate in pressure situations recognizing that body language and tone of voice are important.
- I discuss internal issues with the right person at the appropriate place and time.

Compassion

- I value all members of the health care team.
- I demonstrate respect, open communication, and constructive feedback.
- I listen and then respond appropriately.

Excellence

- I continue to learn, teach, and seek new knowledge.
- I have a sense of ownership in the workplace environment.
- I strive to maintain personal well-being and balance.

Service

- I take concerns seriously and seek understanding, resolution, and learning.
- I support team members in their professional endeavors.
- I embrace the diversity of our health care team and community.

Adapted with permission of Summit Health. (2008) Copyright by Summit Health.

mind. The organizational culture needs to support healthcare professionals who say no to inflicting painful interventions on dying patients and support managers in saying no to kickbacks in contracts from a vendor. Zimbardo created the following 11 steps for supporting a virtuous climate (pp. 156–157).

1. Openly acknowledge errors in judgment.

2. Encourage mindfulness by focusing on the situation and ethical implications before acting.

3. Promote a sense of responsibility and accountability for all one's actions.

4. Do not allow minor transgressions, such as bullying, lying, or gossiping.

5. Distinguish between just and unjust authority; do not tolerate obedience to authority in unethical actions.

6. Support critical thinking; evaluate credibility of evidence and moral justification.

7. Reward moral behavior with public recognition.

8. Respect human diversity to reduce in-group biases and prejudices.

9. Change social conditions that promote anonymity; make people feel special to reinforce self-worth.

10. Challenge pressures for conformity to support people maintaining their moral compass.

11. Refuse to sacrifice crucial freedoms for elusive promises of security; verbal dissent is needed.

Zimbardo uses other examples, like Abu Ghraib Prison and suicide bombers, to illustrate circumstances in which situational forces overwhelmed an individual's dispositional tendency. An anonymous quotation comes to mind—"Evil prevails when good people fail to act, but we rarely hold good people responsible for evil." Sensitivity to the situational determinants of behavior, such as force of group pressure, social modeling, and authoritarian directives, aid us to see the importance of having an organizational culture that consistently supports moral actions and consistently condemns violations of ethical codes of conduct. Zimbardo's 11-step plan provides a framework for creating an ethical organizational culture, one that supports considering ethical implications before acting, rewards moral behavior, and allows verbal dissent. If employees are not provided with role modeled ethical behavior and if there is no internal fair means to resolve ethical and/or legal disputes, then employees have no choice but to leave or become whistleblowers.

Whistleblowing Is an Act of Moral Courage

There are numerous definitions of whistleblowing in the healthcare and business literature, but all point to the importance of advocacy—the need to protect the whistleblower from harm. Whistleblowing is an effort by a member or former member of an organization to release a warning to the public about a serious wrongdoing or danger created or hidden by the organization (Ahern & McDonald, 2002; Bolsin, Faunce, & Oakley, 2004; Davis & Konishi, 2007; Dougherty, 1995). My definition is consistent with differentiating between reporting the problem within the organization and whistleblowing the problem to some external agency (Fletcher, Sorrell, & Silva, 1998; Sellin, 1995). Whistleblowing is the action taken by a healthcare professional or manager who goes outside the organization to protect the public's best interest when the organization is indifferent to the exposure of the danger through the proper organizational channels. Reporting is the action taken by an individual inside the channels of the organization to correct a dangerous situation. Examples of reporting include disclosures of errors, incident reports, and verbal reporting to frontline managers of illegal or unethical actions (Firtko & Jackson, 2005).

Based on these definitions, one can see that whistleblowing results from a failure of the ethical culture of the organization to address its accountability for the safety and welfare of the patients and/or employees. The healthcare professional feels compelled to take a stand against wrongdoing in the organization.

Davis (2003) summarizes the standards theory and explains when whistleblowing is morally required for the greatest good of society:

1. The organization to which the would-be whistleblower belongs will, through its product or policy, do serious and considerable harm to the public (whether to users of its product, innocent bystanders, or the public at large);

2. The would-be whistleblower has identified the threat of harm, reported it to her immediate supervisor, made clear the nature of the threat and the objection to it, and concluded that the superior will do nothing effective;

3. The would-be whistleblower has exhausted all internal procedures within the organization. Any further action would present a danger to herself and others.

4. The would-be whistleblower has accessible evidence that would convince a reasonable, impartial observer that her view of the threat is correct; and

5. The would-be whistleblower has good reason to believe that revealing the threat will probably prevent the harm at reasonable cost (all things considered) (pp. 89–90).

Sometimes, the threat to the safety or health of patients is so immediate that going through all the layers of a hierarchical structure could cost patient lives. If the immediate supervisor is the cause of the problem, the healthcare professional has no option but to leap up a level in the organization. Unfortunately, this failure to follow the proper chain of command could become the focus of retaliation, thereby diverting attention from the identified ethical issue. If the blindness to the danger extends to the next level in the hierarchy, the individual's loyalty to the organization must end. Whistleblowing challenges the amoral view of the organization; it says the healthcare professionals were unable to resolve the ethical concerns internally (Grant, 2002).

Whistleblowers are generally seen as brave individuals, who take a stand against the unethical practices of an organization. Whether in business or health-care, the cases are similar to the examinations of 64 whistleblowers in *The Whistle-blowers: Exposing Corruption in Government and Industry* (Glazer & Glazer, 1991). They are parallel to *The Insider* (Mann, 1999), which depicts the tactics of the tobacco industry to hide the addictiveness of its product.

Iliffe (2002) sees whistleblowing as a mandatory, rather than a selected behavior. From her perspective, whistleblowers must choose to articulate a stance or remain silent about an injustice. In such instances, the situation and the virtue of courage collide. Some choose to sustain the standards they perceive as personal and/or professional. They are not average performers; they are above-average performers who are dedicated to the organization, but have strong convictions grounded in moral principles (Grant, 2002).

Understanding the public character of whistleblowing is vital to valuing the risks connected with the action. Whistleblowing requires moral courage. I am not interested in lecturing to malcontents who file frivolous lawsuits or draw attention to themselves in public media. These individuals demoralize those courageous healthcare professionals who jeopardize so much to honor their codes of conduct.

The list of negative consequences seems endless. It includes broken assurances to correct the problem, disappointment, isolation, dishonor, formation of an "antiyou" group, and loss of job. Sometimes individuals resort to questioning the whistleblower's mental health and character, resulting in formal reprimands and finally in difficult court proceedings (Ahern & McDonald, 2002; Brodie, 1998; Fletcher et al., 1998; Wilmot, 2000).

In the end, the healthcare professional needs to ask, "Am I comfortable with this decision?" Some questions can further assist the person in making a decision (MacDonald, 2001). This individual might not be "comfortable" because situations requiring the virtues of integrity and courage are often difficult, but the healthcare professional or manager needs to raise subsequent questions to determine if, in the long term, they can live with themselves without guilt and a loss of integrity.

Questions to ask oneself could include:

1. If I carry out this decision, would I be comfortable telling my family about it?

2. Would I want my children to take my behavior as an example?

3. Is this decision one that a wise, informed, and virtuous person would make?

4. Can I live with my decision?

These questions are designed to help healthcare professionals, managers, and executives critically reflect on the ethical decisions they confront. Whistleblowing can be avoided if the culture of the organization supports moral actions.

Conclusion

The organizational culture either drives an ethical climate, where moral courage to "do the right thing" is not needed, or it drives an unsafe and unsatisfying healthcare environment through a series of conscious and unconscious strategies and tactics. Rest (1984) guides us in conceptualizing a moral culture, while the ACHE Code of Ethics (2007) gives us more specifics on the role of the executive in creating an ethical environment for patients, employees, and the public. One assessment was presented to help begin this journey: the Organizational Courage Assessment. Although often overlap exists between compliance programs and codes of conduct, an easily remembered code may help organization move toward mutual respect among all members. Zimbardo's (2006) 11-step plan to support a virtuous climate provides the stage needed to support moral courage. Without the framework of Rest, ACHE, and Zimbardo, the organization lays itself open to having employees use whistleblowing to solve the ethical and legal problems they encounter. Davis (2003) clearly outlines when this is necessary, but it is only required if the internal reporting systems in the culture fails to support resolution of the problem. Sections III and IV outline the ingredients needed to create a moral culture, based on what has worked in organizations that are nationally recognized as moral cultures.

Key Points to Remember

1. The phrase organizational culture refers to the personality of the organization. Organizational culture is a set of beliefs and values which, over time, are validated by the organization and transformed into shared underlying assumptions about the organization.

2. Healthcare organizations need to create a moral culture that supports accountability, patient safety, and quality patient care.

3. The organiganizational courage assessment points out the differences among the four types of organizations: courageous, quantum, fearful, and bureaucratic.

4. Ethical codes of conduct are statements of organizational norms against which an actual or proposed action is evaluated, standards to which action must conform, or values/principles we are asked to follow.

5. Organizations must not only be conscientious in identifying criminal conduct, but they must promote an organizational culture that encourages ethical conduct and a commitment to compliance with the law.

6. Whistleblowing is an act of moral courage. It results from a failure of the ethical culture of the organization to address its accountability for the safety and welfare of the patients and/or employees.

References

Ahern, K.M., & MacDonald, S. (2002). The beliefs of nurses who were involved in a whistleblowing event. *Journal of Advanced Nursing, 38*(3), 303–309.

American College of Healthcare Executives Code of Ethics. (2007). Retrieved July 15, 2008, from http://www.ache.org/abt_ache/code.cfm

Bolsin, S., Faunce, T., & Oakley, J. (2005). Practical virtue ethics: Healthcare whistleblowing and portable digital technology. *Journal of Medical Ethics, 31*(1), 612–618.

Brodie, P. (1998). Ethics. Whistleblowing: A moral dilemma. *Plastic Surgical Nursing, 18*(1), 56–58.

Collins, J.C. (2005). *Good to great: Why some companies make the leap . . . and others don't.* New York: HarperCollins.

Davis, M. (2003). Some paradoxes of whistleblowing. In W.H. Shaw (Ed.), *Ethics at work* (pp. 85–99). New York: Oxford University Press.

Davis, A.J., & Konishi, E. (2007). Whistleblowing in Japan. *Nursing Ethics, 4*(2), 194–200.

Dougherty, C.J. (1995). Whistleblowing in health care. In W. T. Reich (Ed.), *Encyclopedia of Bioethics* (Rev. ed.). New York: Simon & Schuster Macmillan.

Firtko, A.J., & Jackson, D. (2005). Do the ends justify the means? Nursing and the dilemma of whistleblowing. *Australian Journal of Advanced Nursing, 23*(1), 51–57.

Fletcher, J.J., Sorrell, J.M., & Silva, M.C. (1998). Whistleblowing as a failure of organizational ethics. *The Online Journal of Issues in Nursing. 3*(3). Retrieved January 27, 2008, from http://www.nursingworld.org/MainMenuCategories/ANAMarketplace/ANAPeriodicals/ OJIN/TableofContents/Vol31998/No3Vol31998/Whistleblowing.aspx

Glazer, M.P. & Glazer, P.M. (1991). *The whistleblowers: Exposing corruption in government and industry.* New York: Basic Books.

Grant, C. (2002).Whistle blowers: Saints of secular culture. *Journal of Business Ethics, 39,* 391–399.

Iliffe, J. (2002). Whistleblowing: A difficult decision. *Australian Nursing Journal. 9*(7),1.

Kidder, R.M. (2005). *Moral courage.* New York: HarperCollins.

Kilmann, R.H., O'Hara, L.A., & Strauss, J.P. (2004). *Organizational courage assessment.* Retrieved July 15, 2008, from http://www.kilmann.com/courage.html

Lee, F. (2004). *If Disney ran your hospital: 9 1/2 things you would do differently.* Bozeman, MT: Second River Healthcare Press.

MacDonald, D. (2002). *A guide to moral decision making.* Retrieved January 27, 2008, from http:// www.ethicsweb.ca/guide/

Mann, M. (Director). (1999). *The Insider* [Motion picture]. Touchstone Pictures.

McDaniel, C. (1997). Development and psychometric properties of the Ethics Environment Questionnaire. *Medical Care, 35*(9), 901–914.

Milgram, S. (1974). *Obedience to authority.* New York: HarperCollins.

Rest, J. (1984). The major components of morality. In W. M. Kurtines & J.L. Gewirtz (Eds.), *Morality, moral behavior, and moral development* (pp. 24–38). Hoboken, NJ: John Wiley and Sons.

Samuel, M. (2006). *Creating the accountable organization: A practical guide to improve perfor mance execution.* Katonah, NY: Xephor Press.

Schwartz, M.S. (2002). A code of ethics for a corporate code of ethics. *Journal of Business Ethics, 41,* 1–2.

Sellin, S.C. (1995). Out on a limb: A qualitative study of patient advocacy in institutional nursing. *Nursing Ethics, 2*(1), 19–29.

Stubblefield, A. (2005). *The Baptist healthcare: Journey to excellence.* Hoboken, NJ: John Wiley and Sons.

Studer, Q. (2008). *Results that last: Hardwiring behaviors that will take your company to the top.* Hoboken, NJ: John Wiley & Sons.

Summit Health. (2008). *Code of mutual respect.* Chambersburg, PA: Summit Health.

Trevino, L.K., & Weaver, G.R. (2003). *Managing ethics in business organizations.* Palo Alto, CA: Stanford University Press.

U.S. Sentencing Commission Guidelines. (2006). Chapter eight, *Sentencing of organizations,* Section 8B2.1, as amended November 1, 2004. Retrieved August 5, 2008, from http:// www .ussc.gov/2006guid/APPC2006.pdf

University of Medicine and Dentistry of New Jersey. (2004). *Maintaining an ethical and compliant environment: A guide to University Hospital's compliance program and code of conduct.* Retrieved August 5, 2008, from http://www.umdnj.edu/uhcomweb/pdf/Code_of_Conduct .pdf

Wilmot, S. (2000). Nurses and whistleblowing: The ethical issues. *Journal of Advanced Nursing, 32*(5), 1051–1057.

Zimbardo, P.G. (2006). Psychology of power: To the person? To the situation? To the system? In D.L. Rhode (Ed.), *Moral leadership* (pp. 129–158). San Francisco, CA: Jossey-Bass.

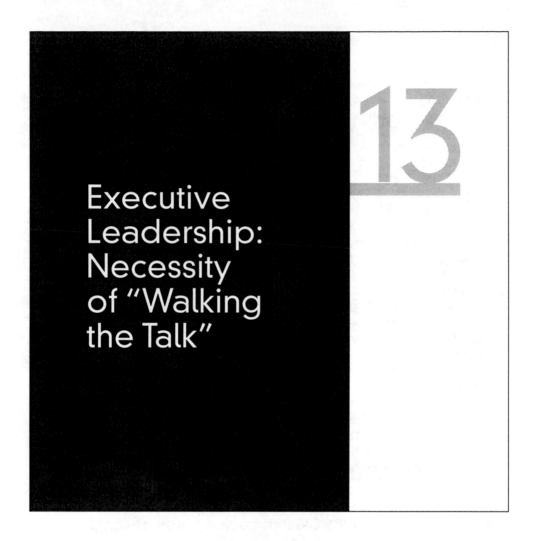

Executive Leadership: Necessity of "Walking the Talk"

Servant-leadership is more than a concept, it is a fact. Any great leader, by which I also mean an ethical leader of any group, will see herself or himself as a servant of that group and will act accordingly.
—M. Scott Peck, psychiatrist and spiritual writer

Defining Moral Leadership

There is a lack of research and consensus on the definition of moral leadership. In fact, a wide-ranging review of leadership publications reveals that two-thirds do not even define the term leadership (Yost & Plunkett, 2009). We often do not define words because we believe we know the meaning. The Old English definition for leadership is "to lead" or "to guide" or "to show the way." Today's definition focuses on the reality that leadership is about having reciprocal relationships with your followers.

The adjective "moral" in moral leadership derives from the Latin word for morality or *mores,* which refers to character, custom, and habit. To be moral is to be ethical. The term value-driven, or authentic leadership, indicates the importance of reaching decisions based on principles outside of oneself or to focus on the importance of acting with integrity (George, 2004).

The concept of value-driven leadership has been periodically watered down since Peters and Waterman's (1982) initial focus on the moral dimensions of leadership. They believed that the main role of executives is to manage an organization's values by articulating an inspiring vision of excellence, service, and integrity. Regrettably, in the 1990s, this perspective was diluted by the addition of other tasks, such as teamwork and customer satisfaction. It is time to end the fortune-cookie homilies included in some leadership and management books. Instead, the focus should be on the importance of the character of the individual who is leading the organization and the need to align organizational practice with principles. Rest (1994) provides a model for ethical decision making. A case illustrating moral leadership will begin this discussion; other examples will be presented as well.

George (2004) frankly describes his experiences as chair and CEO of Medtronic, a medical technology producer. He argues that we need new and authentic business leaders. He outlines five essential dimensions of "authentic" leaders, including purpose, values, heart, relationships, and self-discipline. Moral leaders have a sense of purpose in their vision and values; they will not compromise them because they have self-discipline. Authentic leaders are guided by heart, passion, and compassion, as well as by analytical qualities of the mind. Leaders are under a microscope, as they are constantly being observed and critiqued by employees and outsiders. To have successful relationships with their followers, leaders need to be consistent and not let stress affect their judgment. People follow authentic leaders because they know where those leaders stand. The following case is an example of authentic leadership in a very difficult situation.

Moral Leadership in the Case of Legionnaires' Disease

Case 13.1

It began in July 1995 with a conversation between a pulmonary physician and the Chief Executive Officer (CEO), Mr. Norm Epstein, about some very sick patients in the ICU who remained undiagnosed. Within 48 hours, the Department of Health and the Center for Disease Control were on site. As they investigated, the probable cause was uncovered: *Legionella pneumophila* in the hospital cooling towers. This bacteria produces a pneumonia, commonly called Legionnaires' disease, because it was first identified in July 1976 when an outbreak occurred among people attending an American Legion convention in Philadelphia.

Now the organizational leader had to decide whether to go public with the fact that the hospital was the source of the infection or to remain silent about the origin of the bacteria. Advice from attorneys guided him in the direction of silence. However, as Mr. Epstein states, "we had to take responsibility and be honest with the community and our employees, because this was the right thing to do." He was aware of the short-term consequences on the organization, such as patients staying away and employees not coming to work. The news conference that followed was difficult because, as Mr. Epstein acknowledged, "people died on my watch." But as he also says, "the organization that is moral has to take responsibility to acknowledge an error that causes harm to people who trusted that the organization would do them no harm."

"This was the hardest thing to deal with in my career, up to this point" he states, "but dealing with crisis adds to the moral character of the person and because as the CEO I represent the organization, it adds to the moral character of the organization." When asked about lessons learned, he said "get the facts first, get the best advice from multiple sources that you can trust, and keep people informed with honest information." When asked if, in retrospect, he would do anything differently in this demonstration of moral courage, he said "no, I did not see my actions as courageous; I was raised to do the right thing and to take responsibility and that is what I did. Just like I have a responsibility for my behavior, as a CEO I have responsibility for the actions of the organization I lead to the community we serve" (Epstein, N., personal communication, August 21, 2008).

As this case illustrates, ethically neutral leadership is impossible (Treviño, Brown, & Hartman, 2003). All leadership is value driven, and effective, but sustained leadership requires a commitment to higher levels of principles, such as honesty, fairness, and social responsibility.

Leadership cannot seek an end that cannot be justified morally. This is why contemporary writers on leadership identify certain individuals, such as Hitler and Saddam Hussein, as rulers and not as leaders (Gardner, 1987; Safty, 2003). But even the 1991 U.S. Sentencing Commission Guidelines, or codes of conduct, are not enough to prevent the negative activities of Enron or the Allegheny Health, Education, and Research Foundation (AHERF).

Leaders in AHERF clearly violated many significant legal and ethical principles. Its filing papers for bankruptcy, they cited $1.3 billion in debt owed to 65,000 creditors, making this the largest healthcare bankruptcy (Stevens, Rosenberg, & Burns, 2006). This bankruptcy was the result of many internal and external factors, but only the internal ethical issues will be addressed here. "AHERF had many internal problems, such as weak governance structure, the lack of board member involvement, unethical management and, lastly, their domineering CEO Sherif Abdelhak" (Smailagic, 2006). The lack of oversight by the Board, executives, and even external stakeholders (government and grant funders) suggests a significant lack of accountability at the highest levels. Clearly the CEO and executives dominated a Board that was inexperienced in its understanding of financial matters (Stevens et al., 2006). AHERF lacked internal regulation, as executives used restricted assets and charitable endowment funds for operating costs. The multiple conflicts of interests and unethical actions by executives led the state to charge three executives with multiple felonies and misdemeanors (Stevens et al., 2006). This classic case should make us all consider the consequences of unethical actions on healthcare organizations.

U.S. law and the practices of boards of directors have been far too slow in recognizing the potential conflicts of interest and incidental benefits inherent in gifts to board members' favorite charities (Berenbeim, 2002). Charles Le Maistre, president emeritus of the University of Texas M. D. Anderson Cancer Center, was a director on Enron Corporation board from 1985 to 2001; he was also chairman of Enron's Compensation Committee. His successor at M. D. Anderson Cancer Center, John Mendelsohn, joined the board in 1999 and left in 2001 (Enron Page, 2003). Between 1996 and 2002, Enron donated more than $600,000 to the M. D. Anderson Cancer Center (Berenbeim, 2002). Even if no wrongdoing occurred, the public perception is one of gifts and side deals rather than one of values-based leadership.

For the purpose of this book, moral leadership means leading an organization to accomplish its moral purpose while inspiring ethical conduct in its followers. The purpose could be excellent healthcare for the community or respect for self-determination in India. "Moral leadership entails exemplary conduct in attending to the rights and needs of others, even when it is inconvenient and extracts a personal cost" (Rhode, 2006, p. 90). It requires the ability to exercise control over one's choices and subsequent behaviors, as was seen in the Legionnaires' case. Moral leadership advocates the most basic of values—honesty, fairness, responsibility, and compassion. The Johnson & Johnson story below demonstrates how these values can be balanced while maintaining the organization's financial viability.

State of Perceived Business Ethics

Empirical evidence is mixed on the state of perceived business ethics. The Ethics Resource Center's (ERC) National Business Ethics Survey (2007) analyzed ethics in the workplace from the perspective of employees. Compared to similar ERC surveys from for-profits and government sectors, nonprofits have a somewhat higher standing—58% had a strong culture/strong-leaning culture compared to 52% in the for-profit sector and 50% the government sector. "Nonprofits are also stronger in the four components of ethical culture: ethical leadership, supervision reinforcement of ethics, peer commitment to ethics, and embedded ethical values" (National Business Ethics Survey, 2007, p. 1). The bad news is that misconduct in nonprofit organizations is at the highest level since the ERC began measuring in 2000. The percentage of employees observing one or more acts of misconduct rose from 49% in 2005 to 55% in 2006. The ERC Survey has found that fraud in nonprofits (e.g. alteration of documents and financial records, lying to external stakeholders and employees, and misrepresenting hours) has become more prevalent than in business or government. Nonprofit employees are the least positive about the future of ethics in their organizations when compared to business and government employees.

Furthermore, this same study yielded some disturbing results relevant to moral courage. Forty-one percent of nonprofit employees had failed to report safety violations and 55% failed to report misuse of confidential information. They remained silent because they believed that it would do no good (50%) or would not stay confidential (33%) or that they would suffer retaliation from management or coworkers (42%). What was different in organizations that addressed these concerns? The ERC (2007) survey revealed two important ingredients for reduction of ethics violation risks: (1) a well-implemented ethics and compliance program and (2) a strong ethical culture (p. 9). Ethical culture was discussed

13.1 Recommendations for Nonprofit Leaders and Boards of Directors

1. Make no assumptions—assesses your organization
2. Implement an ethics and compliance program with high-level oversight
3. Implement internal controls to prevent financial fraud
4. Grow your program and culture with your organization

National business ethics survey: An insider's view of private sector ethics. (2007). Arlington, VA: Ethics Resource Center, p. 26.

in Chapter 12, therefore the focus here is on reporting and on the elements of an ethics and compliance program.

Supervisors are the reporting method of choice for ethical and compliance violations. In addition, nonprofits use hotlines as a method of reporting ethics violations more often than businesses or governments. Four of the six elements of an ethics and compliance program are on the increase: (1) a hotline for reporting, (2) a code of conduct, (3) discipline for violators, and (4) ethics training. The two that have been on a steady decline are (1) evaluation of ethical behavior during performance appraisals and (2) a mechanism for ethics advice. Advice for both of these is included in Chapters 14 and 15. Exhibit 13.1 presents recommendations from this survey for nonprofit leaders and boards of directors.

While there is a paucity of research on whether ethics pays, only 4 out of 95 surveys found a purely negative relationship between financial performance and social performance (Margolis & Walsh, 2001). Companies with stated commitments to ethical behavior had a higher mean financial performance than companies lacking such commitments (Procario-Foley & Bean, 2002).

The penalty to an organization's reputation as a result of criminal or unethical conduct can be dramatic declines in market values for both nonprofit and for-profit organizations. The substantial cost is not just in fines or liability damage, but in the long-standing damage to the company's reputation. The way Johnson & Johnson leadership handled the Tylenol recall is an example of "putting the customer first and your positive reputation will follow."

Case 13.2

In 1982, James Burke, President of Johnson & Johnson, faced a corporate crisis of monumental proportions (Ettorre, 1996). Someone had tainted bottles of Johnson & Johnson's pain reliever Tylenol with cyanide. The cyanide-laced Tylenol killed seven people in the Chicago area. Rather than trying to cover up the story, Burke quickly put out the word across the media and even appeared on several television programs. He warned the public to avoid all Tylenol products until the company had more information about the tampering. Johnson & Johnson quickly recalled 31 million bottles of Tylenol. Within six weeks, Burke had devised a plan to institute tamper-proof packaging on all Tylenol products. Despite the fact that his decision cost the company as much as $150 million, its reputation for integrity was reinforced. Johnson & Johnson remains a well-respected company because management recognized that you cannot buy public confidence. You have to show that you will put safety above profits.

Moral Leadership: Personality and Social Influences

It might make us more comfortable to believe that personality is the prime predictor of ethical conduct—after all, it is more predictable than social influences. This is based on the psychological cognitive bias of humans called "fundamental attribution error" (Doris, 2002), which is our tendency to overvalue the importance of individual moral fiber and undervalue the situational causes that determine our behavior.

Another cognitive bias is cognitive dissonance (Harmon-Jones & Mills, 1999). Whenever our behavior and values are at odds with each other and threaten our positive image of ourselves, we experience dissonance or conflict. Fifty years of experimental research tells us that we resolve these conflicts by swinging our beliefs to match our conduct. Integrity does not help when all of this self-delusion is going on unconsciously. Some would call this rationalization. The possible moral problem for a leader is that a rationalizing employee might discount the harm of his or her conduct or the extent of his or her responsibility for it.

Add to this mix the fact that our judgments are profoundly affected by the people who surround us. If I am sitting next to you when an emergency bell goes off, and you do nothing, chances are that I will do nothing either. The presence of the other diffuses the sense of personal responsibility. If I am alone, I am more likely to respond (Latané & Nida, 1981). Apparently, the human mind takes its cues from the situation and from others in the situation. The mind processes these cues in conjunction with previous experiences. If you have no past experience to guide you, and everyone around you is acting as if a situation is acceptable, then you are likely to lose your moral compass and not even know it. This fact speaks to the importance of executive role modeling for managers in moral conduct. Social pressure affects conscience to a degree that most of us would not think (Lubban, 2000).

As a leader, it is also important to understand that people of different socioeconomic levels will look at issues of morality from different perspectives. Haidt, Koller, and Dias (1993) studied various levels of infractions in Philadelphia and Brazil. Participants in both cultures preferred to punish those who inflicted harm on others. However, for every violation studied, individuals in the lower socioeconomic strata had a greater sense of moral offense and were more inclined to punish. They were more prone to describe morality in terms of duties, obligations, and attending to the needs of others. This fact points to the importance of the issue of fairness for employees at the lower pay levels of an organization. Higher socioeconomic individuals define morality more in terms of freedoms and individual rights. For them, fair means the opportunity to individually pursue self-interests (e.g., physicians).

13.2 Mechanisms of Moral Disengagement

1. Perception of the reprehensible conduct (engaging in moral justification, making palliative comparisons and using euphemistic labeling)
2. Sense of detrimental effects of the conduct (minimizing, ignoring, or misconstruing the consequences)
3. Sense of responsibility for the link between reprehensible conduct and its detrimental effects (displacing or diffusing responsibility)
4. View of victims (dehumanizing or blaming them)

Bandura, A. (1990). Mechanisms of moral disengagement. In W. Reich (Ed.). *Origins of terrorism: Psychologies, ideologies, theologies, states of mind* (pp. 161–191). Cambridge, UK: Cambridge University Press.

Ethical self-deception is possible for all leaders, but all rational adults are still accountable for the choices they make. Moral leadership requires thoughtful reflection on values and principles, careful analysis of the situation, and navigation between convenience and principle. Leaders are pressured every day with competing demands from multiple players. They are called on to make decisions without a grounding in nonnegotiable principles, time carved out for self-reflection, and a willingness to receive honest feedback from trusted colleagues. Under such circumstances, it is easy to understand how a leader could rationalize actions.

What we want to avoid is the moral disengagement described by Bandura (1990). This model describes how a person, who usually has a high ethical standards, can end up behaving immorally. The model outlines four cognitive mechanisms that need to be altered for this to occur: (1) the individual's perception of his or her conduct, (2) detrimental effects of the conduct, (3) sense of responsibility, and (4) view of victims (see Exhibit 13.2). Leaders need to guard against the use of any of these cognitive mechanisms. For example, my experience is that these mechanisms are in play when the discussion turns to people who are uninsured or to cheating insurance companies.

Rest (1994) articulated four components of moral development when he examined ethical decision making (pp. 26–29). These four components will help us examine moral courage:

1. Moral awareness: recognition that situations raise ethical issues.
2. Moral reasoning: determining what course of action is ethically sound.
3. Moral intent: identifying which values should take priority.
4. Moral behavior: acting on ethical decisions.

Moral Awareness

Moral awareness of an ethical situation requires the ability to see the problem in an ethical context. This is affected first by the definition of an ethical problem and second by an individual's capacity for empathy or sensitivity to the stakeholders in the situation. For example, the massive closings of maternity services in this country could simply be seen as a prudent financial decision, particularly since the reimbursement rate is so low and it is next to impossible for obstetricians to make money. Organizations with this bottom-line mentality encourage individuals to become blind to the ethical implications of decisions, as did Enron. The company's nose dive from the nation's seventh largest corporation to bankruptcy is partially attributed to its ruthless motto of "profits at all costs" (Sims & Brinkmann, 2003, p. 247).

A hospital CEO may distance or devalue maternity services to the point where moral responsibility for closings was denied, as he did not identify with the group and was not motivated by altruistic action. However, a woman CEO, who had directly experienced this injustice, is more likely to be morally aware of the implications of this decision. Therefore, education should also build awareness of others' needs. Recently, a board of a community hospital evaluated the possibility of closing its maternity services for a second time. Although 18 units had already closed in the City of Philadelphia (George, 2008), the board voted to maintain the service because the members believed they had a moral responsibility to the women of the community.

Moral Reasoning

Moral reasoning is affected by an individual's ability and social context. Considerable evidence points to the fact that organizational reward systems can play a role in lowering the level of an organization's moral reasoning. If bonuses are tied to decisions that support only short-term actions, chances are the individual's moral reasoning will be affected.

The most recent examples of such short-term thinking are the collapse of the subprime housing market, the disintegration of Lehman Brothers, and the continued fall of the stock market. Lehman Brothers filed for Chapter 11 bankruptcy protection on September 15, 2008 (Mamudi, 2008). It is the largest bankruptcy filing in U.S. history, with Lehman holding more than $600 billion in assets. On December 28, 2008, the *New York Times* published five graphs that illustrated the financial crisis (Menna, p. 25). Sales tax collections, sales income tax withholding, the number of airline passengers, and the number of building permits all declined as unemployment rose to 8.7%. Market analysts complained about the lack of regulation by the Federal Reserve and the government. Too many business leaders have loss their moral compasses.

Kohlberg (1983) posits three primary stages of moral reasoning: (1) preconventional, (2) conventional, and (3) postconventional. The preconventional stage focuses on furthering self-interests and analyzes the situation in terms of right or wrong. At the conventional stage, the individual attempts to find a socially acceptable solution and to avoid disapproval. In the postconventional stage, the goal is to maintain self-respect and to judge the situation based on abstract principles that reflect universal concerns. In Chapter 15, all six stages of this model are given, along with the appropriate HR polices to reinforce each level of moral development.

However, this impartial view of morality has been challenged by Carol Gilligan, Nel Noddings, and others (Paley, 2006). These writers believe that morality should allow for a special interest in the welfare of specific others. They believe that the only way we can truly act ethically is when we are in a caring relationship with another. Only then will we truly know what is best for them. Many authors describe leadership in this relational context (Autry, 2004; Baker & O'Malley, 2008; George, 2004; Kouzes & Posner, 2002; Peters & Waterman, 1982; Stubblefield, 2005).

Moral Intent

Moral intent involves identifying what values should take priority in decision making. For those healthcare professionals at the patient's bedside, the focus is on the values of autonomy, beneficence, nonmaleficence, veracity, and fidelity. Successful executives realize that attention needs to be paid to the perpetual balancing of these values in complex business decisions. Executives must *understand* the power and influence dynamics in their organizations, *weigh* competing values, and *determine* where the zone of acceptability rests (Paine, 2003). Experienced executives know the importance of managing interdependent relationships, but at times they too will struggle with the effects of these relationships on ethical considerations. The small rural hospital needs two surgeons, but they hate each other. Both expect complete loyalty, and the CEO is left to balance these delicate egos to ensure care for his or her community. This skill was not taught in management school, but the executive who keeps an eye on the mission of the organization will more likely stay focused on the values important to its viability and success. Effective leadership requires the ability to examine not only the first-order consequences of such decisions, but the third- and fourth-order consequences on all stakeholders.

Moral Conduct

Moral conduct is the ability to follow through and act on your intentions. Do you have the confidence and a strong enough ego to resist situational pressures, such as a lack of time and obedience to authority? A famous experiment by Darly and Batson (1973) with seminary students addresses the influential variable of time. They concluded that a bystander's decision to assist a person in distress depending on whether they had sufficient time. With a production-oriented mentality competing with a patient safety and patient satisfaction mentality, lack of time is the battle cry of frontline staff. Moral leadership necessitates managing time and assuring that those who care for vulnerable patients have the time to make the correct moral decision.

Stanley Milgram's classic obedience-to-authority experiment gives us all pause. We could use Abu Ghraib Prison as an example in which a multitude of independent investigations determined that the soldiers in charge were indisputably normal, but lacked supervision. Leaders approved behavior patterns that encouraged abuse and humiliation of the detainees (Rhode, 2006, pp. 153–155). Are there examples of such blind obedience in healthcare facilities? The answer is yes. Examples of such obedience that can lead to patient safety errors include failing to take time-outs in surgery, taking medication instructions verbally (instead of in writing) without read back from an unknown physician or resident, or continuing to perform procedures on a dying patient as ordered by an attending physician.

Once individuals yield to group pressure in situations where the moral cost seems negligible, the desire to reduce cognitive dissonance ensnares the person in more serious misconduct. We get cooked just like the legendary frog, who does not notice that he is being boiled as the water slowly heats up. Your small alteration to the budget or failing to wash your hands just this once or your need to belong to this "in-group" can lead you down the path of misconduct.

We have four basic options when faced with immoral demands: (1) exhibit moral courage and deal with the consequences; (2) leave the organization; (3) follow orders and do what seems wrong; or (4) try to negotiate around the orders and find another way to resolve the issue. This fourth solution may be a compromise, but it may also be more effective for the patients. For example, rather than fire the verbally abusive chairman of surgery, it may be more constructive to look for solutions that the board, nursing staff, and chairman can accept. If an executive has a strong moral compass, he or she will know which option to pick. This fourth solution may require as much moral courage as the first. Let us look in-depth at stories illustrating strategies for moral leadership.

Strategies for Moral Leadership

Two stories will illustrate the importance of capturing people's hearts if you are to lead from a moral basis of leadership. One is from South Africa and one is from Baptist Healthcare.

Case 13.3

> Irene Charnley believed in Nelson Mandela's vision (Business Women's Association, 2003). The cornerstone of her leadership approach was the advancement of marginalized groups through employment, skill transference, and leadership development. Her conduct during and after apartheid as a successful executive speaks to the leadership skills one needs when using a business to advance social change, while ensuring value for shareholders. Charnley created a successful service in an environment of limited capital and talent, poor infrastructure, and a large population of poor people. This situation is similar to the work required in the educational or healthcare systems of poor urban poor neighborhoods. Charnley understood that powerful leaders could use their ideals to liberate the hearts of people. For her accomplishments, she was named as one of the world's most powerful women by *Fortune Magazine* (Business editors, 2001). She was also the subject of a three-part Harvard Business school case study on leadership (African Business Club at Harvard Business School, 2008).

At Baptist Healthcare, leaders know the power of stories to inspire people, reinforce the culture of the organization, and recognize champions (Stubblefield, 2005). When employees exceed customer expectations in providing excellent care, these employees are identified as *champions*—their stories are highlighted in board meetings, orientation sessions, leadership retreats, and leadership devel-

---

13.3 Hospital Went Beyond Call of Duty

On the morning of April 5, my wife suffered both respiratory failure and a heart attack.

She was rushed to Chestnut Hill Hospital and, in the emergency room, the doctors and nurses there were able to resuscitate her. They performed professionally, even heroically. My wife was then taken to the intensive care unit of the hospital where she remained in a coma for the next 13 days. My wife passed away on the evening of April 18, with her family and the medical staff of the ICU by her bedside.

I want your readers to know that all of the doctors and nurses, working in the ICU at the hospital, attended to my wife with the utmost professional and personal care for almost two weeks, caring for her in a manner that genuinely comforted my family. Our children were treated with warmth, sensitivity and kindness. All of our questions and concerns were addressed honestly and patiently. The ICU staff consistently went out of their way to make sure that we were comfortable and well informed about my wife's condition.

Obviously, it was a heartbreaking ordeal for my entire family. On many occasions, I told the ICU staff and Dr. Kenneth Patrick, my wife's physician, their thoughtful, professional and compassionate attention to my wife's physical needs, as well to the emotional needs of my family, enabled us to find enormous comfort, simply by being with her during the final days of her life. They helped us to remain comfortably close with my wife as she died with genuine dignity.

For their consummate professionalism, their personal dedication and their tireless attention to both my wife and our family, the staff of the Intensive Care Unit at Chestnut Hill Hospital has earned our utmost respect and admiration, as well as our deep and enduring gratitude.

Peter C. McVeigh, Oreland

McVeigh, P.C. (2008, July 24). Hospital went beyond call of duty. *Chestnut Hill Local*, p. 3. Reprinted with permission of *Chestnut Hill Local*.

---

opment education. Champions' stories are posted on communication boards and shared in employee forums. Thank you notes are sent to the homes of these champions. As a trustee for a community hospital, I recently noticed one such letter in our local paper. Such stories "As hospital goes beyond call of duty" remind leaders why they are healthcare executives (McVeigh, 2008) (see Exhibit 13.3).

Conclusion

Dedication to moral leadership requires the incorporation of ethical concerns into all organizational activities. This means incorporating moral considerations into planning, resource allocation, hiring, promotion, compensation, performance evaluations, communications, public relations, and philanthropic activities (Paine, 2003). Why is the commitment of leaders necessary for an ethical culture? Because they set the moral example through their behavior. Employees watch and take cues on expected ethical conduct from organization's leaders. Consistency between words and actions in the day-to-day interaction with managers sends a message about the importance of moral conduct. Hypocrisy will destroy safety and the moral climate. No code of conduct or corporate compliance program will mean anything if leaders play favorites, withhold information, or make it clear that bad news is not wanted. Ethical leaders promote transparency in all communication.

Moral leaders ask tough questions and are open to answering them. Because of the power differential between leaders and employees and the potential toward obedience, leaders also need to solicit differing perspectives and nonconforming views. Any employee, executive, or physician needs to have a safe place to report misconduct. If reporting channels are not seen as effective, the organization opens itself to whistle blowing.

Ethical misconduct, racism, and repetitive violation of patient safety goals are the results of the lack of crucial conversations between leaders and employees. Candid dialog within the organization on these subjects can only occur if leaders provide a safe environment for such discussions. Openly discussing values conflicts helps employees understand the complexities of leadership decisions involving moral responsibility.

Another strategy is to end the incentive for leaders to focus on short-term profits. Recently, in one for-profit hospital chain, the nurse managers were unable to hire new employees. They were told that the budget needed to "look good" to corporate officers at the end of the third quarter. This was the final straw for two managers, who decided to leave the organization.

Key Points to Remember

1. Moral leadership is defined as leading an organization to accomplish its moral purpose while inspiring ethical conduct in its followers.
2. Moral leaders have a sense of purpose in their vision and values; they will not compromise them because they have self-discipline.
3. Moral leadership cannot seek an end that cannot be justified morally.
4. "Moral leadership entails exemplary conduct in attending to the rights and needs of others, even when it is inconvenient and extracts a personal cost."
5. State of perceived business ethics—Misconduct in nonprofit organizations is at the highest level since the Ethics Resource Center (ERC) began measuring in 2000. Nonprofit employees are the least positive about the future of ethics in their organizations when compared to business and government employees.
6. ERC reports that 41% of nonprofit employees failed to report safety violations and 55% failed to report misuse of confidential information.
7. An ERC (2007) survey revealed two important ingredients for reduction of ethics violation risk: (1) a well-implemented ethics and compliance program and (2) a strong ethical culture.
8. ERC states that four of the six elements of an ethics and compliance program are on the increase—hotline for reporting, code of conduct, discipline for violators, and ethics training.

9. Companies with stated commitments to ethical behavior had a higher mean financial performance than companies lacking such commitments.

10. "Fundamental attribution error" is our tendency to overvalue the importance of individual moral fiber and undervalue the situational causes that determine our behavior.

11. Fifty years of experimental research teaches us that we resolve the conflict between our beliefs and behavior by swinging our beliefs to match our conduct.

12. Once individuals yield to group pressure to resolve conflicts in which the moral cost seems negligible, the desire to reduce cognitive dissonance ensnares the person in more serious misconduct.

13. The presence of another person diffuses our sense of personal responsibility. If I am alone, I am more likely to respond to an emergency situation.

14. *Moral awareness* of an ethical situation requires the ability to see the problem in an ethical context.

15. *Moral reasoning* is affected by an individual's ability and social context.

16. *Moral intent* involves identifying what values should take priority in decision making.

17. Executives must *understand* the power and influence dynamics in their organizations, *weigh* competing values, and *determine* where the zone of acceptability rests.

References

African Business Club at Harvard. (February 15, 2008). Retrieved August 9, 2008, from http://www.hbsafricaconference.com/custpage.cfm/frm/13148/sec_id/13148

Autry, J.A. (2004). The servant leader: *How to build a creative team, develop great morale, and improve bottom line performance.* New York: Crown.

Baker, W.F., & O'Malley, M. (2008). *Leading with kindness: How good people consistently get superior results.* New York: AMACOM.

Bandura, A. (1990). Mechanisms of moral disengagement. In W. Reich (Ed.). *Origins of terrorism: Psychologies, ideologies, theologies, states of mind* (pp. 161–191). Cambridge, UK: Cambridge University Press.

Berenbeim, R.E. (February, 2002). The Enron ethics breakdown. *The Conference Board, 15,* 1–6. Retrieved August 9, 2008, from http://www.infoedge.com/samples/CB-EA15free.pdf

Business Editors (October 1, 2001). Carly Fiorina tops FORTUNE's list of 50 most powerful women in business for fourth year. *Fortune Magazine,* 1–12. Retrieved August 9, 2008, from http://www.allbusiness.com/population-demographics/demographic-groups/6177054-1.html

Business Women's Association. (December 19, 2003). *SA's most powerful businesswoman.* Retrieved August 9, 2008, from http://www.bwasa.co.za/Research/SAsMostPowerfulBusinesswomen/Top20Businesswomen/tabid/5348/Default.aspx#charnley

Darly, J.M., & Batson, C.D. (1973). From Jerusalem to Jericho: A study of situational and dispositional variables in helping behavior. *Journal of Personality and Social Psychology, 27*(1), 100–108.

Doris, J.M. (2002). *Lack of character: Personal and moral behavior.* Cambridge, UK: Cambridge University Press.

Enron Page. Retrieved August 9, 2008, from http://www.smokershistory.com/Enron.htm

Ettorre, B. (1996). James Burke: The fine art of leadership. *Management Review, 85*(10), 13–16.

Gardner, J. (1987). *The moral aspect of leadership.* Washington, DC: Independent Sector.

George, J. (April 4, 2008). Delivery of aid for OB Units. *Philadelphia Business Journal.* Retrieved August 9, 2008, from http://www.momobile.org/DeliveryofAidforOBUnits.html.

George, B. (2004). *Authentic leadership: Rediscovering the secrets to creating lasting value.* San Francisco, CA: Jossey-Bass.

Haidt, J., Koller, S., & Dias, M. (1993). Affect, culture and morality, or is it wrong to eat your dog? *Journal of Personality and Social Psychology, 65,* 613–628.

Harmon-Jones, E., & Mills J. (1999). *Cognitive dissonance: Progress on a pivotal theory in social psychology.* Washington, DC: American Psychological Association.

National Nonprofit Ethics Survey. (2007). Arlington, VA: Ethics Resource Center. Retrieved August 9, 2008, from http://www.ethics.org/research/nbes.asp.

Kohlberg, L. (1983). *Moral stages: A current formulation and a response to critics.* New York: Karger.

Kouzes, J.M., & Posner, B.Z. (2002). *Leadership challenge* (3rd ed.). San Francisco, CA: Jossey-Bass.

Latané, B., & Nida, S. (1981). Ten years of research on group size and helping. *Psychological Bulletin, 89*(2), 308–324.

Luban, D. (2000). The ethics of wrongful obedience. In D.L. Rhode (Ed.), *Ethics in practice: Lawyers role, responsibilities and regulation* (pp. 95–97, 102–105). New York: Oxford University Press.

Mamudi, S. (September 15, 2008). *Lehman folds with record $613 billion debt.* Retrieved December 30, 2008, form http://www.marketwatch.com/news/story/story.aspx?guid={2FE5AC05-597A-4E71-A2D5-9B9FCC290520}&siteid=rss

McVeigh, P.C. (2008, July 24). Hospital went beyond call of duty. *Chestnut Hill Local,* p. 3.

Menna, M. (December 28, 2008). A pinch becomes a squeeze. *New York Times,* p. 25.

Margolis, J.M., & Walsh, J.P. (2001). *People and profits? The search for a link between a company's social and financial performance.* Mahwah, NJ: Lawrence Erlbaum.

National business ethics survey: An insider's view of private sector ethics. (2007). Arlington, VA: Ethics Resource Center, 1–48.

Paine, L.S. (2003). *Value shift: Why companies must merge social and financial imperatives to achieve superior performance.* New York: McGraw-Hill.

Paley, J. (2006). Past caring. The limitations of one-one-ethics. In A.J. Davis, V. Tschudin, & L. de Raeve (Eds.), *Essentials of teaching and learning in nursing ethics* (pp. 149–164). New York: Elsevier.

Peters, T.H., & Waterman, R.P. (1982). *In search of excellence: Lessons from America's best-run companies.* New York: HarperCollins.

Procario-Foley. E.G., & Bean, D.F. (2002). Institutions of higher education: Cornerstones in building ethical organizations. *Teaching Business Ethics, 6*(1), 101–102.

Rest, J. (Ed.) (1994). *Moral development: Advances in research and theory.* New York: Praeger.

Rhode, D.L. (Ed.) (2006). *Moral leadership: The theory and practice of power, judgment and policy.* San Francisco, CA: Jossey-Bass.

Rost, J.C. (1991). *Leadership for the twenty-first century.* New York: Prager.

Safty, A. (2003). Moral leadership: Beyond management and governance. *Harvard International Review, 25*(3), 84–85.

Sims, R.R., & Brinkmann, J. (2003). Enron ethics (or culture matters more than codes). *Journal of Business Ethics, 45*(243), 247.

Smailagic, G. (2006). *Analysis of the bankruptcy of the Allegheny Health, Education, and Research Foundation (AHERF).* Retrieved December 30, 2008, from http://www.contrib.andrew.cmu.edu/~gsmailag/portfolio/healthcare%20paper.pdf

Stevens, R.A., Rosenberg, C.E., & Burns, L.R. (Eds.) (2006). *History and health policy in United States.* New Brunswick, NJ: Rutgers University Press.

Stubblefield, A. (2005). *The Baptist Healthcare: Journey to excellence.* Hoboken, NJ: John Wiley and Sons.

Treviño, L.G., Brown, M., & Hartman, L.P. (2003). A qualitative investigation of perceived ethical executive leadership: Perceptions from inside and outside the executive suite. *Human Relations, 56*(1), 23–26.

Yost, P.R., & Plunkett, M.M. (2009). *Real time leadership development.* Hoboken, NJ: John Wiley and Sons.

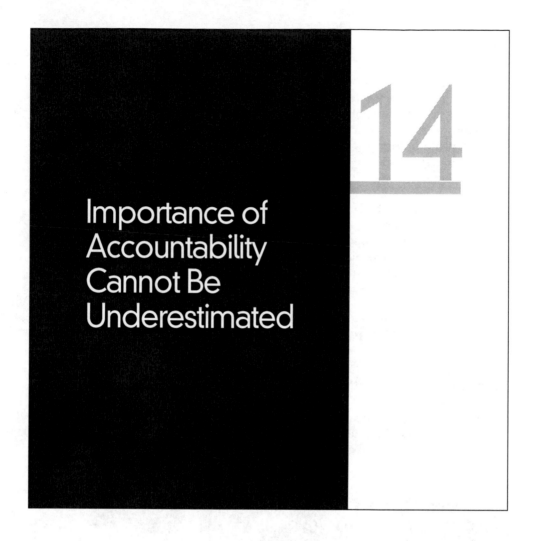

14

Importance of Accountability Cannot Be Underestimated

Whereas most organizations hide problems and keep unresolved conflicts underground, accountable organizations have the courage and processes to address issues.

—Mark Samuel, author and consultant

Personal accountability is the willingness to be responsible for the consequences of one's actions. Without this value, you will not be considered reliable, dependable, or trustworthy. All of these characteristics coexist in a person of integrity. Without the motivation to follow through on your promises or obligations, your word will not be viewed as honorable. Moral individuals believe they have a responsibility to tell the truth (veracity) and to keep promises (fidelity). Without these basic interpersonal behaviors, relationships have no foundation on which to develop.

Developing an accountable organization requires the moral courage to have many crucial conversations. Managers must role model this courage by questioning the effects of executive decisions on operations. Leaders need to create safe environments for these conversations by providing clear direction, timely decisions, coaching to improve performance and, when necessary, firing people. If they do not, the organizational environment will be ensnarled in victimization, conflict, and power plays. Employees feel like victims when they waste time on meaningless paperwork, are required to redo work because someone failed to think, wait for approval of a decision, or recover from the latest verbal abuse. When leadership fails to stand up and hold people accountable, employees respond in kind.

This chapter centers on the principles, steps, and processes that exist in organizations that take accountability seriously. Equal emphasis will be placed on the crucial conversations necessary for employees to buy into the new culture, the importance of continuous efforts to resolve conflicts, and the need to always strive to improve performance. The goal is an overview of how to create a culture in which people at all organizational levels can be depended on to meet their professional obligations.

Entitlement to Organizational Accountability

In Samuel's (2006) five-step model, there is an increasing breadth of accountability across the organization (see Exhibit 14.1). Level one is entitlement, a level at which workers are paid regardless of their performance. There are no expectations for performance and effort. Performance depends on whether it is convenient. When she finishes her personal phone call, the receptionist will look up from her computer to greet the next patient at the registration desk.

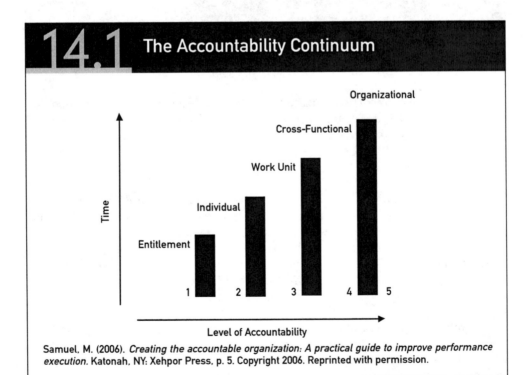

14.1   The Accountability Continuum

Samuel, M. (2006). *Creating the accountable organization: A practical guide to improve performance execution.* Katonah, NY: Xehpor Press, p. 5. Copyright 2006. Reprinted with permission.

Level two is individual accountability. Here, individuals complete their own assignments, but without regard for team priorities. Because you cannot count on others to coordinate efforts, time is wasted and resources are not used wisely. The nurse's aid may fulfill her job expectations and get the patient out of bed, but the physical therapy department may actually need the patient in bed for exercises. High resistance to changing unit routines arises because every person views his or her tasks in isolation.

Level three is work unit accountability. The emergency room team may be a well-oiled machine, but it is not working effectively with critical care units in co-ordinating patient transfers. This often leads to a "we-they" attitude. Silos occur throughout the organization making it difficult for work units to communicate and coordinate activities.

Level four is cross-functional accountability. Operational effectiveness is significantly improved when outcomes are the focus. Getting the patient transferred from the ER to the ICU in a timely manner is the outcome desired. However, conflicts can still occur between levels in the organization.

Level five is organizational accountability. This is a fluid organization with everyone focused on the desired outcome. As a result, any individual can step in, take charge, and direct the process. High involvement of executives, middle management, and staff is the norm.

Increasing Organizational Accountability

Three principles guide an organization's efforts to move toward higher and higher levels of accountability. Samuel (2006) suggests that it takes six months to a year to achieve each level of accountability. Of course, organizations can move more quickly in a crisis situation. Therefore, *principle one* is that accountability increases one level at a time.

Principle two focuses on simultaneously increasing performance expectations and the level of accountability. If the present focus is on improving accountability in work units, then the organization needs to reward work units, not individuals. If the goal is functional unit coordination (level 4), you create quality improvement teams from the different units. To construct teams focused on outcomes, it is necessary to communicate, coordinate, and cooperate.

The *third principle* is not immediately obvious—the farther removed an individual is from the organization's current level of accountability, the greater the pressure will be for that person to leave the organization. For example, when you want to increase the level of team accountability in radiology, you hire new employees and focus on team standards to improve turn-around time. Most employees get on board, but those who are unable to improve efficiency and collaborate with others may choose or be asked to leave the organization. Some employees are not able to reach the new level of team accountability, which demands a higher level of cooperation and communication. Low morale and performance are the results of low accountability (level 1), but another result is the loss of frustrated top performers who accepted individual accountability (level 2). If "new hires" enter an organization at a level of individual accountability (level 2) that does not match their own, they will become a turnover statistic. It is equally true that if the level of required accountability is cross-functional (level 4) and the individual is only at level one accountability, that person will often become frustrated and leave.

Five Steps for Creating Organizational Accountability

Before taking the steps necessary for improvement, first examine the present state of your organization. Look at the characteristics describing high and low organizational accountability (see Exhibit 14.2). An obvious difference is how poor performers and high performers are treated. Another is the need to clearly align values with measurable business results. The resolution of problems and conflicts is also normative in high accountability cultures. Thus, crucial conversations are of vital importance. Samuel's organization, IMPAQ, actually allows you to take an online assessment of organizational and individual accountability (http://www.impaqcorp.com).

To create organizational accountability, there needs to be an unrelenting attack on the dysfunctional habits of individuals, teams, and organizational processes and policies. Everyone needs to join in the search for ineffective and inefficient habits that have developed over time. Some of these habits will be work-arounds that threaten patient safety. Nothing can be off-limits to improvement, but priorities need to be created to keep the organization in line with the

---

14.2 How Accountable Is Your Organization?

Low Organizational Accountability	High Organizational Accountability
1. Poor performers are ignored, transferred or promoted	1. Poor performers are coached, job aligned or out-placed for success
2. Territorialism and functional silos	2. Cross-functional team leadership
3. Low recognition or formal/structured awards	3. Informal and spontaneous recognition of people and success
4. Project failures, delays and over budget	4. Projects on-time and on-budget and successful
5. Blame and finger pointing or hiding from taking responsibility	5. Problem ownership, forgiveness, learning and action
6. Problem and conflict avoidance	6. Openly surface problems and conflicts
7. Fragmented, overwhelming or competing priorities	7. Clear and aligned direction with continual focus and tracking
8. Only business outcomes are measured	8. Performance execution and business outcomes are measured
9. Values are ignored or taken for granted	9. Values are clear, linked to business results and measured
10. Resist change	10. Initiate and execute change

Adapted from "How accountable is your organization?" by IMPAQ. Retrieved August 11, 2008, from http://www.impaqcorp.com/resources/polls/poll1/poll1a.php. Copyright 2006 by IMPAQ. Reprinted with permission.

14.3 Summary of the Five Steps for Creating Organizational Accountability

1. Introduce a new mind set
2. Identify and reverse dysfunctional habits of performance
3. Measure the effectiveness of the new habits of performance execution
4. Establish recovery systems prior to implementation
5. Recognize results and people

Samuel, M. (2006). *Creating the accountable organization: A practical guide to improve performance execution*. Katonah, NY: Xehpor Press, pp. 25–28.

accomplishment of desired outcomes. Samuel (2006) describes five steps for creating organizational accountability (see Exhibit 14.3).

Step One—Introduce a New Mind Set

A new way of thinking is needed if habits are to change. Habits are designed to minimize the need to think about routine activities. As destructive as some habits may be, they become comfortable routines. It requires courage to change mindsets, because most people resist changing routines. Therefore, people cannot just drop a habit; they need to replace it with a new habit. For example, in adopting a patient-focused care model, functional departments will need to work closely with each other to coordinate their efforts. Without the addition of the mind set of "no blame," the departments could slip back into fear and bickering. Therefore, the new mindset must be accompanied by *clear expectations for new and expanded roles and responsibilities.* A lack of clear expectations leads some people to do more and some to do less. Second, employees need to understand how *relationships will be altered* because of the change in expected outcomes. For example, the ICU nurse will now be receiving a patient report directly from the OR nurse, as the open-heart surgery patient will be going directly to the ICU. Third, *clarify any new expectations for improved performance.* What do we expect to improve as a result of this change? All of these changes in mindset and expectations must arise from a clear vision from the top. The captain (board and executives) decides the direction of change and prioritizes activities for a successful voyage. If the direction remains vague, individuals, departments, and cross-functional teams can not be expected to change their behaviors.

Vision statements provide direction and are meant to inspire people; they are supposed to represent the organization's intention. Vision statements are necessary to change mindsets. While the mission statement expresses the purpose of the organization, a vision statement focuses on how to accomplish this goal. Value statements should be designed to support the organizational culture by helping people understand what behaviors are expected. These include values, such as integrity, excellence, compassion, and service, as well as the support behaviors of honesty, high performance, caring, and customer focus. Finally, employees need to know why this vision and its supporting values were chosen. With this information, they can connect the dots to their role in making the vision a reality. This can only be done if employees are aware of the external factors (e.g., competition, reimbursement) and internal drivers (e.g. patient safety, employee diversity) driving the organizational changes. Understanding the organization's mission, values, and response to external/internal drivers helps people make sense of the vision. The vision is the context; it is the picture on the cover of the puzzle box. The vision is the why behind the goals. A patient-focused vision is not attainable without patient safety goals and cross-functional accountability.

Step Two—Identify and Reverse Dysfunctional Habits of Performance

Because organizational accountability requires coordinated and cooperative linkages among people, start by examining present connections. For example, what is the present process for resolving conflicts among mid-level managers across the organization? If managers do not feel safe enough to have the crucial conversations necessary to improve collaboration across departments, they will not achieve cross-functional accountability (level 4). When accountability is at the organizational level (level 5), we would expect managers to be able to resolve issues by speaking to each other to resolve the problem. They should only go to senior management if cannot reach a resolution.

Both Samuel (2006) and Patterson, Grenny, McMillian, and Switzler (2002) focus on the importance of creating a climate of safety for behavior change. People do not change when they are comfortable, but they also find it extremely difficult to change when they are afraid. The adrenaline rush that accompanies fear makes it almost impossible to think through a problem with the frontal cortex. People are ready to avoid or fight, but safety provides space for the risk taking associated with behavior change. When people resist change, they have a small safety zone. They view the required change as a punishment, rather than an opportunity for growth. Remember, the ideal goal is to create an organizational culture in which moral courage is not needed to confront ethical- and performance-related issues.

Leaders need to support an employee's courage in making changes by first helping the person understand the reason why the change is required. The employee needs to know the leader and appreciate that they share a mutual purpose. When we have the same goal, we trust the other person's motives. Mutual respect allows us to continue the dialog of a crucial conversation about new performance expectations. As soon as people perceive disrespect in a conversation, the interaction is no longer about the original topic. It is now about defending dignity.

The safety zone is not without discomfort. But we stay because we recognize that the crucial conversation will improve accountability and, therefore, team performance. The courage to tell the truth in a behaviorally descriptive way is the first step toward accountability. Say, for example, "Sarah, we both want to reduce the falls in this organization. This is the second meeting that you missed for the falls prevention project." The second step is helping the individual deal with the gap between the expected and present performance. You might say, "You made a commitment to attend every meeting. What happened?" Because the person may not know how to change, guidance for specific actions is the third step. ("Let us discuss how you will approach your manager to get the release time for the meeting.")

Unfortunately, many organizations replaced the dysfunctional habit of blaming people with a new tendency to blame the processes. Before the quality movement began, we focused on skill development. Therefore, when a problem occurred, additional training was seen as the solution. The number of hours spent on process improvement has yielded benefits, but teams still need practice to reach higher levels of performance. Individual stars on a team are fun to watch, but when the entire orchestra plays or the open-heart team effortlessly moves from one task to another, one is struck by the synergy of effort. Leaders need to focus on outcome, not process. Dysfunctional habits include dysfunctional processes, all of which cause patient safety errors. To achieve organizational accountability, all employees need to answer the question, "Did you achieve the desired outcome for which you planned?"

Samuel (2006) sees performance execution as the missing piece in achieving breakthrough results. To obtain the highest level of performance, the team must examine the actions, interactions, behaviors, and communication necessary to achieve safe and quality care for all patients. Work-unit and cross-functional teams must determine the communication and coordination needed to achieve this result. They will uncover habits that need to be changed. Teams, not individuals, are the basic learning unit in organizations today. Teams supply the means for creating true accountability.

Improving team performance will be most affected through coaching rather than through teambuilding retreats and training programs. These raise awareness, but they rarely change performance execution. Samuel (2006) argues that once the team has a vision of excellence, the team needs to develop success factors that support the vision. The vision answers the question, "What kind of team do we want to be?" The success factors are specific behaviors that reflect the highest level of performance in coordination and communication. Furthermore, these success factors are criteria from which objectives/benchmarks can be developed. These benchmarks can cover such topics as efficiency, customer service, quality, decision making, and outcomes. For example, a success factor could be, "We continually evaluate the needs of our customers through surveys and focus groups so that we might better anticipate and exceed their needs." The teams prioritize their top three success factors, develop action plans, and measure results again in six months. This focus forms the basis for accountability. Equally important is continuous feedback and coaching for performance improvement. Put together, these create the mechanism for creating sustainability. A new culture of accountability could then be born.

Step Three—Measure the Effectiveness of the New Habits of Performance Execution

Changing habits requires repeated enactment of the new habit until it becomes automatic. It is important to remove processes that create the likelihood of regression to old habits (e.g., the ability to circumvent computerized physician order entry with verbal orders). To rise to organization accountability (level five), all individuals in all departments and at all levels are required to communicate and cooperate. It is at this level that moral courage becomes unnecessary. This transition requires the elimination of outdated bureaucratic structures, long-standing conflicts between departments, and barriers to engaging staff in organizational decisions. Outcome-oriented performance execution requires "Olympic-style" team performance. For this level of performance, teams need to practice, practice, and practice some more. But it also requires identifying areas where refinement is needed to ensure that the same mistakes are not made in practice. In a system of shared accountability, the linkages between departments and levels are consistently improved because new key performance executions are tracked.

These cross-functional teams are the mechanism for creating true accountability. Peter Senge, in his famous book, *The Fifth Discipline* (1990), calls attention to the importance of teams: "Team learning is vital because teams, not individuals are the fundamental learning unit in modern organizations. This is where the 'rubber meets the road'" (p. 23). As teams learn and grow, so do the individual team members, as they take personal accountability for the changes required for success.

Because all habits can not be changed at once, everyone needs to be clear what the focus is and how success will be measured. Samuel (2006) calls these "success factors," and I call them the ground rules by which the team operates. As Samuel says, "they are the desired habits to achieve successful results" (p. 108). In general it will take a team approximately two hours to map out the 20 or so criteria needed for success. Two examples would be: (1) "We will speak directly to the person with whom we have a problem and seek a resolution satisfactory to all concerned" and (2) "We will respond to all patient feedback with openness, action to correct the problem, and follow-up to determine what process or structure change could prevent the problem in the future."

Step Four—Establish Recovery Systems Prior to Implementation

Even the best laid plans do not always work. This is the reason why contingency planning is part of effective leadership. "Plan B" and sometimes "Plan C" need to be thought through. Too often, with the first major push-back against the new plan, it is abandoned or the crisis comes as a surprise, and everyone reverts to business as usual. Being prepared with a recovery strategy allows you to continue making progress when flaws or mistakes are encountered.

Planning to the point of perfection never works. Learning organizations recognize if you demand perfection, you eliminate the safety to make mistakes, take risks, and create breakthrough results. It is important to have enough safety in the organization that people can admit mistakes, raise concerns, and hold others accountable.

A shared accountability model is much better for recovery than a vertical model, as it is more efficient and promotes team accountability. Sometimes we recognize we have made a mistake; at other times, we cannot see the mistake and need feedback from a coworker or manager. In an environment of mutual accountability, the coworker is not viewed as interfering or overstepping his or her bounds when providing guidance or coaching. The manager has the ultimate accountability for organizational effectiveness. Coaching may be a daily need. If the manager lacks the moral courage to have the crucial conversation surrounding performance, the team's performance will slip into mediocrity. When the leader fails to deal with performance problems, everyone loses. The individual performer never improves and the morale of the unit suffers, as teammates attempt to compensate and, of course, complain. The leader also loses because the team loses respect for the leader.

Step Five—Recognize Results and People

If people are to repeatedly assume individual accountability for the success of the organization, they need to know when they have made a difference. Without feedback, they are left to conclude that the results were not important. Recognition of cost savings and improvements in patient satisfaction or patient safety are cause for celebration. To eliminate dysfunctional habits and solidly set the new mind set, the organization needs to recognize successes in achieving its new accountability goals.

Conclusion

Samuel (2006) provides a roadmap for leaders and for teams to follow in creating an accountable organization. He recognizes that it takes time to move along the accountability continuum from entitlement to full organizational accountability. To move through the five levels of accountability, he offers five steps to embed accountability in the organizational culture. This kind of evolutionary process begins by introducing a new mindset that ties values and business outcomes together in a vision clearly articulated by leaders. This new way of operating includes clarifying performance expectations and identifying how the relationships in the organization will be altered. In step two, the dysfunctional habits of performance execution are identified and rectified. Silos are forced to disappear, as it becomes evident that patient care outcomes can not be achieved without the cooperation of cross-functional teams. Step three focuses on measuring the effectiveness of new habits. These habits have to stay aligned with the organization's vision and desired business outcomes. In step four, Samuel entreats us not to waste time on perfection, but instead to spend time on establishing recovery systems prior to implementation. Finally, in step five, we celebrate results and the people who created the success. Effective recognition highlights the purging of dysfunctional habits and the development of new ones that are important.

Key Points to Remember

1. Personal accountability is the willingness to be responsible for the consequences of one's actions.
2. Developing an accountable organization requires the moral courage to have many crucial conversations.
3. Five-step model for increasing breadth of accountability across the organization—entitlement > individual accountability > work-unit accountability > cross-functional accountability >organizational accountability.

4. It takes six months to a year to achieve each level of accountability.
5. Three principles should guide the effort to move the organization toward higher levels of accountability.
   A. *Principle one*—accountability increases one level at a time.
   B. *Principle two*—simultaneously increase performance expectations as you increase the level of accountability.
   C. *Principle three*—the farther removed an individual is from the organization's current level of accountability, the greater the pressure will be for that person to leave the organization.
6. Examine the present state of your organization by utilizing the online accountability assessment.
7. There are five steps for creating organizational accountability
   A. Introduce a new mind set with clear expectations for new and expanded roles and responsibilities.
   B. Identify and reverse dysfunctional habits of performance.
   C. Measure the effectiveness of the new habits of performance execution.
   D. Establish recovery systems prior to implementation.
   E. Recognize results and people.
8. Performance execution is the missing piece for breakthrough results. To obtain this breakthrough, the team must examine the actions, interactions, behaviors, and communication necessary to achieve the business outcome of safe, quality care for all patients.

References

IMPAQ. *How accountable is your organization?* Retrieved August 11, 2008, from http://www .impaqcorp.com/resources/polls/poll1/poll1a.php

Patterson, K., Grenny, J., McMillian, R., & Switzler, A. (2002). *Crucial conversations: Tools for talking when stakes are high.* New York: McGraw-Hill.

Samuel, M. (2006). *Creating the accountable organization: A practical guide to improve performance execution.* Katonah, NY: Xehpor Press.

Senge, P.M. (1990). *The fifth discipline.* New York: Doubleday.

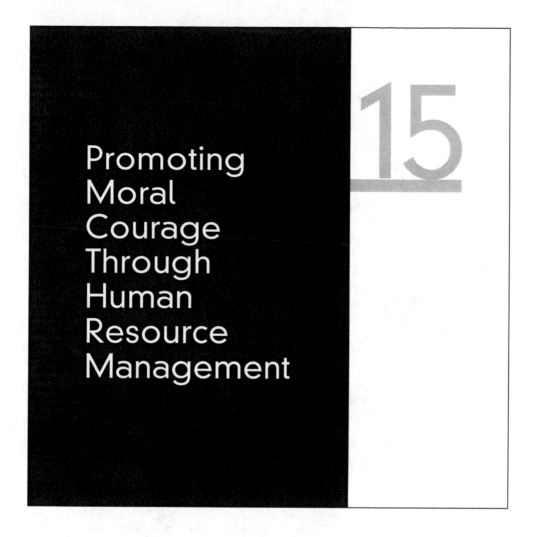

Promoting Moral Courage Through Human Resource Management

15

Baptist excels at building a well-managed brand; the company ranks #6 among large companies on the Fortune best-place-to-work list. They are number one in recruiting and retention in an industry that has some of the most backward recruiters and recruiting practices on the planet.

—Dr. John Sullivan, a leader in Human Resources

Dr. John Sullivan has been called the "Michael Jordan of Hiring" by *Fast Company* magazine. The only healthcare organization included in his list of the top 25 firms in recruiting and talent management is Baptist Health Care (Sullivan, 2005, p.1). Joining Baptist on the center stage of excellent HR practices in this chapter will be Disney. In addition, this chapter also explores the HR strategies put forth by both Jim Collins (2001) and Quint Studer (2008). We begin with a discussion of hiring practices that support employing only people of integrity and moves to an orientation process that begins the hardwiring of values orientation into the organizational culture. The chapter ends with the right reward and recognition strategies to sustain excellence in patient care and retain desired employees. As Collins (2001) says, to build great organizations you have to ". . . get the right people on the bus (and the wrong people off the bus) before you figure out where to drive it" (p. 41). Great organizations know it is the ability to get and keep enough of the right people that determine their destiny.

Hiring the Best

Sullivan (2008) says recruiting videos can entice people by allowing potential recruits to better "see, feel, and hear" the passion and the excitement of the organization. Videos allow an outsider to "meet" the employees, see the technology, and sometimes even tour the facilities. Such visual representations allow the viewer to decide if this organization has values that they have the courage to support.

Videos on the Internet are one of the hottest trends, especially among the younger generations. With the growth of the Internet and mobile phone technology, videos can be viewed almost anywhere by almost everyone. In fact, 56% of Americans with Internet access have viewed a video or listened to audio online, making it important for organizations to consider getting their message out via recruiting videos (Sullivan, 2008). When using videos to exemplify the values of the organization, they can help screen people, as does the Disney video that all potential employees are required to view before filling out an application (Lee, 2004).

Recruiting the best employees, especially younger employees, requires online application systems. These sites can provide the videos and standards of performance expected. Because the research suggests that employee referrals are most likely to yield the best employees for that organizational culture, a section for referral would be helpful (Sullivan, 2005). These employees know what values will need to be supported and would be unlikely to refer someone who lacked the integrity to sustain them.

Benchmarking the job is another strategy used by almost all the organizations on Sullivan's top ten list (2005). A job benchmark identifies the real needs of the job and helps distinguish candidates who are a natural fit to succeed in the position from less desirable applicants. McKenna (2005) uses benchmarking strategy and discusses strategies to prevent hiring the wrong candidate: (1) *Define the "hard" needs of the job*. These include type and quantity of experience, knowledge of industry, training and education, and special skills, such as proficiency in a particular software program or interpersonal skill. To support moral courage, the interpersonal skills need to include assertiveness and negotiation. (2) *Develop a list of three-to-six key accountabilities or goals that apply to this job*. These are other activities that must be accomplished and will impact the business. Key accountabilities are the rationale for the job's existence. The outcomes must be measurable and the key accountabilities should occupy approximately 80% of the employee's time. (3) *Benchmark the job*. The job benchmarking process begins by compiling a list of "key accountabilities." Once defined, these key accountabilities serve as the foundation for producing a guideline for the specific talents necessary for successful performance of the benchmarked job. (4) *Assess your top job candidates (internal and external) against the benchmark*.

You can have the candidates complete assessments from anywhere there is Internet access. In assessment areas that are marginal, the candidate's reports can guide you in asking interviewing questions that target the behaviors most important for success. Mason (2005) benchmarked the critical success factors that led to the development of specific interview questions that determine the soft-skill competencies of a candidate's job success. These ensure that the candidate will be the "right fit" for the organization. Mason believes you need to develop your interview process to adequately assess candidates' necessary soft skills. Kent Sherwood, CEO of Sutter Medical Center of Santa Rosa, emphasized the need for "integrity" as one of the highest soft-skill competencies for leadership candidates (Mason, 2005).

Baptist Health Care and Disney both require any person seeking employment read and agree to comply with its standards of performance. Baptist Health Care standards can be seen in Exhibit 15.1. These standards act as an early filter for admission to the organization, because people can recognize a culture in which they will be required to exceed the customer's expectations. They may decide this organization is not be for them. The Baptist Standards team, which included its own employees, developed these performance standards. Because employees developed the standards, they know what behavior is needed in the culture to achieve organizational excellence. Many of these behaviors will require moral courage and will need reinforcement by leadership.

The Standards Team is one the committees recommended by Quint Studer (2008). These standards are not developed in a vacuum. Committee members obtained feedback from customers and other employees and benchmarked other organizations. The list of standards focuses on key interaction points between staff members and between staff members and patients. Just like at Disney, there is tremendous peer pressure to adhere to these standards, and they are helpful in coaching individuals who need reminders.

Studer is a strong advocate of peer interviewing, in which employees hire their coworkers. Leaders first interview the candidate and decide whether to pass a candidate on to a peer interview. Leaders then select the highest performing employees to be part of the interview process. Employees go through two-hour training on the interview process and learn how to ask behavioral-based questions. Leaders and employees then complete a "decision matrix" that describes the key elements the employee should have for a particular position. This matrix generates questions and provides for an objective comparison of all candidates. This assures that new hires fit the organizational culture of integrity and excellence.

Behavioral-based questions use past behaviors to help predict future performance. Examples of behavioral-based questions that could assess candidates for integrity and courage are given in Exhibit 15.2 (on page 186). Behavioral-based questions ask how candidates have actually performed rather than how they *feel* or what they *think* they would do. They begin with phrases such as, "Tell me about a time when you . . ." or "Describe for me. . . ." Individuals are instructed to probe until they get all parts of the story—description of the event, the action the candidate took, and the results of the action. They close the interview with two questions: (1) What value would you bring to us? and (2) What questions do you have for us?

15.1 Baptist Health Care Standards

Attitude

Our job is to serve our customers and provide high quality service with care and courtesy. Always thank customers for choosing Baptist Hospital. Exceed expectations.

Acknowledge a customer's presence immediately. Smile and introduce yourself at once.

Appearance

Be clean and professional.

Follow dress code policies and wear your identification badge correctly at all times.

Pick up litter and dispose of it properly. Clean up spills and return equipment to its proper place.

Communication

Listen to customers. Be courteous. Don't use jargon. Keep patient information confidential.

When someone appears to need directions, escort that person to his or her destination.

Know how to operate the telephones in your area. Provide the correct number before transferring a call. Get the caller's permission before putting him or her on hold and thank the caller for holding.

Answer calls within three rings. Identify your department and yourself and ask, "How may I help you?"

Call Lights

All employees are responsible for answering patient call lights.

Acknowledge call lights by the fifth ring and respond to requests within three minutes. Always address the patient by name.

Anticipate patients' needs so they will not have to use their call lights.

Ensure continuity of care by reporting to relief caregivers before leaving the floor. Return promptly from breaks.

Check on patients one hour before shift change to minimize requests during report.

Commitment to Co-workers

Treat one another as professionals deserving courtesy, honesty and respect. Welcome newcomers.

Avoid last-minute requests and offer to help fellow employees whenever possible.

Cooperate with one another. Don't undermine other people's work; praise whenever possible.

Do not chastise or embarrass fellow employees in the presence of others.

Address problems by going to the appropriate supervisor.

15.1 Continued

Customer Waiting

Educate families about processes and provide a comfortable atmosphere for waiting customers.

An acceptable waiting time for scheduled appointments is ten minutes; it's one hour for non-scheduled appointments.

Offer refreshments and an apology if a wait occurs. Always thank customers for waiting.

Update family members periodically—at least hourly—while a customer is undergoing a procedure.

Elevator Etiquette

Always smile and speak with fellow passengers; hold the door open for others.

When transporting patients in wheelchairs, always face them toward the door and exit with care. If transporting a patient in a bed or stretcher, politely ask others to wait for another elevator.

Pause before entering an elevator so you do not block anyone's exit. Step aside or to the back to make room for others.

Walk departing guests to the elevator.

Privacy

Make sure that patient information is kept confidential. Never discuss patients and their care in public areas.

Knock before entering. Close curtains or doors during exams and procedures. Provide a robe or second gown if the patient is ambulating or in a wheelchair. Make sure all gowns are the right size for the patient.

Safety Awareness

Report all accidents or incidents promptly.

Correct or report any safety hazard you see.

Use protective clothing, gear and procedures when appropriate.

Sense of Ownership

Take pride in this organization as if you own it. Accept the responsibilities of your job.

Adhere to policies and procedures. Live the values of this organization. Do the right thing.

15.2 Sample Behavioral-Based Questions

Tell me about the most difficult patient service experience that you have ever had to handle. Be specific and tell what you did and what the outcome was (Courage).

Tell me about a situation where you had to risk speaking up because a negative response was likely (Courage).

Describe a situation in which you felt it might be justifiable to break organizational policy or alter a standard procedure (Integrity).

Adapted from StuderGroup and Studer, Q. (2008). *Results that last.* Hoboken, NJ: John Wiley and Sons, Inc.

Orientation to the Culture

Baptist Health Care has been included on *Fortune* magazine's list of "The 100 Best Companies to Work For" for the last six years. This would not have happened if management did not have a commitment to *hire* and *retain* an excellent workforce. Using an adapted version of the Disney *Traditions* orientation model (Lee, 2004), Baptist Health Care requires all new employees to go to *Traditions,* a two-day hospital orientation. This is not the dry, boring orientation that is the hospital industry standard. It begins with a two-hour presentation by the administrator on organizational culture. In fact, 8 out of the 16 hours are allocated to culture orientation activities. The purpose of the orientation is to educate, but also to inspire employees to exceed customer expectations.

Since receiving the Baldridge National Quality Award in 2004, Baptist Health Care has received awards each year for quality, patient satisfaction, and staff satisfaction. Clearly, this focus on the culture and this early alignment to the "five pillars of focus" have made a difference. The five pillars are people, service, quality, financial performance, and growth. Stubblefield provides more detailed description of *Traditions,* the half-day refresher, *SerU,* that occurs within six months, and the quarterly town-hall-style forums in his book, *The Baptist Health Care Journey to Excellence* (2005). All of these activities are designed to help keep the employee's moral compass aligned with the integrity and excellence the organizational culture demands.

"More than 25 percent of employees who leave their positions do so in the first 90 days of employment" (Studer, 2008, p. 180). Therefore, Studer (2008) recommends 30-day and 90-day meetings between the leader and employee. The focus of these meetings is to discover what is going well and what is not. In other words, the manager/executive needs to discover what issues in the organization still require moral courage to address. "New employee turnover can be reduced by 66% if these meetings are conducted according to question guidelines" (Studer, 2008, p. 180). Since leadership is about the quality of the relationship, these meetings serve to further bond the employee to the organization. In the 90-day meeting, the leader can also use one of the best forms of recruiting by asking the newly oriented employee, "Is there anyone you know who might be a valuable addition to our team?" It is at this 90-day point the leader will know if the organization would want more of this type of employee, and the employee is likely to still be in touch with former coworkers.

15.3 The Top Five Workplace Incentives

1. Personal thanks from manager
2. Written thanks from manager
3. Promotion for performance
4. Public praise
5. Morale-building meetings

From *Motivating today's employees* (p.16) by B. Nelson. (1996). San Diego, CA: Nelson Motivation, Inc. Copyright 1996 by Bob Nelson. Reprinted with permission.

Recognizing and Rewarding the Behavior You Want

How do you reinforce desirable behaviors? You do so by consistently rewarding and recognizing them. Recognized behaviors get repeated. When you act as a partner with employees in the success of the organization, employees will begin to look at their jobs differently. When you recognize significant contributions to the mission, vision, and values of an organization, you reinforce the values espoused. "Integrity is the first of the Baptist Health Care values—integrity is maintaining the highest standards of behavior. Integrity encompasses honesty, ethics, and doing the right things for the right reasons" (Stubblefield, 2005, p. 24). This means actions, such as disclosing patient errors, honoring advance directives, and telling the truth about prognoses, would be normative. The goal is to create an organizational culture in which moral courage will not be needed because the culture so honors its patients and the employees.

To select and retain great people, an organization needs a persistent and unfailing commitment to recognizing and rewarding individuals and teams. It is important to be specific in the behavior you recognize, so the person will know exactly what to repeat. StuderGroup is a big advocate of handwritten thank-you notes sent to the employee's home. This is number two on the list of the top five workplace incentives. The others can be seen in Exhibit 15.3.

Another place to hardwire in recognition is in daily rounding. Studer (2008) outlines the reasons and process for rounding, in which the focus is again on the five pillar outcomes, establishing personal connections, and recognizing achievements. It also helps leaders get a handle on a potential problem and to follow up with employees on identified problems. This gives employees two out of the five critical elements employees want from their leaders: (1) a manager who cares about them and (2) recognition for doing good work (Studer, 2008, p. 33). The other three are (3) working systems with tools and equipment to do the job; (4) opportunities for professional growth; and (5) no low-performers as coworkers. Baptist Health Care has another recognition program that keeps goals and culture aligned. It is the *Bright Ideas* program that harvests any idea that can better serve the patients, employees, or community (Stubblefield, 2005). The idea must save time or money or both, represent a positive change for the organization, and be within the capacity of the organization's resources to implement. Based on the Baptist experience, initiating a flourishing *Bright Ideas* program could provide your organization with the opportunity to capture the untapped pool of knowledge in your organization (Baptist Health Care Leadership Institute, 2004). Baptist Health Care now makes available the software to manage the program. This program also fulfills the principle of rewarding ideas that support the values of the organization and encourages a sense of ownership in employees. The following is one example of a "bright idea":

> Pillar: Service
> Idea: Provide free flu vaccine to community service organizations, including Health Department and Community Clinic. We have not-returnable flu vaccine left over.
> Benefit: Utilize excess flu vaccine for indigent care.
> Department: BHC Towers Pharmacy

There are many ways to recognize and reward individuals and teams. With excellent front-line leadership, most employees will meet expectations. It is important to repeatedly recognize those who exceed expectations, so you can retain high performers. However, there are times when the organization will hire the wrong people, even with the strategies discussed.

Coaching, Counseling, Disciplining, and Firing

All employees in an organization focused on excellence receive periodic coaching in the continuing effort for further improvement. This coaching is made easier because standards of expected performance are reinforced by orientation, additional training, performance evaluations, and reward and recognition programs. But can you teach compassion, kindness, and caring, which are the adjectives linked to patient loyalty? These are all rooted in the capacity for empathy, the ability to sense and understand someone else's feelings as if they were your own. Without empathy, you also will not have moral courage. Such courage was found in the study of Holocaust rescuers, in whom "the only common characteristic that could be found was a capacity for empathy that was strong enough to overcome the primitive fear for one's own safety" (Lee, 2004, p. 139).

Lee shows that the way to teach empathy is by introducing us to the skills of great actors. Acting is not pretending. A patient can tell when a person is pretending to care, and they will find it patronizing. So how do you show sincerity? Actors do it by re-creating the intense emotions of anger, sadness, humiliation, joy, and betrayal that they have experienced. When shared, these "sensory choices" have the ability to stimulate the imaginations of others. For example, if I was to describe to you the saddest event in my life, you too might experience the same depth of sadness. Your pain and empathy would be real. When I put my arm around a sobbing mother in an emergency department who is holding her dead eight-month-old baby, tears are likely to roll down my cheeks. This baby may still be alive if the mother had received the correct advice from her pediatrician. Health care is a sterile and impersonal stage, and healthcare professionals need to remember to ask a fundamental question, "What is the reality of this patient's experience, and how can I make it real to me?" In this way, imagination creates empathy, which leads to compassion, which leads to the courage to do the right thing for this patient. We can teach people to be polite, and we can have zero tolerance for rudeness, but compassion and courage come not from policies but from the ability to empathize.

Unfortunately, sometimes a person will not respond to the coaching, and the leader needs to implement more counseling or even more discipline to let the person know that this organization takes its values and standards of performance seriously. So how do you know when you have the wrong person on the bus? The moment you feel a need to closely manage someone because the person/employee has not responded to coaching, you need to help that person off the bus. Allowing the wrong people to stay is unfair to the right people, as they lose time and become disillusioned as they try to compensate for the wrong people. Worse, it will drive away the best people. How do you know when it is time? Ask yourself, "Would I hire this person again?" and "Would I be secretly relieved if the person came and told me he or she is moving on to another opportunity?"

Sometimes "the square peg in the round hole" can be moved to a place in the organization where he or she can thrive. I have seen this over and over again. If these individuals support the values of the organization and meet the standards of performance, then look for another spot where they can blossom. Collins (2001) found that "whether someone was the right person has more to do with character traits and innate capabilities than with specific knowledge, background or skills" (p. 64). If an employee is not meeting the standards and failing to uphold organizational values, then do the right thing and let the person find another bus.

Conclusion

An organizational culture that supports everyone's integrity and excellence in patient care requires hiring the best people. The interviewing process begins with the act of advertising for a position. It is clear that if we want to attract younger people, we need to provide Internet access and online videos. In addition, the most successful referrals come from employees, because they know the values and performance standards of the organization. HR Department staff begins the actual interviewing process by screening the person using video and/or standards of performance. Next, the leader interviews the candidate and refers the best people to the candidate's prospective coworkers for an interview. After a person is hired, orientation needs to focus on the values of the culture, as well as the organizational systems designed to help the employee succeed. Because the behavior that gets rewarded gets repeated, several ideas for recognition and rewards are offered. If the employee does not fit into the organization, the leader needs to counsel and perhaps fire the individual. When excellence is the goal, low performers cannot be tolerated. Baptist Health Care and the StuderGroup are used throughout this chapter as a model for the human resource activities because they have produced high patient quality, patient satisfaction, and employee satisfaction results.

The next section will focus on organizational opportunities for demonstrating moral courage—patient safety and disruptive physicians. In addition, the importance of organizational ethics committees and clinical ethics committees will be emphasized. Section IV will end on the importance of leadership development at all levels of the organization. Leaders sustain organizational values and support organizational culture. Without a knowledgeable and dedicated effort by front-line managers and supervisors, the organization will never be at its best.

Key Points to Remember

1. Recruiting videos can entice people by allowing potential recruits to better "see, feel, and hear" the passion and the excitement of the organization.
2. Employee referrals are most likely to yield the best employees for that organizational culture.
3. Benchmarking the job is a strategy used by top organizations in recruiting. A job benchmark identifies the real needs of the job and helps distinguish candidates who are a natural fit to succeed in the position from less desirable applicants.
4. Baptist Health Care and Disney both require that any person seeking employment read and agree to comply with its standards of performance.
5. Leaders first interview the candidate and decide whether to pass a candidate on to a peer interview. Employees in actual fact hire their own coworkers.
6. Behavioral-based questions ask how candidates have actually performed rather than how they *feel* or what they *think* they would do.
7. Eight out of the 16 hours of two-day orientation (Traditions) is allocated to culture orientation activities. The purpose of the orientation is to educate, but also to inspire employees to exceed customer expectations.
8. *Traditions,* the half-day refresher, *SerU,* and quarterly town-hall-style forums are designed to help keep the employee's moral compass aligned with the integrity and excellence the organizational culture demands.
9. The focus of 30-day and 90-day meetings between the leader and the employee is to discover what is going well and what is not going well.
10. When you recognize significant contributions to the mission, vision, and values of an organization, you reinforce the values espoused.
11. Baptist Health Care has recognition programs that keeps goals and culture aligned.
12. The five critical elements employees want from their leaders are (1) a manager who cares about them; (2) recognition for doing good work; (3) working systems with tools and equipment to do the job; (4) opportunities for professional growth; and (5) no low-performers as coworkers.
13. Healthcare is a sterile and impersonal stage and upon it healthcare professionals need to ask a fundamental question, "What is the reality of this patient's experience, and how can I make it real to me?"
14. Compassion and courage come not from polices but from the ability to empathize, as with Holocaust rescuers among whom "the only common characteristic that could be found was a capacity for empathy that was strong enough to overcome the primitive fear for one's own safety."
15. "Whether someone was the right person has more to do with character traits and innate capabilities than with specific knowledge, background or skills."
16. Sometimes "the square peg in the round hole" can be moved to a place in the organization where they can thrive, as long as they support the values of the organization.

17. How do you know when it is time to ask the person to leave? Ask yourself, "Would I hire this person again?" and "Would I be secretly relieved if the person came and told me he or she is moving on to another opportunity?"

References

Baptist Health Care Leadership Institute. (2004). *Bright ideas.* Retrieved August 23, 2008, from https://www.baptistleadershipinstitute.com/Store/Item.aspx?ContentID=100049

Collins, J. (2001). *Good to great.* New York: Harper Business.

Lee, F. (2004). *If Disney ran your hospital: 9 1/2 things you would do differently.* Bozeman, MT: Second River Healthcare Press.

Mason, J.L. (2005, November 10). *Strategies for hiring winners: Executive summary.* Retrieved August 23, 2008, from http://ezinearticles.com/?Strategies-for-Hiring-Winners:-Executive-Summary&id=94639

McKenna, J. (2005). *Hire the best candidate, not the best interviewer.* Retrieved August 23, 2008, from http://www.kennacompany.com/articles/HiretheBestCandidate.htm

Stubblefield, A. (2005). *The Baptist Health Care journey to excellence: Creating a culture that wows!* Hoboken, NJ: John Wiley and Sons.

Studer, Q. (2008). *Results that last: Hardwiring behaviors that will take your company to the top.* Hoboken, NJ: John Wiley and Sons.

StuderGroup. (2006, May 24). *Behavioral based interview questions.* Retrieved August 23, 2009, from http://www.studergroup.com/dotCMS/knowledgeAssetDetail?inode=515

Sullivan, J. (2005, February 28). *The top 25 benchmark firms in recruiting and talent management* (p. 3). Retrieved August 23, 2008, from http://www.ere.net/2005/02/28/the-top-25-benchmark-firms-in-recruiting-and-talent-management/

Sullivan, J. (2008, August 11). *Recruiting videos allow potential candidates to feel the passion.* Retrieved August 23, 2008, from http://www.ere.net/2008/08/11/recruiting-videos-allow-potential-candidates-to-feel-the-passion/

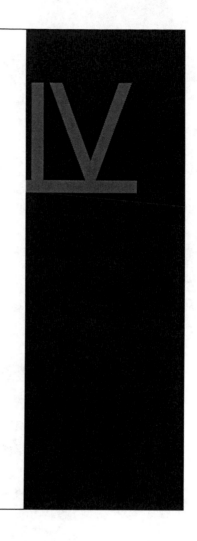

Organizational Opportunities for Moral Courage

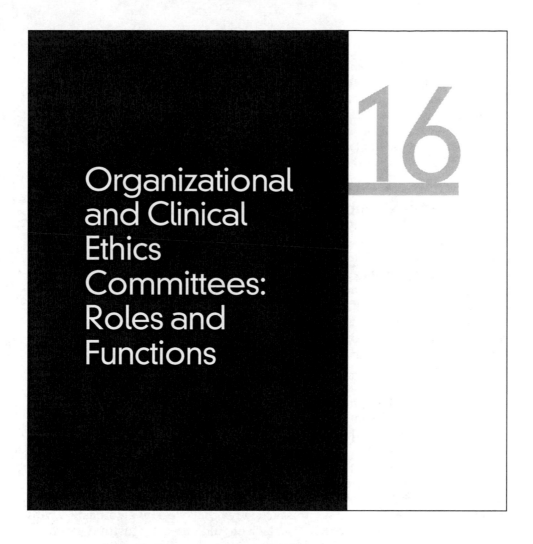

16

Organizational and Clinical Ethics Committees: Roles and Functions

To give real service you must add something which cannot be bought or measured with money, and that is sincerity and integrity.

—Douglas Adams, British author and satirist

Case 16.1

Mrs. Jones, a 92-year-old patient with severe dementia, has an advance directive indicating that she desires no aggressive care at the end-of-life, including no artificial hydration or nutrition. Her daughter has said, "I know my mother would not want to live like this, but I cannot let her die. Put in the PEG tube." The nurse caring for the patient shows the physician the advance directive. Later, she calls an ethics consultant because she sees the physician writing an order for the insertion of the PEG tube.

Clinical ethics committees accept the obligation of nonmaleficence and function to protect patients from violations of their autonomy. Advance directives act as the voice of the patient when the person is no longer able to speak. This nurse had the moral courage to speak up and act as this patient's advocate. She knew that the ethics consultant would also give this daughter the needed resources to deal with her grief over the impending loss of her mother.

Clinical Ethics Committees

The Joint Commission (1995) demanded clear evidence that mechanisms for ethical resolution of dilemmas be in place in all hospitals. The need for these mechanisms to provide guidance in difficult situations involving ethical issues became obvious during the case of Karen Ann Quinlan.

Clinical ethics committees became an obvious answer. In the beginning, they spent most of their time reviewing decisions to limit or withdraw life-sustaining treatment for dying or persistent vegetative state (PVS) patients (Gostin, 1979). Since its inception, the purpose of the clinical ethics committee was seen as threefold—education, policy formation, and case consultation.

The education focus begins with the establishment of ethical decision making principles that help the committee resolve dilemmas. The committee members then participate in or recruit other healthcare professionals and bioethicists to educate employees and administrative staff. As most cases involve communication problems between parties, education includes how to deliver bad news, discuss advance directives, and obtain a do-not-resuscitate (DNR) order.

Policy formation includes drafting and reviewing such policies as withholding and withdrawing treatment, cardiopulmonary resuscitation, and advance directives. As you will see, this is the area that overlaps significantly with organizational ethics. When there is a lack of guidance from institutional policies, you often find ambiguous situations, communication conflicts, and fears of retaliation against healthcare providers who might choose to speak out. If we are to support the moral courage of professionals who choose to advocate for patient autonomy, then the organization's ethical environment needs monitoring.

Three models exist for case consultation: (1) an individual consultant who reports to the entire committee on the results of a consultation; (2) a team of committee members; and (3) the entire committee. All of these models have advantages and disadvantages. The first affords flexibility and timeliness, but it loses the diversity of different perspectives. The second offers the advantage of having people with experience in different disciplines examine the problem, such as an ethicist and a healthcare professional. The third model—the entire committee meets—offers significant expertise to the individual requesting the consultation, but it lacks efficiency and probably timeliness. After all, to get that many busy professionals together at one time is a challenging task. A meeting of the entire committee is usually reserved for postanalysis of the case, when the individual who did the consultation reviews his or her findings with the committee. This provides an opportunity for the committee to learn and the consultant(s) to receive feedback.

16.1	Differentiating Clinical and Organizational Ethics

Clinical Ethics	Organizational Ethics
Involves clinicians	Involves executives → frontline staff
Bedside decisions	Business issues impacting patients
Arena of illness, dying, and research	Arena of business, financial, and contractual issues

Whatever model is chosen, the ethical issues of justice (fairness) and confidentiality need to be addressed. Consultants must be prepared to voice recommendations, but these must be based on knowledge of health care law, bioethics, and organizational polices. Although the consultation is often requested to support the viewpoint of the person who requested it, the consultant's authority is only advisory. Because most case consultations focus primarily on end-of-life ethical dilemmas, patient capacity, and informed consent, the consultant must also be versed in these issues. I serve on two ethics committees and have found that most issues revolve around conflicts between the provider and families. Therefore, a key skill of a consultant is the ability to act as a mediator for all parties.

Exhibit 16.1 shows the key areas of difference between clinical and organizational ethics. While clinical ethics focuses on clinicians at the patient's bedside, organizational ethics focuses on how business issues impact patients. The focal point of organizational ethics is primarily the administration's financial, business, and contractual decisions.

Organizational Ethics Committees

Unfortunately, healthcare facilities did not respond with the same specificity to the 1994 Joint Commission organizational standard calling for mechanisms to ensure ethical integrity in a number of management arenas (Schyve, 1996). While the Commission did not call for the creation of an organizational ethics committee, it did require the creation of a code of conduct (Talone, 2006). Around this same time, organizations were beginning to develop corporate compliance programs. Unfortunately, many thought ethics and compliance were interchangeable; they viewed organizational ethics as more the purview of legal counsel than as behavior connected with mission and/or ethics (Talone, 2006).

A compliance focus assumes that the organization knows right from wrong and relies on auditing, sanctions, and hotlines to enforce the correct choice. In contrast, an organizational ethics view is reflective in nature, discussing competing ethical alternatives and the development of values and polices that support the right choices (Khushf & Tong, 2002). Exhibit 16.2 provides a comparison between compliance and organizational ethics.

16.2 Differentiating Compliance and Organizational Ethics

Compliance Ethics	Organizational Ethics
Enforcement	Reflective in nature
Use of authority to punish	Reinforcement of values
Penalties for violations	Reliance on integrity
Rules	Principles

The Health Insurance Portability and Accountability Act of 1996 triggered the development of corporate compliance programs in the healthcare industry (McDaniel, 2004). This Act gives the Department of Health and Human Services' Office of the Inspector General and the U.S. Department of Justice increased funding for investigations and the authority to increase penalties for healthcare fraud and abuse. Healthcare providers shield themselves from such liability by implementing corporate compliance programs that incorporate the seven elements outlined in the U.S. Sentencing Guidelines for Organizations. These elements provide the backbone of a well-designed compliance program by informing employees about the proper steps to follow in reporting ethical infractions. As a result, employees know that they can report violations of standards without fear of retribution (McDaniel, 2004). In this way, these compliance mechanisms can actually support the moral courage of employees.

Basically, compliance with regulations is necessary, but not sufficient, for creating an ethical organization. Codes of conduct and policies for enforcement are good starting points, but organizations must move beyond compliance to developing a process for addressing situationally unique challenges. An organizational ethics committee provides an opportunity to step back from a situation, reflect on mission statements and values, and examine the appropriate conduct for each situation.

The Joint Commission (1995) standards focused only on economic issues, but healthcare institutions are no longer "silent partners" that simply provide space and manage financial arrangements. Healthcare is no longer practiced only by individuals. Instead, the type and intensity of clinical services in an organization are determined by leaders of the institution, as well as by other organizations unconnected to the fabric of the community the institution serves (e.g., AHQR, managed care organizations). The outcome-management and evidence-based practice (EBP) focus of these organizations exercises considerable control over the clinical practice of healthcare professionals. The traditional separation of clinical and organizational ethics no longer exists. Organizations are now agents deeply involved in healthcare transactions; each organization has its own integrity, norms, and culture (Khushf, 1998). Therefore, it is crucial that an organization make known the norms and values that guide its decisions.

Organizational ethics is a thoughtful deliberation on an organization's values, principles, and goals for the purpose of guiding managerial decisions that affect patient care. It is an intentional use of values to guide decisions for the system and is a disciplined approach to resolving value-laden business issues impacting patient care. With this reflection comes the development of processes and structures that promote the collaborative pursuit of organizational values. In summary, organizational ethics is an ethical analysis of managerial decision-making. For example, moral courage may be necessary to alert management to the pressing issues that are in conflict with the values of excellence or compassion.

In many academic medical centers, the triple focus of patient care, education, and research can compete for attention and dollars. Which should receive the highest priority? Sometimes, the mission statement can help us see what value might trump another. What follows are the mission statements of two premier healthcare organizations in the United States. The Mission Statement of the University of Pennsylvania Health System is "Creating the future of medicine through: Patient Care and Service Excellence, Educational Pre-eminence, New Knowledge and Innovation, and National and International Leadership." The mission of Johns Hopkins Medicine is to improve the health of the community and the world by setting the standard of excellence in medical education, research, and clinical care. Diverse and inclusive, Johns Hopkins Medicine educates medical students, scientists, healthcare professionals and the public; conducts biomedical research; and provides patient-centered medicine to prevent, diagnose, and treat human illness. In the University of Pennsylvania mission statement, patient care is listed first; at Johns Hopkins, it is listed last. In an organizational ethics committee meeting, this would be food for conversation.

The purpose of an organizational ethics committee is to assure that all decisions are in keeping with the organization's mission and vision. For example, most organizations have formal mechanisms reaching such significant strategic decisions as closing or initiating service lines. The typical issues that come to organizational ethics committees include how to downsize, when and how to discuss medical errors, what is just or fair compensation for entry-level employees, and what are appropriate requirements for diversity (O'Toole, 2006). But competing values can arise when a healthcare organization provides maternity services to a community (mission), while simultaneously assuming responsibility for the financial stability of the organization (margin).

Because of the conflict between clinical and financial needs in such a situation, attention to organizational ethics is critical (Khushf & Tong, 2002). Business ethics topics include finance, marketing, human resources, materials management, managed care contracting, billing, and information technology. With the rise of managed care, the line between clinical and administrative polices has become blurred. Financial mechanisms, such as capitation, cash bonuses, generalist gatekeepers, and hospitals' purchasing physician practices, all could result in people using fewer hospital services or the organization passing on financial incentives.

Case 16.1

On June 29, 2006 Tenet Health Care, the nation's second largest for-profit hospital chain, announced a settlement of about $900 million to resolve a variety of allegations, including the accusations that it had overcharged Medicare and had improperly offered doctors financial incentives to move to certain cities where the chain hospitals were located.. To finance the settlement, Tenet plans to sell 11 hospitals in four states. Although Tenet did not admit to any illegal practices, Company officials admitted that they made mistakes in conduct. "What ultimately matters is that the company's actions did not meet the highest ethical standards that the public expects," said Tenet CEO Trevor Fetter.

This announcement by Tenet offers us a case example of a perceived lack of ethical conduct in the financial aspects of business. Whether or not Tenet was guilty, as the CEO said, "the company's actions did not meet the public's ethical expectations" (Department of Justice, 2006). What we do know is that some members of this organization used accounting strategies that led to overbilling. We do not know if this came to light through whistleblowing or through detection of the problem by Medicare. Healthcare executives must scrutinize the administrative practice of "aggressive accounting" for ethical conflict just as they would investigate conflict of interest or diversity (Boyle, Dubose, Ellingson, Guinn, & McCurdy, 2001).

Several studies point to the conflict between administrative practice and the nursing professional's responsibility to advocate for patients (Borawski, 1995; Cooper, Frank, Gouty, & Hansen, 2002; Silva, 1998). Borawski's study of nurse managers found 28% experienced this conflict. Cooper et al. found, in a study of 325 members of the American Organization of Nurse Executives, that the perceived failures of healthcare organizations to provide service of the highest quality were the four top-rated concerns. The nurse executives reported that the key reason for this failure was economic restraints. Other highly rated items indicated that these nursing executives also were failing to manage effectively the conflict between organizational and professional philosophies and standards. In this author's experience as an organizational development consultant, little has changed since these studies. Organizational ethics committees could serve to assist and support healthcare institutions in meeting the challenging task of reducing the gap between what is ethical and what is desirable for business.

Cook, Hoas, and Joyner's (2000) study of rural nurses supported Lipp's (1998) finding that nurses seldom have the moral courage to act against the organizational power structure that controls their professional and economic destiny. The nurses in this rural study especially questioned their abilities to respond appropriately to ethical issues if organizational factors were involved. Numerous participants mentioned the possible loss of a job or retaliation. They also noted the lack of organizational resources to help them maintain their professional obligations. Clearly, there is an obvious need for clinical and organizational ethics committees. But without courageous leadership, these committees are not likely to tackle the tough issues that need addressing.

As discussed in Chapter 12, the organizational culture is a key factor in determining the amount of moral courage generated by staff and management. When conflicts between administrative practice and patient advocacy arise, courageous leaders will use the values of the organization to argue for the right action. For example, an organization recently added bariatric surgery to its offerings, but failed to budget for needed equipment and staff education on the appropriate use of this surgery for morbidly obese patients. Lucrative financial reimbursement for these surgeries trumped the stated organizational value of compassion. The nurse executive in this situation saw the need to advocate for the patient and the staff. He used ethical (nonmaleficence) and financial (cost of work injuries) arguments to create a safer implementation of this new program.

Structure of an Organizational Ethics Committee

Should an organizational ethics committee be a subcommittee of a clinical ethics committee or a separate committee? Often members of a clinical committee are professionals who have little understanding of operational goals and have no direct responsibility for achieving those goals (O'Toole, 2006). Committee members take a case-based approach to frame the issue, resulting in resolution only of the specific case. Often, they do not examine the underlying processes or systems that contribute to the problem. If a subcommittee model is chosen, it should include supplementary representatives from administration and finance, along with people committed to developing knowledge in business ethics (American Academy of Pediatrics, 2001). If, in addition to resolving the problem, the subcommittee also seeks to prevent the reoccurrence of the problem, then the committee members need to examine the problem through both a macro and micro lens.

The experience of the clinical ethics committee at M. D. Anderson Cancer Center provides a good example of the expanding responsibility to include organizational ethics. Cost-effectiveness and justice were listed as important ethical considerations in only 6% of their ethics consultations from 1993 to 1996, but this jumped to 21% in 1997 (Prentz, 1998). The committee first added a financial officer and, on request, created "Ethical Principles for Allocating Clinical Resources." Since then, the members have reviewed advertising, because it affects both present and future patients, and have had a representative on the billing and collections task force. The bulk of the committee's caseload is still the primary need for responding to end-of-life case consultations. However, any clinical ethics committee today needs to be aware of the effects of cost-containment efforts on patient care. For example, this author recently brought to the hospital ethics committee of a 100-bed hospital a concern that between January to May 2008, 147 patients were restrained, with the majority of these patients being over 70 years of age. Sitters were not being hired because of budget restrictions. The clinical ethics issue of tying down elderly patients so that they could not pull out tubes suddenly became an organizational ethics issue of cost allocation.

Seeley and Goldberg (1999) proposed an integrated organizational-clinical model, as they thought a dichotomy between clinical and organizational ethics prevented development of effective systems-level responses. Foglia and Pearlman (2006) believe these macro responses aim to make ethical responses easier. For example, both electronic reminders to update advance directives or discuss possible DNRs when APACHE scores reach a certain level help the practitioner to stay current with ethical responsibilities. Foglia and Pearlman believe that systems-oriented ethics consultants understand the power of organizational culture to negatively affect a healthcare professional's ability and willingness to demonstrate moral courage. These authors want to support the healthcare professionals in doing the right thing by fixing factors extrinsic to them. Second, their approach is similar to a quality management viewpoint—the gap between how healthcare professionals should act and actually act is profoundly affected by organizational systems. This fosters an "upstream" examination for predisposing issues that add to an increase of ethical problems. Both Seeley and Goldberg and Foglia and Pearlman would likely argue for one committee with an integrated approach to clinical cases, because such cases are influenced by the organizational context.

Whatever model is chosen, the first step would be determining the highest priority issues. To achieve this goal, an intranet survey could be conducted among frontline and management personnel in the organization. Another option might be to conduct focus groups, as healthcare professionals know where the conflicts of interest lie and where they feel unprotected and fear retaliation.

Choosing Committee Members

St. Louis Sisters of Mercy System developed an approach for integration of ethics and operations in a separate Corporate Ethics Committee (O'Toole, 2006). They recognized that leaders must constantly prioritize and reach decisions between competing values. They believe their Corporate Ethics Committee is an effective way to address ethical and operational concerns. In the restructuring of the committee, they included ethical experts and individuals with organizational authority to assure follow through.

They believe the skills of the members of this ethics committee are similar to those of the clinical ethics committee. The difference in membership will be addressed in the last two items of the list below (O'Toole, 2006; Talone, 2006).

1. Knowledgeable, experienced, and competent in their own field of expertise.
2. Willing to do preparatory work necessary for deliberations (reading and education).
3. Capable of ethical discourse, as distinguished from argumentative or passive acceptance of other's stance.
4. Informed of the organization's mission, vision, values and, if applicable, code of conduct.
5. Recognized for honesty and integrity.
6. Chair should be someone in a senior leadership position, but not the CEO or executive in charge of mission.
7. Members should include an ethicist and representatives of management and healthcare professionals.

A nonhospital attorney familiar with health care ethical issues, especially organizational ethics, could also be beneficial (American Academy of Pediatrics, 2001). A hospital attorney or risk manager might experience a conflict of interest between protecting the patient and protecting the institution.

This Corporate Ethics Committee developed position papers or policies on joint ventures, care of the indigent, socially responsible investing, and privacy and confidentially in information services. The committee also assists the leaders of the organization in keeping the mission and values of the organization in the forefront of their decision making.

In this author's experience, religious organizations are most likely to have an executive with grounding in religious doctrine and ethics and the authority to speak out in the decision-making process. Therefore, this author disagrees with Talone and would recommend such a person chair the committee.

If such a person does not exist in the organization, then an investment in ethical training for an executive would be worthwhile. There are numerous on-line ethics certificate courses (e.g., University of New Mexico Business Ethics Certificate) and week-long in-person training (e.g., Kennedy Institute of Ethics). Training should also to be offered to other committee members. Attendance at any training as a whole committee would support discussion about the relevance of the information and cases for their institution.

Conclusion

Though the focus of clinical ethics committees and organizational ethics committees are different, both support the maintenance of the ethical environment of the organization. The original primary mission of the clinical committees should be the same for the organizational committees—education, policy formulation and case consultation. Models for organizational ethics include a separate committee or a subcommittee of clinical ethics committees. Whatever model is chosen to support organizational ethics, the advisory recommendations need serious consideration. Even though these recommendations will not have the authority of compliance regulations, they will be seen as important if they support the integrity of the organization. Healthcare professionals need the help of these organizational resources to support the ethical culture and effective reporting mechanisms.

Key Points to Remember

1. The purpose of the clinical ethics committee is threefold—education, policy formation, and case consultation.
2. Three models exist for provision of case consultation: (1) an individual consultant who reports to the entire committee on the results of a consultation; (2) a team of committee members; and (3) the entire committee.
3. Clinical ethics focuses on clinicians at the bedside; organizational ethics focuses on how the business issues impact patients.
4. The focal point of organizational ethics is primarily the administration's financial, business, and contractual decisions.
5. A compliance focus assumes that the organization knows the obvious right and wrong and relies on auditing, sanction, and hotlines to enforce the right choice.
6. An organizational ethics view is reflective in nature, discussing competing ethical alternatives to resolve specific situations, as well as the development of values and policies.

7. Codes of conduct and polices for enforcement are a good starting point, but compliance to regulations is necessary, but not sufficient, for achieving an ethical organization.
8. An organizational ethics committee provides an opportunity for stepping back from a situation, taking time for ethical reflection on mission statements and values, and examining appropriate conduct in each situation.
9. Healthcare executives must scrutinize the administrative practice of "aggressive accounting" for ethical conflict, just as they scrutinize conflicts of interest or diversity.
10. Organizational ethics committees could assist and support healthcare institutions to meet the challenging task of reducing the gap between what is ethical and what is desirable for business.
11. An integrated organizational-clinical model reduces the dichotomy between clinical and organizational ethics and facilitates the development of effective systems-level responses.
12. Members of clinical ethics committee should be competent in their own fields of expertise; willing to do preparatory work necessary for deliberations; capable of ethical discourse, as distinguished from argumentative or passive acceptance of other's stance; informed of the organization's mission, vision, values, and code of conduct; and recognized for honesty and integrity. Members should include an ethicist.
13. Chair of organizational ethics committee should be a leader with a focus on the organization's mission or someone else in a senior leadership position. Committee members should include representatives of management and healthcare professionals.

References

American Academy of Pediatrics, Committee on Bioethics. (2001). Institutional ethics committees. *Pediatrics, 107*, 205–209.

Borawski, D. (1995). Ethical dilemmas for nurse administrators. *Journal of Nursing Administration, 27*, 60–62.

Boyle, P.J., Dubose, E.R., Ellingson, S.J., Guinn, D.E., & McCurdy, D.B. (2001). *Organizational ethics in health care: Principles, cases and practical solutions.* San Francisco: Jossey-Bass.

Cook, A., Hoas, H., & Joyner, J. (2000). Ethics and the rural nurse: A study of problems, values and needs. *Journal of Nursing Law, 7*(1), 41–51.

Cooper, R.W., Frank, G.L., Gouty, C.A., & Hansen, M.C. (2002). Key ethical issues encountered in healthcare organizations. *Journal of Nursing Administration, 32*(6), 331–337.

Department of Justice. *Tenet Healthcare Corporation to pay U.S. more than $900 million to resolve False Claims Act allegations.* June 29, 2006. Retrieved July 1, 2008, from http://www.usdoj.gov/opa/pr/2006/June/06_civ_406.html

Foglia, M.B., & Pearlman, R.A. (2006). Integrating clinical and organizational ethics. *Health Progress, 87*(2), 31–35.

Gostin, L.O. (1997). Deciding life and death in the courtroom from Quinlan to Cruzan, Glucksberg and Vacco: A brief history and analysis of constitutional protection of the "right to die." *JAMA, 278*, 1523–1528.

Joint Commission on Accreditation of Healthcare Organizations. (1995). *Accreditation manual for hospitals.* Oakbrook Terrace, IL: JCAHO.

Kennedy Institute of Ethics. Retrieved July 1, 2008, from http://kennedyinstitute.georgetown.edu/

Khusf, G. (1998). The scope of organizational ethics. *HEC Forum, 10*(2), 127–135.

Khusf, G., & Tong, R. (2002). Setting organizational ethics within a broader social and legal context. *HEC Forum, 14*(2), 77–85.

Lipp, A. (1998). An inquiry into a combined approach for nursing ethics. *Nursing Ethics, 5*(2), 122–138.

McDaniel, C. (2004). *Organizational ethics: Research and ethical environment.* Surrey, UK: Ashgate Publishing.

O'Toole, B. (2006). St. Louis system has a corporate ethics committee. *Health Progress, 87*(2), 42–45.

Prentz, R.D. (1998). Expanding into organizational ethics: The experience of one clinical ethics committee. *HEC Forum, 10*(2), 213–221.

Schyve, P. (1996). Patient rights and organizational ethics: The Joint Commission perspective. *Bioethics Forum, 12*(2), 13–20.

Seeley, C.R., & Goldberg, S.L. (1999). Integrated ethics: Synecdoche in healthcare. *Journal of Clinical Ethics, 10*(3), 202–209.

Silva, M.C. (1998). Organizational and administrative ethics in healthcare: An ethics gap. Online *Journal of Issues in Nursing.* Retrieved June 30, 2008, from http://www.nursingworld.org/ojin/topic8/topic8_1.htm

Talone, P.A. (2006). Starting an organizational ethics committee. *Health Progress, 87*(6), 34–37.

University of New Mexico Ethics Certificate program. Retrieved July 1, 2008, from http://www.e-businessethics.com/Ethics.htm

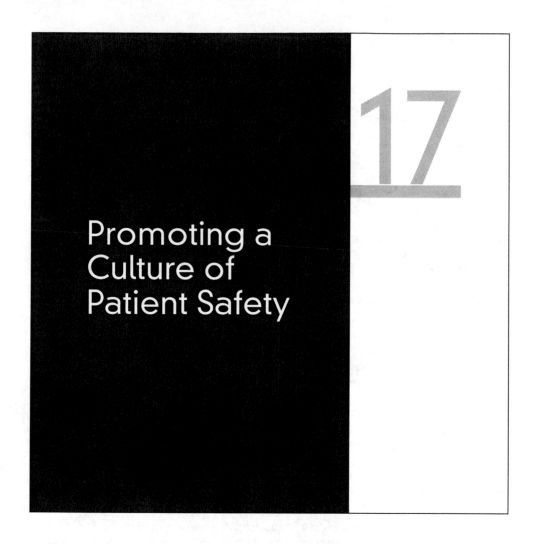

Promoting a Culture of Patient Safety

The safety of the people shall be the highest law.
—Marcus Tullius Cicero, one of the greatest Roman philosophers and
orators

The Institute of Medicine (IOM) released two reports that changed the way the public and members of the healthcare system think about patient safety and quality of care. The first report was *To Err is Human: Building a Safer Health System (1999)* and second was *Crossing the Quality Chasm: A New Health System for the 21st Century* (2001). This second report recommends a sweeping redesign of the healthcare system to improve quality of care and provides a suggested framework and key steps to accomplish this goal. Recommendations from these reports, as well as from the Joint Commission (2008a,b), are included in this chapter.

The recommendations are based on questions such as "What do organizations do differently to keep their infection and patient falls rates low?" Benchmark data from organizations that are successful in meeting these and national patient safety goals are also presented. To meet the nationally acknowledged benchmark of Magnet Recognition, a program that recognizes excellence in nursing, high standards of quality patient care must be met. Several examples from organizations that focus on patient safety will be offered as well. Finally, the key components necessary for a culture of patient safety are outlined. Thus, this chapter focuses on the macrolevel of reducing medication errors and not on the microlevel already addressed in Chapter 10.

Institute for Medicine Recommendations

Crossing the Quality Chasm: A New Health System for the 21st Century, published in March 2001, explains the perfect storm that has been created in health care by arguing that "Health care today is characterized by more to know, more to manage, more to watch, more to do and more people involved" (p. 25). Therefore, many opportunities exist for healthcare professionals to overlook the information necessary for making treatment decisions. Perhaps something distinctive about a particular patient's condition is missed—some information that might have been significant to the diagnosis or treatment decision (IOM, 2000). To the information about this perfect storm, I can add the fact that more patients than ever lack coordinated care for a chronic illness. Among the issues:

1. "Baby boomers," an aging population whose members want a say in the kind and location of their care.
2. Modern technology with its benefits, but also its abuses—particularly of terminally ill patients.
3. Fragmented health care insurance coverage or lack of access to coverage.
4. The complexity of our healthcare system.

A culture of safety focuses on systems and the reduction of individual blame, on data collection and reporting, and on leadership involvement. What responsibilities do the executive and management teams have to make the culture of safety a reality? They need to (1) articulate and model the importance of patient safety to all employees and physicians; (2) provide direction on eliminating barriers to success; (3) be open to the recommendations for quality improvement (QI) teams; and (4) ensure support of frontline staff when members demonstrate moral courage in the face of noncompliance by physicians. The primary focus for executives needs to be on the systems, policies, and strategies of benchmark organizations. "Employees need to see their superiors and peers demonstrate ethical behavior in the work they do and the decisions they make every day" (Seligson & Choi, 2006).

As described in *To Err Is Human* (Institute of Medicine, 1999), designing healthcare processes for safety requires a three-part strategy: (1) designing systems to prevent errors, (2) designing procedures to make errors visible when they do occur, and (3) designing procedures that can mitigate the harm to patients from errors that are not detected or intercepted. This is based on an engineering principle that can be stated as—*design for the usual, but recognize and plan for the unusual* (Institute of Medicine, 2001, p. 120). Process design should be explicit for the usual case, which is 80% of the work. For the remaining 20%, contingency plans should be assembled as needed.

Crossing the Quality Chasm specifies that the healthcare system must continue to support improvements with six aims in mind—safety, effectiveness, patient-centeredness, timeliness, efficiency, and equity. The Institute of Medicine defines six key challenges to support these aims:

1. Redesigning care processes.
2. Making effective use of information technologies.
3. Managing clinical knowledge and skills.
4. Developing effective teams.
5. Coordinating care across patient conditions, services and settings over time.
6. Incorporating performance and outcome measurements for improvement and accountability. (IOM, 2001, p. 117)

Redesigning the Care Processes

First, care processes must be reliable and should promote a strong relationship of trust among the caregiver, patient, and family. Reliability can be achieved by standardization, as shown in the following example. Duke University's pediatric emergency department uses a color-coded tape to measure a child's length and approximate weight range (IOM, 2001, p. 121). Then color-coded supplies, such as IV tubing and syringes, correspond to the four weight ranges. Standardizing equipment for each color zone ensures that dosages and equipment are appropriate and safe for children in each range.

Effective Use of Information Technologies

Health care delivery has been relatively untouched by the revolution in information technology. An example of the second challenge to make effective use of information technology is using pharmaceutical software to alert the prescriber to an incorrect dose or possible interaction with another medication. The internet has enormous potential to transform through information technology applications such as consumer health, clinical care, and biomedical research.

Managing Clinical Knowledge and Skills

The third challenge is managing clinical knowledge and skills. The flood of new information that is relevant to a medical practice can no longer be adequately managed by individual clinicians. It is impossible to keep up with the literature or with new developments by attending conferences or lectures. Clinicians need evidence-based guidelines that make clear which steps are well founded and which are based on expert consensus.

Developing Effective Teams

The fourth challenge is assuring that all healthcare professionals are operating as a team. Donaldson and Mohr (2000) emphasized that the team should be the base for quality improvement work. The team needs to recognize the contributions that all members of the group could make, with various individuals taking leadership roles for specific improvement activities.

Coordinating Care Across Patient Conditions. Services. and Settings Over Time

The fifth key challenge for organizations is coordination (or clinical integration) of work across services. Most baby boomers will have at least one chronic disease, and this will call for integration of services. For example, coordination may involve nurse case managers transmitting information to both a primary and a specialty care practitioner about a patient's unmet needs. Coordination of care across clinicians and settings has been shown to result in greater efficiency and better clinical outcomes (Shortell et al., 2000).

Incorporating Performance and Outcome Measurements for Improvement and Accountability

The sixth challenge is holding everyone accountable for incorporating performance and outcome measurements. Clinical practices that participated in the IOM study of exemplary practices described how routine performance measurement has become part of their production process (Donaldson & Mohr, 2000). Quality can be measured with a degree of scientific precision equal to that of most of the measures used to take care of patients today.

Growing Complexity of Health Care

In a follow-up report from IOM, *Health Professions Education: A Bridge to Quality* (2003), the Committee on the Health Professions Education stated, "All health professionals should be educated to deliver patient-centered care as members of an interdisciplinary team, emphasizing evidence-based practice, quality improvement approaches, and informatics" (p. 3). Nurses who combine a doctoral education with clinical, organizational, economic, and leadership skills will be most successful at critiquing nursing. They are also best able to analyze clinical scientific findings, design programs for the delivery of care, and foster a culture of patient safety.

The growing complexity of health care, the burgeoning growth in scientific knowledge, and the increasing sophistication of technology has changed nursing education. APNs now need a master's degree that requires hours of study and training far beyond that required in virtually any other field (American Association of Colleges of Nursing [AACN] & National Organization of Nurse Practitioner Faculties, 2002).

In March 2002, the American Association of Colleges of Nursing (AACN) Board of Directors charged a task force with the responsibility to examine the current status of clinical or practice doctoral programs, compare various models, and make recommendations regarding future development. As a result, the AACN made 12 recommendations. Its position statement affirmed that practice-focused doctoral nursing programs should include seven essential areas of content. Of the seven, two focus directly on the skills needed to improve the culture of safety: (1) organization and system leadership/management, quality improvement, and system thinking and (2) analytic methodologies related to the evaluation of practice and the application of evidence for practice (AACN, 2004).

Joint Commission and Magnet Recognition System Approaches

The Joint Commission (2008a) defines *Patient Safety Solutions* as "Any system design or intervention that has demonstrated the ability to prevent or mitigate patient harm stemming from the processes of health care." The development of Patient Safety Solutions is a joint initiative of the Joint Commission and the Joint Commission International in its role as a WHO Collaborating Center for Patient Safety. In April 2007, they published nine inaugural patient safety solutions. Each creates responsibilities for the individual healthcare provider, but the evidence-based suggested actions for the organizational system are many.

These solutions are driven by the need to redesign care processes so that foreseeable human errors are prevented. For example, the continuing failure to correctly name patients leads to medication, transfusion, and testing errors, as well as wrong person procedures. Organizations can hold each employee accountable for checking the identity of the patient and encouraging patients to "speak up" (Joint Commission, 2008b), but system approaches, such as clear organizational protocols for identifying patients (e.g., name and date of birth) or biometrics, will be more effective and are likelier to reduce patient risk.

For those who are unfamiliar with The Magnet Recognition Program® for excellence in nursing, it is based and administered by the American Nurses Credentialing Center (ANCC, 2009). Magnet hospitals have embarked on a far-reaching review and methodical evaluation of nursing practice. They must meet rigorous quantitative and qualitative standards that delineate the highest quality of nursing practice and patient care. Becoming a Magnet hospital means that the organization has met more than 65 standards developed by the ANCC. The standards must be demonstrated in an extensive written document and validated and clarified by a site visit. The Magnet designation signifies that the hospital has crafted an environment that sustains professional nursing practice and focuses on professional autonomy, decision making at the bedside, nursing involvement in determining the nursing work environment, professional education, career development, and nursing leadership. This can only be accomplished in a hospital that always puts patient care first.

A hospital must meet 14 standards of care and practice, including categories such as clinical skill and leadership, to receive a rating of Magnet status Force 6 for Quality of Care and a Force 7 for Quality Improvement. In a Magnet hospital, quality is the systematic driving force for nursing and the organization. Nurses serving in leadership positions are accountable for providing an environment that influences patient outcomes. There is a persistent perception among nurses that they provide high-quality care to patients. The organization has structures and processes for the measurement of quality and programs for improving the quality of care and services within the organization. Together, these forces promote an organizational culture of safety.

Magnet hospitals must document their commitment to patient safety, quality care, and support for nurses. The process for achieving Magnet recognition requires years of effort and collaboration among hospital departments and physicians. A Magnet hospital functions well as a team. Research has also shown that

Magnet hospitals achieve higher levels of patient satisfaction and lower mortality and complication rates.

The empowerment seen in Magnet hospital cultures correlates well with the culture of patient safety. Lake (2002) identified five aspects of the work environment that define a Magnet hospital's nursing settings: nurse participation in hospital affairs; nursing foundations for quality of care; nurse manager ability, leadership, and support of nurses; staffing and resource adequacy; and collegial nurse-physician relations. Laschinger and Leiter (in press) found that these characteristics were significantly related to staff nurse burnout and patient safety outcomes. Armstrong and Laschinger's (2006) study attempted to understand how organizational structures interrelate to create a culture of safety that enables nurses to provide the highest quality of patient care possible. Greater staff nurse workplace empowerment was associated with higher ratings of patient safety. Other models can coexist with The Magnet Recognition Program® to assure patient safety.

Human Factors and Reliability Science

Over the past 20 years, many models have been proposed for redesigning operational and clinical processes to improve quality, reduce cost, improve patient satisfaction, and now, advance patient safety. Work transformation and reengineering were replaced by Kaizen (Kaizen Institute, 2007) and Six Sigma (Six Sigma, 2007). A review of the literature shows that progress has been made, but significant concerns regarding patient errors reveal that we still need to find a better way. Two disciplines offer possibilities for further improvements in effectiveness, efficiency, and safety—human factors engineering and reliability science.

Human Factors Engineering

Human factors engineering is the discipline that studies human capabilities and limitations and applies that knowledge to the design of safe, effective, and comfortable products, processes, and systems (Bosten-Fleischhauer, 2008). Human factors engineering, which is sometimes called ergonomics, is a scientific discipline attempting to appreciate the interactions among humans and the other essentials in the work system.

All components of a work system designed for patient safety must be considered equally to design an effective, efficient, and safe admission, transfer, and discharge system. For example, some people have limitations, such as short-term memory capacity, fatigue, and stressful organizational conditions, that could affect the person's ability to cooperate. If these limitations are not considered, they could impact the "hand-off" in these systems. If the system design fails to pay attention to human limitations, standardization will not occur. Every human interacting with the process will adapt it to his or her needs. This will lead to workarounds, shortcuts, and a propensity for error.

SBAR, discussed in Chapter 10, is a positive example of human factors application. This model provides for effective physician-nurse communication because it follows the normal flow of physician thinking. Unfortunately, many computerized physician order entry (CPOE) systems are inefficient, and design flaws create too much of a reliance on human memory and involve many isolated steps. The logic that physicians use in thinking through a diagnosis and then treatment implications is too often lacking.

Crew Resource Management, a human factors process also mentioned in Chapter 10, has found that pilots who were superior leaders shared some traits in common that are relevant to the teamwork required in healthcare crew members (Pizzi, 2001). These traits include:

- Encouraging crew members to question decisions.
- Acting sensitive to other crew members' problems.
- Recognizing the need to communicate plans and strategies.
- Providing training to fellow team members.

Team members who lack the moral courage to question leaders (physicians or managers) could cause serious communication breakdowns leading to patient harm.

Reliability Science

The goal of *reliability science* is to create a failure-free operation. It is a scientific method of evaluating, calculating, and improving the overall reliability of a complex system. The Institute for Healthcare Improvement (IHI) has defined reliability as "the measurable ability of health-related process, procedure, or service to perform its intended function in the required time under commonly occurring conditions" (Nolan, Resar, Haraden, & Griffin, 2004, p.4). To calculate reliability, the number of actions taken that achieve the intended results are divided by the total number of actions. They are reflected in parts per 10, 100, 1000, and 10,000. For example 10^{-6} generally compares to Six Sigma performance. These metrics can provide executives with concrete guidelines of reliability. Reliability science advocates an achievement rate of 90% (10^{-1}) reliability as the threshold performance metric for health care. This means that for every 100 times the process is done right, 10 times it is done wrong.

According to reliability science, if the process, product, or system exhibit less than 80% reliability, the operation is totally unreliable. In a recent Joint Commission survey, an organization's remediation plan required that medications be reconciled across the continuum of care 80% of the time (#8 patient safety goal) for three months. In theory, this organization, which initially had a 60% rating, should be celebrating if it achieved a 75% rating, but the improved process is still chaotic according to reliability science. HealthPartners Regions Hospital designed a project to ensure the accuracy of the electronic medication reconciliation (EMR) medication list and the patient's understanding of medications in the week following discharge for congestive heart failure (Averbeck, 2006). The results were that for 6 out of 79 patients, as clinically significant medications were identified not reconciled, even though this procedure was able to potentially mitigate a readmission for these patients. Executives and managers clearly need to rethink organizational benchmarks if they want to create a culture of safety.

An example of a reliable design (10^{-1}) is summarized below to provide a point of reference (IHI, 2006). It requires:

- Standardization of process.
- Common equipment and standard order sheets.
- Personal checklists.
- Policies/procedures that are documented.
- Awareness of policies/procedures and training.
- Feedback on user compliance with policies and procedures.
- Feedback that shows less than 100% performance means more training, awareness building, and harder work.

Unfortunately, we frequently still see a number of ineffective approaches to achieving reliability, such as different colored constraints with flags or warnings, no overrides, and visual cues. Although these are necessary at earlier stages in the development of a safety culture, standardization of the process should evolve as systems need to support healthcare professionals in doing it right all of the time.

High reliability organizations achieve success because of their systematic approach. The High Reliability Organizations (HRO) model has five elements:

- *process auditing*—a system of on-going checks to monitor hazardous conditions.
- *a reward system*—expected social compensation to reinforce correct behavior or disciplinary action for incorrect behavior.
- *quality assurance*—policies and procedures that promote high-quality performance.
- *risk management*—how the organization perceives risk and takes corrective action.
- *command and control*—policies, procedures, and communication processes used to mitigate risk (Roberts, 1993).

When these elements are in place, they serve as a check to the pressure in hospitals to work quickly and efficiently with few delays. Left unchecked, such pressure can encourage overrides of safety procedures.

Two significant studies in the perioperative area used the Hospital Survey on Patient Safety Cultures created with funding from AHRQ (Marshall & Manus, 2007; Scherer & Fitzpatrick, 2008). This survey has 12 key dimensions of patient safety and can be accessed from the AHRQ Web site. Marshall and Manus (2007) studied five sites ranging from 50 to 1,700 beds using a prepost survey. The familiar obstacle of gaining physician buy-in was surmounted by recruiting physician champions. Specific changes for the staff from this study were shared in Chapter 10. From an organizational perspective, it was disappointing that the least improvements occurred in "organizational learning/continuous improvement," "feedback and communication about the error," and "communication openness" (only a 3%–4% improvement). It sounds as if better mechanisms need to be put in place for feedback and for evaluation of effectiveness of the changes to reduce errors. The arena of "communication openness" is specifi-

cally relevant to moral courage. Below are the three items from the questionnaire specific to "communication openness":

- Staff will speak up freely if they see something that may negatively impact patient care.
- Staff feels free to question the decisions or actions of those in authority.
- Staff is afraid to ask questions when something does not seem right (re-
  versed).

Surgeons and anesthesiologists thought communication openness was very good,
while RNs/surgical technologists rated it much lower. However, among certified
registered nurse anesthetists (CRNAs), the lack of "communication openness"
was the only item in the survey ranked in the negative. No explanation was given
for this result. As a result of the survey, several procedures were put in place in
the surgical suite to make it safer for staff to speak out.

In their 2008 study at a 172-bed hospital, Scherer and Fitzpatrick compared
the views of 40 physicians and 43 RNs on a hospital survey assessing perceptions of safety in the perioperative setting. Although the majority of respondents
answered positively, significant differences between physician and RN perceptions occurred in the areas of "supervisor/manager expectations and actions
promoting safety" and "feedback and communication about error." Nurses rating these two items lower than did the physicians. These researchers found that
clinicians were more negative in their responses than nonclinicians. Although
the nursing management team had been in place for less than a year, there was
clearly need for improvement in those arenas. High uniformity of a safety mind
set is crucial to bring to fruition a safety culture (Singer et al., 2003).

Zohar, Livne, Tenne-Gazil, Admi, and Donchin (2007) studied the results
of a hospital climate and unit climate survey on the ability to predict nursing-
related medication and emergency safety six months after implementation of
new policies in three tertiary hospitals in Israel. Results indicated that the
higher the climate strength (strong), the greater the agreement among employees regarding the priorities of patient safety. This study supports the expectation
that technical and administrative changes must be accompanied by a change
led by organization executives and managers. These changes must make patient
safety a front-and-center priority. A positive unit climate led by nursing managers was able to compensate for the injurious effect of the overall hospital climate. The researchers concluded that when there is high agreement among the
unit staff, the level of unit climate better predicts safety outcomes. These results
support the extensive evidence gathered over more than 20 years and the recommendation of IOM that patient safety initiatives be designed to affect the
organizational context.

Nurse-Physician Communication and Collaboration for Patient Safety

Nurse-physician collaboration not only results in improved outcomes for patients
but also in a reduction in actual mortality rates (Baggs et al., 1999; Knaus, Drape,
Wagner, & Zimmerman, 1986). However, collaboration is defined differently by

17.1 AACN Standards for Establishing and Sustaining Healthy Work Environments

1. Skilled communication: nurses must be proficient in communication skills as they are in clinical skills
2. True collaboration: nurses must be relentless in pursuing and fostering true collaboration
3. Effective decision making: nurses must be valued and committed partners in making policy, directing and evaluating clinical care and leading organizational operations
4. Appropriate staffing: staffing must ensure the effective match between patient needs and nurse competencies
5. Meaningful recognition: nurses must be recognized and must recognize others for the values each brings to the work of the organization
6. Authentic leadership: nurse leaders must fully embrace the imperative of a healthy work environment, authentically live it and engage others in its achievement

Reprinted from "AACN standards for establishing and sustaining healthy work environments: A journey to excellence. Executive Summary," by American Association of Critical-Care Nurses. Retrieved December 31, 2008, from http://www.aacn.org/WD/HWE/Docs?ExecSum.pdf. Copyright 2005 by American Association of Critical-Care Nurses. Reprinted with permission.

nurses and physicians, with nurses repeatedly less satisfied with quality of collaboration (Thomas, Sexton, & Helmreich, 2004). Two of the American Association of Critical-Care Nurses (AACN) standards identified skilled communication and true collaboration as specific to achieving the goal of patient-focused care and patient safety.

The AACN and the American College of Chest Physicians (ACCP) created two projects that are synergistic in creating true collaboration, quality care, and patient safety improvement (McCauley & Irwin, 2006). AACN (2005) developed "Standards for Establishing and Sustaining Healthy Work Environments: A Journey to Excellence" (see Exhibit 17.1). These six standards resulted from research evidence about what is needed to create a work environment that supports nurse job retention and satisfaction and improves patient outcomes, especially in area of patient safety. The ACCP synergistic project was a patient-focused care initiative that viewed every encounter with a patient as an opportunity to deliver the same care that physicians would want for their own family member. This projected created a pledge that has received remarkably favorable responses in the United States and worldwide (See Exhibit 17.2).

McCauley and Irwin (2006) speak at length about the short- and long-term changes necessary to foster true collaboration. A few of their ideas include interdisciplinary rounds, use of the SBAR model, incorporation of the patient's family as integral member(s) of the decision-making team, and interdisciplinary educational efforts, including adjusting the totally separate medicine and nursing school curriculums. They also addressed the need for a high level of personal integrity for all team members and the need for all to speak up if the patient is affected by incompetence or ineffective systems. They conclude their article with a description of a new design for critical care initiated at the University of Massachusetts Memorial Medical Center that could serve as a model for collaboration even beyond the ICU environment. For example, nurse managers and medical directors are considered peers who are equally accountability for clinical outcomes and the performance of their professional team. They have also incorporated acute-care nurse practitioners and physician assistants into the interdisciplinary team to provide rapid responses to the short-term needs of the patients. This organization obviously took IOM's fourth challenge seriously—developing effective teams.

Conclusion

The Institute of Medicine brought to light patient safety issues with two reports: *To Err is Human: Building a Safer Health System (1999)* and *Crossing the Quality Chasm: A New Health System for the 21st Century* (2001). Since the release of these reports, healthcare organizations have tried a multitude of methods to improve patient safety, with the primary focus on the Joint Commission's patient safety goals. I believe we need to go deeper into the problem and tease out what makes the difference in safety from one organization to another. The use of human factor engineering and reliability science could provide the tools for managing mistakes resulting from human error and lack of reliable design. Because all team members touch a patient on a daily basis, the work of AACN and ACCP provides guidance on some key communication and clinical processes that make intensive care safer. But all the policies, procedures, and processes will fail if the executive and managerial team members do not demonstrate in words and actions that their priority is patient safety. Actions do speak louder than words (Seligson & Choi, 2006).

Key Points to Remember

1. The *Crossing the Quality Chasm—A New Health System for the 21st Century* (2001) report recommends a sweeping redesign of the healthcare system to

improve quality of care and provides a suggested framework and key steps to accomplish this goal.

2. "Health care today is characterized by more to know, more to manage, more to watch, more to do and more people involved."

3. A culture of safety focuses on systems and reduction of individual blame, on data collection and reporting and on leadership involvement.

4. Executive and management team responsibilities that create a culture of safety are the following: (1) articulate and model the importance of patient safety to all employees and physicians; (2) provide direction on eliminating barriers to success; (3) be open to the recommendations of quality improvement (QI) teams; and (4) ensure support of frontline staff when they demonstrate moral courage in the face of noncompliance by physicians.

5. Design healthcare processes for safety in a three-part strategy: (1) designing systems to prevent errors, (2) designing procedures to make errors visible when they do occur, and (3) designing procedures that can mitigate the harm to patients from errors that are not detected or intercepted.

6. Process design should be explicit for the usual case, which is 80% of the work; for the remaining 20%, contingency plans should be assembled as needed.

7. Healthcare system needs to support continued improvement using six aims— safety, effectiveness, patient-centeredness, timeliness, efficiency and equity.

8. Care processes must be reliable and they must also pay attention to building a relationship with a caregiver that meets the expectations of both the patient and the family.

9. Two disciplines offer possibilities for further improvements in effectiveness, efficiency and safety—human factors engineering and reliability science.

10. *Human factors engineering* is the discipline that studies human capabilities and limitations and applies that knowledge to the design of safe, effective and comfortable products, processes, and systems for the human beings involved.

11. Crew Resource Management, a human factors process, has found that pilots who were superior leaders shared some traits in common that are relevant to the teamwork required in healthcare crew members.

12. Reliability science is "The measurable ability of health-related process, procedure, or service to perform its intended function in the required time under commonly occurring conditions."

13. According to reliability science if the process, product, or system exhibit less than 80% reliability, then the operation is totally unreliable.

14. High Reliability Organizations (HRO) model has five elements—process auditing, reward system, quality assurance, risk management, command and control.

15. The results of several studies support the extensive evidence gathered over more than 20 years and the recommendation of IOM that patient safety initiatives be designed to affect the organizational context.

16. Two of the American Association of Critical-Care Nurses (AACN) standards identified that skilled communication and true collaboration are specific to achieving the goal of patient-focused care and patient safety.

17. Short- and long-term changes necessary to foster true nurse-physician collaboration are interdisciplinary rounds, use of the SBAR model, incorporation of the patient's family as integral member(s) of decision-making team

and interdisciplinary educational efforts including rectifying the totally separate medicine and nursing school curriculums.

18. *Patient Safety Solutions* is defined as "any system design or intervention that has demonstrated the ability to prevent or mitigate patient harm stemming from the processes of health care."

19. Greater staff nurse workplace empowerment was found to be associated with higher ratings of patient safety culture in Magnet work settings.

References

American Association of Colleges of Nursing. (2004, October). *AACN position statement on the practice doctorate in nursing*. Retrieved January 2, 2009, from http://www.aacn.nche.edu/dnp/pdf/DNP.pdf

American Association of Colleges of Nursing & National Organization of Nurse Practitioner Faculties. (2002). *Master's-level nurse practitioner educational programs. Findings from the 2000–2001 collaborative curriculum survey*. Washington, DC: AACN.

American Association of Critical-Care Nurses (AACN). (2005). AACN standards for establishing and sustaining healthy work environments: A journey to excellence. *American Journal of Critical Care, 14*, 187–197.

American Nurses Credentialing Center. *The Magnet Recognition Program®*. Retrieved January 2, 2009, from http://www.nursecredentialing.org/Magnet/ProgramOverview.aspx

Armstrong, K.J., & Laschinger, H. (2006). Structural empowerment, Magnet hospital characteristics, and patient safety culture: Making the link. *Journal of Nursing Care Quality, 21*(2), 124–132.

Averbeck, B., Kealey, B., Huebsch, J., Carpenter, J., Lindquist, T., & McCarty, M. (2006). *Medication reconciliation across the continuum*. Retrieved August 1, 2008, from http://www.ihi.org/IHI/Topics/Reliability/ReliabilityGeneral/ImprovementStories/MedicationReconciliationAcrosstheContinuum.htm

Baggs, J.C., Schmidt, M.H., Mushlin, A.I, Mitchell, P.H., Eldredge, D.H., Oakes D., & Hutson, A.D. (1999). Association between nurse physician collaboration and patient outcomes in three intensive care units. *Critical Care Medicine, 27*(9), 1991–1998.

Bosten-Fleischhauer, C. (2008). Enhancing healthcare process design with human factors engineering and reliability science, Part 1. *Journal of Nursing Administration, 38*(1), 27–32.

Donaldson, M.S., & Mohr, J.J. (2000). *Exploring innovation and quality improvement in health care micro-systems: A cross-case analysis*. Washington, DC: Institute of Medicine, National Academy Press.

Hospital Survey on Patient Safety Culture. (2007). *AHRQ*. Retrieved March 7, 2008, from http://www.ahrq.gov/qual/hospculture

Institute of Medicine. (2001). *Crossing the quality chasm: A new health system for the 21st century*. Washington, DC: National Academy Press.

Institute of Medicine. (2003). *Health professions education: A bridge to quality*. Washington, DC: National Academy Press.

Irwin, R. (2004). Patient-focused care: The 2003 American College of Chest Physicians convocation speech. *Chest, 125*, 1910–1912.

Joint Commission. (2008a). *Patient safety solutions*. Retrieved January 2, 2009, from http://www.jointcommission.org/PatientSafety/NationalPatientSafetyGoals/

Joint Commission. (2008b). *Speak up initiatives*. Retrieved January 2, 2009, from http://www.jointcommission.org/PatientSafety/SpeakUp/

Kaizen Institute. (2007). Retrieved August 1, 2008, from http://www.kaizen.com/

Knaus, W.A, Drape, E.S., Wagner, D.P., & Zimmerman J.E. (1986). An evaluation of the outcome from intensive care in major medical centers. *Annals of Internal Medicine, 105*(3), 410–418.

Lake, E. (2002).Development of the practice environment scale of the nursing work index. *Research in Nursing and Health, 25*, 176–188.

Laschinger, H.K., & Leiter, M. The impact of nursing work environments on patient safety outcomes: the mediating role of burnout/engagement. *Journal of Nursing Administration*. In press.

Marshall, D.A., & Manus, D.A. (2007). A team training program using human factors to enhance patient safety. *AORN Journal, 86*(6), 994–1011.

McCauley, K., & Irwin, R.S. (2006). Changing the work environment in ICUs to achieve patient-focused care: The time has come. *Chest, 130,* 1571–1578.

New hospital alliance seeks to address medical errors. Retrieved August 1, 2008, from http://www.medicalnewstoday.com/articles/71497.php

Nolan, T., Resar, R., Haraden, C., & Griffin, F.A. (2004). *Improving the reliability of health care.* IHI Innovation Series white paper. Boston: Institute for Healthcare Improvement. Retrieved January 2, 2009, from http://www.ihi.org/IHI/Results/WhitePapers/Improvingthe ReliabilityofHealthCare.htm

Pizzi, L., Goldfarb, N.I.., & Nash, D.B. (2001). Crew resource management and its application in medicine. In *Making health care safer: A critical analysis of patient safety practices.* Rockville, MD; AHRQ (Publication # 01-E058). Retrieved March 6, 2008 from http://www.ahrq.gov/clinic/ptsafety/

Roberts, K.H. (1993). Cultural characteristics of reliability enhancing organizations. *Journal of Managerial Issues, 5*(2), 165–181.

Scherer, D., & Fitzpatrick, J.J. (2008). Perceptions of patient safety culture among physicians and RNs in the perioperative area. *AORN Journal, 87*(1), 163–174.

Seligson, A., & Choi, L. (2006). *Critical elements of an organizational ethical culture.* Washington, DC: Ethics Resource Center.

Shortell, S.M., Gilles, R.R., & Anderson, D.A. (2000). *Remaking health care in America* (2nd ed.). San Francisco, CA: Jossey-Bass.

Singer, S.J., Gaba, D.M., Geppert, J.J., Sinaiko, A.D., Howard, S.K., & Park, K.C. (2003). The culture of safety: Results of an organization-wide survey in 15 California hospitals. *Quality and Safety in Health Care, 12*(2), 112–118.

Six Sigma. Retrieved August 1, 2008, from http://www.isixsigma.com/sixsigma/six_sigma.asp

Thomas, E.J., Sexton, J.B., & Helmreich, R.L. (2003). Discrepant attitudes about teamwork among critical care nurses and physicians. *Critical Care Medicine, 31,* 956–959.

Zohar, D., Livne, Y., Tenne-Gazil, O., Admi, H., & Donchin, Y. (2007). Healthcare climate: A framework for measuring and improving patient safety. *Critical Care Medicine, 35*(5), 1312–1317.

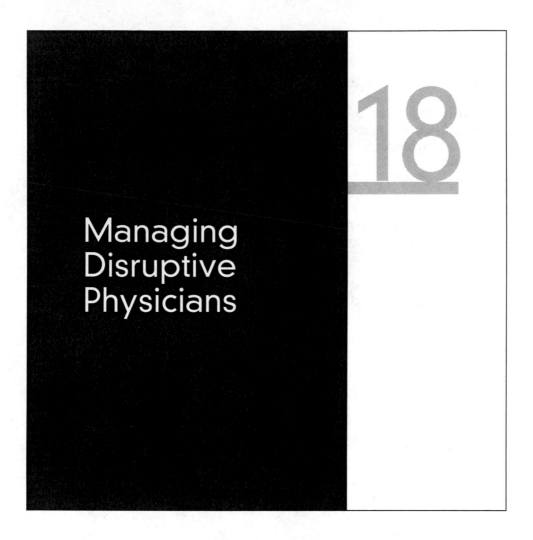

Managing Disruptive Physicians

Disruptive behavior causes stress, anxiety, frustration, and anger, which can impede communication and collaboration, which can result in avoidable medical errors, adverse events, and other compromises in quality care.

—Alan H. Rosenstein, MD, and Michelle O'Daniel, MHA (2008), researchers on quality

Disruptive physicians not only threaten the morale and retention of healthcare professionals and other staff, but newer information indicates that they are a threat to patient safety (Rosenstein & O'Daniel, 2005; Weber, 2004). This chapter analyzes the results of a physician's disruptive behavior on the staff, patients, and organization; strategies for resolving difficulties in reporting such behavior; and, the steps for creating an effective organizational system to prevent and resolve this threat. After defining the types of disruptive behaviors, the focus will be primarily on how to increase the moral courage of all those involved so they can confront and report the disruptive behavior.

Examples of Disruptive Behavior

The American Medical Association (AMA) defines disruptive behavior as "a style of interaction with physicians, hospital personnel, patients, family members, or others that interferes with patient care . . . [and] that tends to cause distress among other staff and affect overall morale within the work environment, undermining productivity and possibly leading to higher staff turnover or even resulting in ineffective or substandard care . . ." (2000, p. 2). It is easy to see how a physician's swearing or use of foul, profane, or crude language would negatively affect patient care, but a physician's unwillingness to adhere to practice/hospital standards can have an equal impact. Exhibit 18.1 lists examples of disruptive behavior, with the most common being disrespect, yelling, insulting others, and a refusal to carry out duties (ACOG Committee opinion, 2007; Bauman, 2006; Lazoritz & Carlson, 2008; Pfifferling, 1999; Weber, 2004). Because the targets of these behaviors are often healthcare professionals and staff with lesser power, the consequence is a distortion of teamwork. The communication goal of teamwork is to treat each other with courtesy and respect. Disruptive behavior fails to demonstrate cooperation and respect for the dignity of all involved.

Occurrence of Behavior

It is estimated that 3% to 5% of physicians engage in disruptive behavior, although the Rosenstein and O'Daniel (2005) study indicated 1% to 3%. Weber sent a survey to 1,600 physician executives, and respondents said they observed problems with physician behavior weekly (14%) or monthly (18%). Fully 70% of Weber's survey respondents stated that physician problems involved the same people over and over again.

Some recent studies lead us to believe that this behavior begins in medical school, where the most common behaviors are irresponsibility and a diminished ability to improve the behavior (Papadakis et al., 2005). Papadakis and colleagues studied 235 graduates from three medical schools who were disciplined by state medical boards and compared them to a matched control group of 469 physicians. Disciplinary action was strongly associated with prior unprofessional behavior in medical school. Examples of irresponsibility were unreliable attendance and lack of follow-up on patient care. Diminished capacity for self-improvement was seen as the inability to accept constructive criticism, argumentativeness, and a poor attitude. Compared to the control group, the physicians who had been disciplined were more likely to have impaired relationships with students, residents, faculty, and nurses. In this case-controlled study, physicians who were disciplined by state medical licensing boards were three times as likely to have exhibited unprofessional behavior in medical school.

The 2005 Stern, Frohna, and Gruppen study was conducted in a medical school in Michigan on 183 graduates. The results reveal that conscientious behavior, as measured by not obtaining the four required immunizations and completing course evaluations in preclinical years, was predictive of lack of professionalism in clinical settings. Feedback to graduates who needed improvement had no effect. The only other preclinical predictor variable that proved accurate

18.1   Examples of Disruptive Behaviors

Yelling/shouting, insulting others or sarcasm and cynicism

Anger outbursts, rudeness and verbal threats

Swearing or using foul, profane or crude language; ethnic or racial slurs

Physical intimidation—throwing objects, charts, etc.; pounding on desk; or invading
    another person's space with pointing finger in face of person or pushing

Offensive sexual humor, sexual innuendo, or sexual harassment

Derogatory comments about nurses, other physicians or hospital

Refusing to do tasks or respond to requests

Chronically late; unable to maintain a schedule

Inappropriate or inadequate chart notes; retaliatory notes in medical record

Unwillingness to adhere to practice/hospital standards

Not responding to call from HCP or pages in timely and appropriate manner

Unprofessional appearance or demeanor

Argumentative (always right, never wrong)

Complaining to patients about other physicians or staff or internal matters

Criticizing other healthcare professionals in front of patients or staff

Threats of retribution, violence, or legal action directed at staff, partners or patients

Exhibit is a summary from behaviors taken from ACOG Committee opinion, 2007; Bauman, 2006; Lazoritz & Carlson, 2008; Pfifferling, 1999; Weber, 2004.

was for students who underestimated their performance as measured against standardized patient evaluations. Perhaps this reflects humility not seen in the arrogance of disruptive physicians.

Rosenstein and O'Daniel (2008) reported the results from a total of 4,530 survey respondents from 2001 to 2006. Seventy-four percent reported witnessing disruptive behavior in physicians. Of interest is the fact that 56% of the physicians reported witnessing disruptive behavior in other physicians. The surgical specialties identified as more inclined to exhibit disruptive behavior were general surgery (31%), cardiovascular surgery (21%), neurosurgery (15%), orthopedic surgery (7%), and obstetrics/gynecology (6%). The repeatedly cited medical specialties were cardiology (7%), gastroenterology (4%), and neurology (4%). All other specialties were mentioned less than 3%. Although this chapter focuses on disruptive physicians, it is also important to mention that many of the respondents (64%) also witnessed disruptive behavior in nurses. Many nurses (70%) witnessed disruptive behavior initiated by other nurses. The regularity of instances of disruptive behavior events varied from never to daily. The most usual responses were that disruptive events occurred 1 to 2 times a month (35%) and 5 to 6 times a year (30%). The percentage of staff that exhibited these types of behaviors was 2% to 4% for both physicians and nurses.

Ultimately this disruptive behavior affects quality of care and patient safety, as healthcare professionals try to avoid the abusive physician. In the Rosenstein and O'Daniel (2008) study, 94% of the respondents thought that disruptive behavior could potentially have a negative impact on patient outcomes. In addition,

66% were aware of an adverse event that had occurred and almost 75% thought these events could have a serious, very serious, or extremely serious impact on patient outcomes. Some respondents (14%) reported that they were aware of a specific adverse event that occurred because of a disruptive behavior episode.

In an earlier study by Rosenstein and O'Daniel (2005), most (78%) of those who reported a disruptive event thought the adverse event could have been prevented. Examples were given of patients who required emergency intubation and transfer to the ICU because the physician did not act on information from a nurse or of a patient who had to be reopened because the physician refused to listen after being told twice that the sponge count was off.

According to a 2000 study conducted by Brigham and Women's Hospital and Harvard School of Public Health, adverse events occurred in 2.9% of hospitalizations (Thomas, Studdert, Burstin, et al., 2000). One is left to wonder how many of these adverse events in these 15,000 medical records in 28 hospitals were the result of disruptive physician behavior. Here are some of the comments from the 2005 Rosenstein and O'Daniel study (p. 25).

- "Adverse event related to med error because MD would not listen to RN."
- "RN did not call MD about a change in patient condition because he had a history of being abusive when called. Patient suffered because of this."
- "Cardiologist upset by phone calls and refused to come in. RN told not her job to think, just follow orders. Rx delayer. MI extended."
- "Communication between OB and delivery RN was hampered because of physician behavior. Resulted in poor outcome for newborn."
- "MD yelled at RN for calling at night, patient condition not addressed, resulting in negative patient outcome."

Other articles also speak to the importance of effective communication in preventing medical errors (Bates & Gawanda, 2003; Blendon, Des Roches, Brodie, et al., 2002). An effective handoff between clinicians and team members can not occur in an environment in which disrespect, yelling, and insults are present. Use of a standard communication strategy, such as the SBAR described in Chapter 10, can help frame a discussion about these concerns. The general public believes that this lack of ability to work as a team is a very important cause of medical errors; 67% of 1,207 survey respondents rated this as a failure causing errors (Blendon et al., 2002).

The Institute for Safe Medication Practice (2004) reported that 7 percent of medication errors could be the result of physician intimidation of nurses. On the whole, pharmacists and nurses register similar occurrences of intimidating behaviors by physicians. In the 12 months of this study, 64% of pharmacists and 34% of nurses reported that they had assumed a medication order was correct and safe rather than check by interacting with a particular physician. While more nurses (62%) than pharmacists (50%) believed that their organizations had defined an effective process for managing disagreements about the safety of an order, both reported equal dissatisfaction (61%) with their organizations' ability to deal successfully with physician intimidation.

But how can an organization deal with this intimidation and other disruptive physician behaviors? It starts at the top with "zero tolerance," but other structures and processes need to be created. Rosenstein and O'Daniel (2005) found that organizations had two main approaches to decreasing disruptive behavior —education and leadership. The education venue was varied; techniques included team collaboration, anger management, and mutual respect. Organizations also emphasized the importance of strong leadership and a commitment to take action.

In the next section, I collated information from multiple sources to create a framework for change based on the literature, personal experience in coaching disruptive physicians, and the use of systems established in organizations that have been successful in reducing this problem. In effecting change, the reader will clearly see the need for moral courage, as healthcare professionals face these difficult situations.

Multifaceted Approach to Dealing With Disruptive Physicians

Effective January 1, 2009 for all accreditation programs, the Joint Commission (2008) has a new leadership standard (LD.03.01.01) that addresses the problems of disruptive and improper behaviors:

> *EP 4: The hospital/organization has a code of conduct that defines acceptable and disruptive and inappropriate behaviors.*

> *EP 5: Leaders create and implement a process for managing disruptive and inappropriate behaviors (p. 2).*

In addition, six core competencies need to be addressed in the credentialing process, including interpersonal skills and professionalism. The Joint Commission believes that each organization is responsible for guaranteeing quality and endorsing a culture of safety; healthcare organizations must deal with the problem of disruptive behaviors that threaten the professional environment of the health care team.

Rosenstein and O'Daniel (2008) recommended the following six strategies for correcting disruptive behaviors (see Exhibit 18.2): (1) raise awareness, (2) develop polices and procedures, (3) education, (4) communication, (5) structure and process, and (6) project champions.

As a result of my experience, I believe even more action is needed and have proposed a full complement of strategies to address the disruptive physician problem (see Exhibit 18.2). The resolution of this problem of disruptive behavior begins and ends with the team member's ability to have the crucial conversation. Strategy #4 (communication) focuses on these skills. Healthcare professionals need to confront the disruptive physician when it happens using the skills outlined in Chapters 3 to 5. An educational program on assertiveness would be useful to healthcare professionals. In the confrontation, individuals could learn to briefly and descriptively state the disruptive behavior and the effect it had on them ("Dr. Jamas, you just yelled at me in front of the patient. I felt humiliated."). Most physicians will apologize and give you some explanation for their behavior. It is important not to accept their justification, but to simply say "I appreciate your apology, and I hope to count on you never treating me that way again." It is

18.2 Recommended Strategies to Deal With Disruptive Physicians

1. Raise awareness
   Internal assessment
   Business case for improvement
2. Develop policies and procedures
   Code of behavior policy
   Disruptive behavior policy
   Confidential reporting system
   Compliance enforcement
   Follow-up and feedback
3. Education
   General education on relationship of disruptive behaviors and communication gaps to
       staff relationships and patient safety
   Specific educational programs and training workshops to include sensitivity training,
       diversity training, and assertiveness training
4. Communication
   Specific educational programs and training workshops on communication skills and
       team collaboration
5. Structure and process
   Nurse-physician-staff relationship committee
6. Project champions
   Executive
   Clinical

From "Managing disruptive physician behavior: Impact on staff relationships and patient care," by A.H. Rosenstein & M. O'Daniel, 2008, *Neurology, 70,* p.1569. Copyright 2008 by Lippincott, Williams and Wilkins. Reprinted with permission.

important to share the results of this interaction with your manager, because the manager will know if this is a pattern and if further action is needed.

However, long-term success with disruptive physicians requires top level leadership commitment to stay the course, no matter how uncomfortable it gets. This is more than Strategy #2 (develop polices and procedures). The policies will be tested, and executives and managers will need the moral courage to stand firm in face of this testing. Weber (2004) reports that survey respondents indicated that physician behavior problems are "only reported when a physician is completely out of line and a serious violation occurs." Some (29.5%) stated that there is underreporting because of fear of staff reprisals. The administration may also be concerned about reprisals. Leadership may fear the loss of physician referrals or a lawsuit for defamation of character. It will not be easy to stay the course. However, leaders must also consider if they want a hostile work environment suit? Are they ignoring the risk of malpractice claims? Do they have the moral courage to tackle this problem that is adversely affecting staff and patients?

How do we know if this is a bona fide problem? Gawande (2000) discussed the four types of behavioral sentinel events that indicate a physician needs help:

(1) persistent poor anger control and abusive behavior; (2) bizarre or erratic behavior; (3) transgression of proper boundaries; and (4) a disproportionate number of complaints or lawsuits. Bauman offers us five questions to help decide if the problem merits attention:

1. Would I tolerate this behavior in a staff member?
2. If I screamed at a patient, was rude to a referring physician, or acted unethically inside or outside the practice, how would I expect my colleagues to act?
3. Would I want to explain this physician's behavior during a deposition?
4. Could this physician's behavior impact the reputation of the practice or my personal reputation?
5. If this physician were to leave the practice, how would the dynamics of the group change? (Bauman, 2006, p. 80)

An effective approach will include the following six components (ACOG Committee Opinion, 2007; Kissoon, Lapenta, & Armstrong, 2002; Rosenstein & O'Daniel, 2008; Simpson, 2007):

Develop a Code of Conduct

A code of conduct provides guidance to clinicians and administrators. These codes should focus on expected behaviors and should be designed by the people who will be responsible for enforcing them. By this I mean the physician leadership in the organization, such as department chairs, the president of the medical staff, and the Chief Medical Officer (CMO), as well as physicians who have informal authority in the organization and who demonstrate the expected behaviors. The code is then taken to Medical Executive Committee (MEC) for approval. The CMO introduces the code at the first available quarterly physician staff meeting. This speaks to the need for project champions, Strategy 6.

In some organizations, this Code of Mutual Respect is separate from the disruptive physician policy that focuses on policy and consequences. I recommend this separation to open the doors to a positive approach to creating a collaborative work climate. This code then becomes the ideal, and positive feedback is based on meeting that ideal. An example of such a code was illustrated in Exhibit 12.2. This organization provided behavioral expectations under each of its values. In its code, education can be conducted at the quarterly physician staff meetings. For example, one value in the code could be discussed at each of the meetings, with positive and negative illustrations.

Some organizations have also created a set of practice expectations that define competent interpersonal behavior. Below is an example of practice expectations (Pfifferling, 1999, p. 60):

- Seek and obtain appropriate consultation.
- Arrange for appropriate coverage when not available.
- Complete patient records within established time frame.
- Disclose potential conflicts of interest.
- Assist in the identification of colleagues who may be in need of assistance.
- Address dissatisfaction with polices through appropriate grievance channels.

- Participate in clinical outcome reviews.
- Maintain professional skills and knowledge and participate in continuing medical education (CME).
- Comply with the practice standards.
- Refrain from fraudulent scientific practices.

Several articles address the importance of having a physician champion for the Code of Conduct and disruptive physician policy (Rosenstein, 2002; OR Manager, 2005). This is because 50% of the survey respondents thought the hospital's policy was ineffective in managing the problem (Rosenstein & O'Daniel, 2005). For the policy to have clout, it needs to be seen as the way the organization does business. In response to the Joint Commission standards, many hospitals have developed disruptive physician policy that is often modeled on guidelines set forth by the AMA (2000). All of their recommendations are included in the guidelines for the policy below.

Develop a Disruptive Physician Policy

A disruptive physician policy should do the following (AMA, 2000; Joint Commission, 2008; Kissoon, Lapenta, & Armstrong, 2002):

- State that the objective of the policy is to ensure high standards of patient care and to promote a professional practice environment.
- Define disruptive behavior.
- Reiterate the behavioral standards found in Code of Conduct.
- State specific examples of unacceptable behavior (see Exhibit 18.1). These are necessary for healthcare professionals to determine if what they are experiencing constitutes disruptive behavior.
- Identify the process for documentation of the event.
- Define a review process to establish the validity of complaint.
- Define the process to notify the disruptive physician of the complaint.
- Provide a mechanism for physician to respond to the complaint.
- Identify a clear delineation as to who will be involved in various stages of the process to address the issues.
- Propose guidelines to protect confidentiality.
- Identify possible corrective actions based on the behaviors.
- State clearly the initial and subsequent consequences if the policy is violated. This may include verbal and written warnings, a formal hearing, suspension and termination without cause provision (if appropriate in your state).
- Articulate the monitoring system used to determine if the behavior improves.
- Specify a mechanism used for initial appointment and subsequent reappointments to medical staff. For example, require the physician to read and sign the Code of Conduct, thereby indicating willingness to honor the defined Code.
- Identify conditions for referral to a medical wellness or equivalent committee.

- Ensure that individuals who report disruptive physicians (or other healthcare professionals) are duly protected.
- Incorporate a "zero tolerance" policy into medical staff bylaws, employment agreements and administrative polices.

The Lazoritz Group (2008) has a sample of 25 different disruptive physician policies on its Web site in which the company also offers consulting services to help organizations deal with the problem physician.

As with the Code of Conduct, dissemination of the disruptive physician policy requires staff and physician education. Combining the dissemination of policy with a physician guest speaker on the subject at a quarterly meeting of the medical staff could underscore the reality of the problem (Barnsteiner, Madigan, & Spray, 2001). In addition, other healthcare professional staff could review issues on disruptive behavior in a professional development seminar on assertiveness training.

Institute a System for Monitoring and Reporting

The policy for monitoring and reporting disruptive behavior should be widely disseminated, and executive leadership should encourage managers to use the policy. Usually the person an employee contacts for discussion of such a problem is the person's manager or the Director/Vice President of Human Resources. The chair of the physician's department would also be involved and, depending upon the severity of problem, the CMO. It is important to have a transparent system that safeguards healthcare professionals and physicians and allows for a dialog that leads to an apology and resolution of the problem. The physician also needs a forum to respond to the complaint.

The formal complaint documentation should include (1) date and time of the incident; (2) incident location; (3) names of everyone involved in the incident; (4) circumstances that precipitated the incident, if known; (5) a description of incident that is limited to factual, objective language; (6) consequences of the incident, if any, to patients or hospital operations; (7) names of witnesses; and (8) any immediate action taken at the time of the incident to remedy the situation, including names and actions done (Lapenta, 2004; Lazoritz Group, 2008).

The person identified in the organization's policy to facilitate resolution of the problem must have the moral courage to deal with senior physicians, physicians of status, and physicians who bring in millions of dollars of revenue. Otherwise, the staff will learn early on when it does not pay to bring forward the complaint. This will lead to mistrust in the process both by healthcare professionals and other physicians in the organization. This complaint can act as a wake-up call for physicians, so that they realize the impact of their behavior on other team members (Kissoon, Lapenta, & Armstrong, 2002).

Provide Assistance to Physician in Changing Behavior

The focus of coaching or counseling sessions is to understand the cognitive, emotional, and social precursors to the incident and help the physician change his/her response to the triggering event. The central aim is behavioral change.

However, some situations require immediate disciplinary action because of the severity of the behavior, such as instances of physical abuse of a patient or staff member. Other forms of serious violations include conduct that violates state or federal law or conduct that creates a serious adverse effect on patient care (Kissoon, Lapenta, & Armstrong, 2002). It is important that the person responsible for providing guidance for an appropriate response reflect appropriate behavior standards and have the skills to coach others to effect the required change. In my experience, physicians in the organization rarely have these coaching skills.

Most physicians *only* conduct an initial meeting to discuss the problem. Few follow up to see if the physician changed behavior after receiving suggestions from the coaching physician. This lack of a contract to change one's behavior often leads to repetitive meetings where the immediate infraction is discussed, but not the unacceptable behavioral pattern.

Most Medical Executive Committees (MECs) suggest three meetings with a chronically disruptive physician before the physician is brought before the credentials committee (Crow, Hartman, Nolan, & Zembo, 2004). In the first meeting, the documented incident is discussed, and the committee determines what the physician will do to ensure that such an incident will not occur again. If a second meeting is required for a repeated offense, the physician must sign a mutually created written plan of action. If a third offense occurs, the meeting should include the department chair, the president of medical staff, and the CMO. At this point, the physician is informed that the situation will be taken before the credentials committee and that the physician can expect at least a letter of reprimand in his/her personnel folder, but that he or she should be prepared for even worse.

Formal counseling recommendations should be given when the pattern is identified in second meeting. This recommendation could include an Employee Assistance Program (EAP), local therapist or, often more palpable, a coach who knows how to tutor in anger management skills. Pfifferling (1999) gives other resources specific to physicians and provides some classic confrontation guidelines. Ludemann and Erlandson (2004) offer hints on how to coach the "alpha male" in a business setting, and many of their ideas are applicable to physicians. Their section on "when strengths become weaknesses" and the defensiveness rating scale could be particularly helpful.

After coaching a dozen chronically disruptive physicians, my experience is that more than half had either a narcissistic personality disorder, obsessive compulsive personality disorder, and/or sociopathic personality disorder. All of these individuals were referred to psychiatrists for treatment. The remainder responded to cognitive and behavioral approaches to managing their anger and stress reduction techniques. Many of these individuals also needed help in changing their lifestyles, because they had put themselves in a pressure-cooker situation; it was little wonder they were losing control of their emotions.

Other specific questionnaires and centers can be used. Several articles discuss the Birkman Method questionnaire (Lazoritz, 2008; Samenow, Siggart, & Spickard, 2008) or the Physicians Universal Leadership Skills survey (Samenow, Siggart, & Spickard, 2008). These studies suggest that physicians often lack awareness of their behavior, and these questionnaires can help them recognize and plan a change strategy. If the individual is resistant to the feedback, then a 360 degree instrument for feedback is recommended. For example, the Vanderbilt Center for Professional Health offers a three-day program with follow-up for distressed physicians (Samenow, Siggart, & Spickard, 2008). This program helps physicians identify specific triggers for their anger, assists them to develop alternative responses to the triggers, engages in role playing, teaches assertiveness, identifies long-standing family of origin issues, and focuses on relapse prevention. Although the program is expensive and the data effectiveness scarce, it has had some initial success.

Highlight Code of Conduct Behaviors During Contract Renewal or Performance Reviews

If the physician has exhibited good citizenship behaviors, then this should be noted during contract renewal or performance reviews. If there have been problems, then review why there has been a lack of success in resolving these continuing problems. There should also be discussions between the CMO and the credentialing committee when it is time to recredential a disruptive physician. It is an opportunity for all to reflect on whether the burden is worth the benefits of the services of this physician. With an effective reporting and monitoring process, the CMO will have the necessary information to guide the credentials committee.

Seek Legal Counsel if Termination Looks Like the Best Answer

This step speaks to the legal implications of the "termination without cause" clause. Legal counsel can reassure the organization of its position at this time of high emotion and pain. The Health Care Quality Improvement Act of 1986 does provide extensive safeguard to peer reviewers if the conduct of the individual physician could adversely affect the health of a patient. In the case of Eden v. Desert Regional Medical Center, the medical center won the case because the administrative records contained significant examples of Dr. Eden's aberrant behavior (Tammello, 2006). This speaks to the importance of codes, policies, and documentation all along the way in the process. In the end, this administrative, ethical, and legal support to executives can help them muster the moral courage to take this one final step in a disciplinary action that they know will affect the physician's career.

Conclusion

There are many reasons why some physicians periodically demonstrate disruptive behavior. The research is clear about the types of behaviors and their effects on healthcare professionals, patients, and other physicians. Administrative and physician leadership in the organization have a responsibility to the staff and patients to prevent and/or eliminate this problem for the sake of staff and customer satisfaction and safety. It will take moral courage to deal with a high status and/or very productive physician, but it is the ethical obligation of leadership to address this problem in a way that honors all parties involved.

Key Points to Remember

1. Disruptive physicians not only threaten the morale and retention of health-care professionals and other staff, but newer information indicates that they are a threat to patient safety.
2. The AMA defines disruptive behavior as "a style of interaction with physicians, hospital personnel, patients, family members, or others that interferes with patient care . . . [and] that tends to cause distress among other staff and affect overall morale within the work environment, undermining productivity and possibly leading to higher staff turnover or even resulting in ineffective or substandard care."
3. The most common examples of disruptive behaviors are disrespect, yelling, insulting others, or a refusal to carry out duties.
4. It is estimated that 3% to 5% of physicians engage in disruptive behavior.
5. The surgical specialties identified as more inclined to exhibit disruptive behavior were general surgery (31%), cardiovascular surgery (21%), neurosurgery (15%), orthopedic surgery (7%), and obstetrics/gynecology (6%).
6. Many nurses (70%) witnessed disruptive behavior initiated by nurses.
7. In the Rosenstein and O'Daniel (2008) study, 66% were aware of an adverse event that had occurred and almost 75% thought these events could have serious, very serious, or extremely serious impact on patient outcomes.
8. The general public believes that this lack of ability to work as a team is a very important cause of medical errors—67% respondents.
9. The Institute for Safe Medication Practice (2004) reported that seven percent of medication errors could be caused by physician intimidation of nurses; 64% of pharmacists and 34% of nurses reported that they had assumed a medication order was correct and safe rather than check by interacting with a verbally abusive physician.
10. The primary strategies to reduce disruptive physician problems are: (1) raise awareness, (2) develop policies and procedures, (3) education, (4) communication, (5) structure and process, and (6) project champions.
11. Long-term success with disruptive physicians requires top level leadership commitment to stay the course, no matter how uncomfortable it gets.
12. Four types of behavioral sentinel events that indicate a physician needs help: (1) persistent poor anger control and abusive behavior; (2) bizarre or erratic behavior; (3) transgression of proper boundaries; and (4) a disproportionate number of complaints or lawsuits.
13. An effective approach to manage the problem will include the following six components: (1) Develop a code of conduct, (2) Develop a disruptive physician policy, (3) Institute a system for monitoring and reporting, (4) Provide assistance to physician in changing behavior, (5) During contract renewal or performance reviews highlight Code of Conduct behaviors, (6) Seek legal counsel if termination looks like the best answer.
14. Develop a disruptive physician policy that clearly indicates "zero tolerance" for defined behaviors, mechanisms for reporting, and consequences for behaviors.
15. A Code of Mutual Respect is separate from the disruptive physician policy that focuses on policy and consequences.

16. The focus of coaching or counseling sessions is understanding the cognitive, emotional, and social precursors to the incident and helping the physician change his/her response to the triggering event.

References

ACOG Committee Opinion No. 366. (2007). Disruptive behavior. *Obstetrics and Gynecology, 109,* 1261–1262.

American Medical Association. (2000). *Physicians with disruptive behavior.* Report of the Council on Ethical and Judicial Affairs. Retrieved May 5, 2008, from http://www.ama-assn.org/ama1/pub/upload/mm/369/ceja_2a00.pdf

Barnsteiner, J.H., Madigan, C., & Spray, T.L. (2001). Instituting a disruptive conduct policy for medical staff. *AACN Clinical Issues, 12*(3), 378–382.

Bates, D.W., & Gawande, A.A. (2003). Improving safety with information technology. *New England Journal of Medicine, 348*(25), 26–34.

Bauman, R.R. (2006). Disruptive physicians . . . and how to deal with them. *Journal of Medical Practice Management, 22*(2), 79–83.

Birkman Method. Retrieved May 3, 2008, from http://www.birkman.com/birkmanMethod/whatIsTheBirkmanMethod.php

Blendon, R.J., DesRoches, C.M., Brodie, M., Benson, J.M., Rosen, A.B., Schneider, E., et al. (2002). Views of practicing physicians and the public on medical errors. *New England Journal of Medicine, 347*(24), 1933–1940.

Center for Professional Health. Retrieved May 3, 2008, from http://www.mc.vanderbilt.edu/root/vumc.php?site=cph&doc=4253

Crow, S.M., Hartman, S.J., Nolan, T.E., & Zembo, M. (2003). A prescription for the rogue doctor. *The Physician Executive, 30,* 6–14.

Gawande, A. (2000, August 7). When good doctors go bad. *The New Yorker.* pp. 60–69.

Health Care Quality Improvement Act of 1986. Retrieved May 5, 2008, from http://www.semmelweis.org/articles/HCQIA%20by%20RChalifoux.pdf

Institute for Safe Medicine Practice. (2004). *Intimidation: Practitioners speak up about this unresolved problem (Part I).* Retrieved May 3, 2008, from http://www.ismp.org/MSAarticles/Intimidation.htm

Joint Commission. (2008, July 9). *Behaviors that undermine a culture of safety. 40.* Retrieved December 31, 2008, from http://www.jointcommission.org/SentinelEvents/SentinelEventAlert/sea_40.htm

Kissoon, N., Lapenta, S., & Armstrong, G. (2002). Diagnosis and therapy for the disruptive physician. *Physician Executive, 1,* 54–58.

Lapenta, S. (2004). Disruptive behavior and the law. *Physician Executive, 8,* 24–26.

Lazoritz, S. (2008). Coaching for insight: A tool for dealing with disruptive physician behavior. *The Physician Executive, 1,* 28–31.

Lazoritz, S., & Carlson, P.J. (2008). Don't tolerate disruptive physician behavior. *American Nurse, 3*(3), 20–22.

Lazoritz Group. *Sample disruptive physician behavior policies.* Retrieved May 5, 2008, from http://www.lazoritz.com/samplebehaviorpolicies.html

Ludemann, K., & Erlandson, E. (2004, May). Coaching the alpha male. *Harvard Business Review, 5,* 58–67.

OR Manager. (2005). Study links disruptive behavior to negative patient outcomes, *21*(3), 1, 20–22.

Papadakis, M.A., Teherani, A., Banach, M.A., Knettler, T.R., Ratter, S.L., Stern, D.T., et al. (2005). Disciplinary action by medical boards and prior behavior in medical school. *New England Journal of Medicine, 353*(25), 2673–2683.

Pfifferling, J.H. (1999). The disruptive physician: A quality of professional life factor. *Physician Executive, 3,* 58–61.

Rosenstein, A.H. (2002). Nurse-physician relationships: Impact on nurse satisfaction and retention. *American Journal of Nursing, 10*(2), 26–34.

Rosenstein, A.H., & O'Daniel, M. (2008). Managing disruptive physician behavior: Impact on staff relationships and patient care. *Neurology, 70,* 1564–1570.

Rosenstein, A.H., & O'Daniel, M. (2005). Disruptive behavior and clinical outcomes: Perceptions of nurses and physicians. *American Journal of Nursing, 105*(1), 54–64.

Samenow, C.P., Siggart, W., & Spickard, A. (2008). A CME course aimed at addressing disruptive physician behavior. *Physician Executive, 1,* 32–40.

Simpson, K.R. (2007). Disruptive clinician behavior. *American Journal of Maternal Child Nursing, 32*(1), 64.

Stern, D.T., Frohna, A.Z., & Gruppen, L.D. (2005). The prediction of professional behaviour. *Medical Education, 39,* 75–82.

Tammelleo, A.D. (2006). Disruptive behavior is grounds for suspension of staff privileges. *Medical Law's Regan Report, 39*(3), 1.

Thomas, E.J., Studdert, D.M., Burstin, H.R., Orav, E.J., Zeena, T., Williams, E.J., et al. (2000). Incidence and types of adverse events and negligent care in Utah and Colorado. *Medical Care, 38*(3), 261–271.

Weber, D.O. (2004). Poll results: Doctor's disruptive behavior disturbs physician leaders. *The Physician Executive, 30*(5), 6–15.

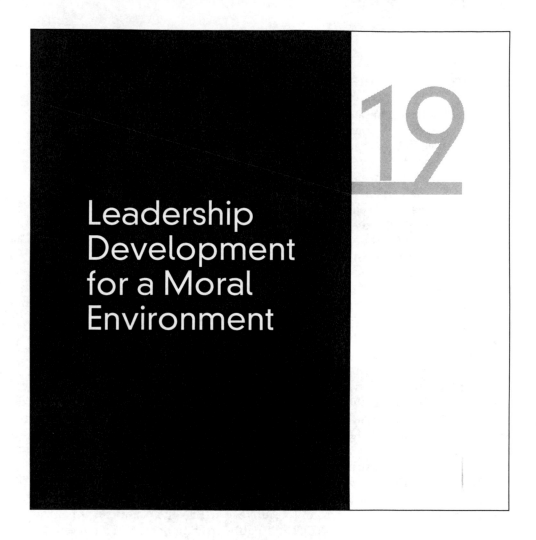

Leadership Development for a Moral Environment

19

Leadership is a combination of strategy and character. If you must be without one, be without the strategy.

—General H. Norman Schwarzkopf, Commander of the Coalition Forces in the Gulf War of 1991 and author

Unfortunately, many leaders in health care only receive on-the-job training (OJT). Even as health care has begun to recognize itself as a business, basically the OJT mentality has persisted everywhere other than in academic medical centers. Successful organizations, however, know that leadership skills need continuous development. Organizations that understand this need are usually recognized for their quality and ethical performance and have high scores in patient and employee satisfaction. There are many leadership and management skills that excellent clinicians lack. This chapter identifies the necessary competencies for executives and managers responsible for leading organizations that have a moral healthcare environment. Of specific concern are the skills needed to sustain an environment that supports integrity and moral courage.

Leadership Competencies Needed in Health Care

Many leaders have competencies that they can overuse, thereby hindering their success. For example, I spent a year coaching a Director of Materials Management for a two-hospital system. Shelia was a bright, experienced, and a strategic thinker, but she lacked the insight to see how her orientation to detail was hampering her work performance. In fact, this orientation actually preventing her from effective delegation of tasks, and it often caused her to harshly criticize her employees rather than coach them to appreciate the importance of detail in specific situations. She lacked the "communications for relationship management" competency identified below. My first step was to help her with what White, Clement, and Nayar (2006) called the "ability for honest self-evaluation." Through the use of self-assessment questionnaires, feedback from interviews of her staff, role playing, and a mentor with excellent communication skills, she was able to see how she was getting in her way of effectively managing her staff. In the following year, she was promoted to Vice President of the same organization and is presently mentoring other people in her field.

Garman and Johnson (2006) define competencies as "characteristics of employees with behavioral implications that are thought to be associated with successful performance of their job" (p. 336). White, Clement, and Nayar (2006) list nine studies identifying the leadership competencies and end with the tenth, the results of their own work. The White et al. list of competencies was remarkably similar to the Healthcare Leadership Alliance (HLA) results, which divided the competencies into the domains of leadership, communication, business skill, and technology. The results also closely parallels the results of the HLA study, which was comprised of representatives from key leadership organizations in health care, including the American College of Health Care Executives (ACHE), the American College of Physician Executives (ACPE), the American Organization of Nurse Executives (AONE), the Healthcare Financial Management Association (HFMA), the Health Information and Management Systems (HIMSS), the Medical Group Management Association (MGMA), and the American College of Medical Practice Executives (ACMPE). HLA produced the *Competency Directory*, which is considered a milestone in the field of healthcare administration. It lists 300 competencies and categorizes them into five domains: (1) leadership, (2) communication and relationship management, (3) professionalism, (4) business knowledge and skills, and (5) knowledge of the healthcare environment. Griffith (2007) criticizes these results on a number of fronts. He finds the list is weakest in its exclusion of any obvious outcomes or process measurement, as excellent healthcare organizations rely on benchmarks and quality indicators. He is also critical of the vagueness of some terms and a focus on the verb "develop" as opposed to "implement." Griffith also does not see the answer for healthcare leadership in the list of exclusively behavioral competencies developed by the National Center for Healthcare Leadership (NCHL). He sees the need for the knowledge competencies as in the HLA *Competency Directory*. The NCHL capabilities could be evaluated in the workplace, but are not scaled for usability in academic settings for training healthcare managers and executives. Finally, he calls for a national consensus panel of currently active healthcare executives and academics to create a usable taxonomy.

Shewchuk, O'Conner, and Fine (2006) conducted a study to do just this, that is, to develop healthcare competencies from the perspectives of practitioners and academicians by using a common framework of critical environmental issues that face healthcare managers. These critical issues were developed by 12 senior level executives in a Nominal Group Technique and yielded a rank ordering of five clusters. The clusters were rank ordered with cluster A (Traditional Management Tasks) and cluster B (Patient's Interests) receiving the same weighted ranking. The same happened for cluster C (Political, Legal and Ethical Concerns) and cluster E (Financial and Economic Issues). Cluster D (Medical Issues) was seen as the least important. The consistent difference in the deeper analysis of these competencies was the pragmatic and specific focus of executives versus the theoretical focus of academics (e.g., public/community knowledge versus the social determinants of health). There was more agreement than disagreement in most clusters on major issues. For example, both groups agree that a strong ethics base and training is the most important competency for cluster C, which focuses on political, legal, and ethical issues.

In the White et al. (2006) study, "professional and managerial ethics" was one of the key factors under leadership, along with the "ability for honest self-evaluation," "leading and managing others," and "planning and implementing change." The focus of the "professional and managerial ethics" domain was organizational business and personal ethics; professional standards and codes of ethics; conflict of interest situations as defined by organizational bylaws, policies, and procedures; and ethics committee's roles, structures, and functions. All of these have been discussed in this book as important components of an ethical organization. In other studies cited by White et al., the ethical component often fell under professionalism. Bennis and O'Toole (2005) charged that business schools "are failing to impart useful skills, failing to prepare leaders and failing to instill norms of ethical behavior . . ." (p. 96). All of these studies still leave us wondering if a true consensus exists in formal education requirements.

Skills Needed by Healthcare Leaders Today

Hartman and Crow (2002) surveyed executives about the top five tasks of healthcare executives (see Exhibit 19.1). Given the turbulence of the industry, strategy

---

19.1 Five Key Tasks Confronting Executives

1. Forming strategic vision of where organization is heading
2. Setting objectives to move from vision to performance
3. Crafting a strategy to achieve desired objectives
4. Implementing and executing the chosen strategy
5. Evaluating performance and implementing corrective adjustments

Hartman, S.J., & Crow, S.M. (2002). Executive development in healthcare during times of turbulence. *Journal of Management in Medicine, 16*(5), p. 362.

implementation skills were seen as more important than strategy formulation. Leaders need to be strategic thinkers, who are flexible and able to read the signs of the times so they can continuously adjust course. There appeared to be two primary lines of reasoning—"real-life" experience supplemented with mentoring and the need for solid business education, especially in finance. Although they see the need for the ability to see the "big picture," they also argue for staying nimble in short-term implementations.

Welton (2004) wrote about the need for a new set of skills in the complex arena of constant change. He spoke to the importance of the skill sets required for successful orchestration of healthcare delivery systems, but he also wrote about providing value-oriented leadership. Executives and the managers must repeatedly strike a balance between profits and investing to meet community needs.

Hartman and Crow (2002) found course content is not all that is needed to develop future health care leaders. Skills are important in balancing quality with the bottom line profit requirement, but future leaders also need mentoring to manage the "white water change" found in the rapid, complex, turbulent, and unpredictable healthcare climate (Lanser, 2000). Mentors can help these developing leaders gain a "real world" perspective, in which they recognize that leadership is a marathon, not a sprint. In this world, leaders think strategically, as in a chess game. They never make a move until they know the consequences of their last move. These mentors can also help leaders understand and learn the people skills necessary for conflict resolution and negotiation.

Peter Drucker, in his classic 1994 *Harvard Business Review* article, states that "Every organization, whether a business or not, has a theory of business—the assumptions on which the organization has been built and is being run" (p. 96). He cautions against a focus on "how-to" strategies and asks leaders to address the vital management challenge—what to do. He goes on to name four conditions for a theory of business:

1. The assumption about the environment, mission, and core competencies must fit reality.
2. The assumptions in all three areas have to fit one another.
3. The theory of the business must be known and understood throughout the organization.
4. The theory of the business has to be tested constantly (p. 96).

Current reality, however, is that our theory of business is being tested and our healthcare performance is not good enough, as indicated by many quality measures. Our healthcare system is not characterized by the six descriptors that the Institute of Medicine put forth in 2001—safety, effectiveness, patient-centeredness, timeliness, efficiency, and equity. Leaders need to know how to design the systems outlined in this report (see Exhibit 19.2). When leaders design the healthcare system with these rules in mind, the patient's autonomy is restored, staff members are supported in advocating for their needs, and obstructive systems are changed. Leaders understand that cross-functional teams are necessary to coordinate care across patient conditions, services, and settings. This kind of leadership requires the skills of conflict resolution, facilitation, collaboration, and cooperation, not command and control. The need for transparency

19.2 Rules for Redesigning the Healthcare System

1. Case based on continuous healing relationships
2. Customization based on patient needs and values
3. The patient as the source of control
4. Shared knowledge and free flow of information
5. Evidence-based decision making
6. Safety as a system priority
7. Need for transparency
8. Anticipation of needs
9. Continue decrease in waste
10. Cooperation among clinicians

Corrigan, J.M., Donaldson, M., & Kohn, L. (2000). *To err is human: Building a safer health system*. Washington, DC: National Academy Press, p. 287.

in this rules list speaks to the need for disclosure of errors and a level of openness between employees and leaders not often seen. Do we have a model that could take our good healthcare system to one that is great?

Collins (2001) and his research team offered a model for taking an organization from good to great. Although none of the organizations they examined are in the healthcare field, there are lessons to be learned. There are seven crucial components in the break-through process; five will be briefly mentioned, but the focus will be on Level 5, *Leadership (First who, then what),* because this encompasses the key ingredients discussed in this chapter (See Figure 19.1).

Collins (2001) offers five levels of leadership, but level 5 is needed for the transformation. It is defined as "building enduring greatness through a paradoxical blend of personal humility and professional will" (p. 20). These two sides of *Level 5 leadership* can be seen in Exhibit 19.3. Collins believes that people can develop the skills to become level 5 leaders. He says that the other findings from his research will help individuals become level 5 leaders. He views these leaders as plow horses, not show horses.

These level 5 leaders must also ensure that the right people are on board to accomplish the goals *(First who . . .).* This is why the interviewing process outlined in Chapter 15 is crucial. If you want a moral organization, you need to hire people with integrity. The companies described by Collins do not hire someone when they are in doubt about that person; they just keep looking. They do not keep people who require a high degree of management. Guided, taught, lead, yes. They want people who reach beyond the expectations of their jobs. They also put their best people on the biggest projects, such as a new building program, a new service line, or acquisition of another healthcare facility. This is all part of their leadership development process that takes an organization from good to great.

Even though the process starts with leadership and getting the right people on board, for the sake of completeness my focus is on the other five components of a breakthrough. *Confront the Brutal Facts (Yet Never Lose Faith)* is an important

19.1

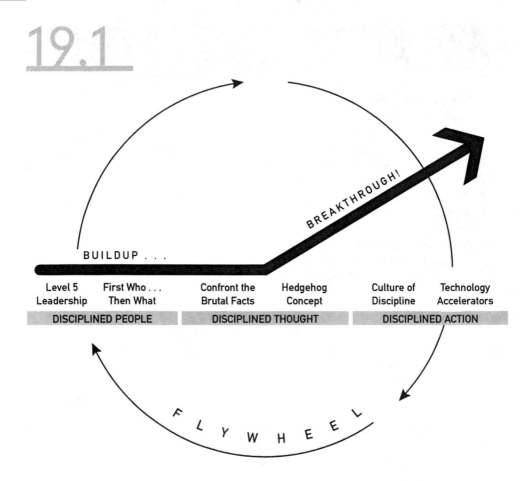

BREAKTHROUGH!

BUILDUP . . .

Level 5 Leadership	First Who . . . Then What	Confront the Brutal Facts	Hedgehog Concept	Culture of Discipline	Technology Accelerators
DISCIPLINED PEOPLE		DISCIPLINED THOUGHT		DISCIPLINED ACTION	

F L Y W H E E L

component of disciplined thought that uses the Stockdale Paradox. This paradox says, "you must maintain unwavering faith that you can and will prevail in the end, regardless of difficulties, AND at the same time have the discipline to confront the most brutal facts of your current reality, whatever they might be" (p. 86). The *Hedgehog Concept* is used to rise above the curse of competence or the philosophy of "that is the way it is." It asks us to answer three questions: (1) What are we deeply passionate about? (2) What can you be the best in the world at? and (3) What drives your economic engine? Once you have the answer to these three questions, you will have your focus. A *Culture of Discipline* centers on the results of the hedgehog questions. Once you have this focus on values, you do not need hierarchy or excessive controls to maintain quality. Disciplined people with an entrepreneurial sprit are unstoppable. Baptist Health Care is such an example because the employees know they make a difference. *Technology Acceleration* is the fourth component for breakthrough results. Technology is used to reach goals, such as improving patient safety by using Pyxis, barcoding, and physician order entry. Finally, the *Flywheel* concept takes all six components and creates the transformation. Baptist Healthcare changes are an example of this task of relentlessly pushing a giant heavy flywheel in one direction and building momentum until the point of breakthrough.

19.3 Summary: The Two Sides of Level 5 Leadership

Professional Will	Personal Humility
Creates superb results, a clear catalyst in the transition from good to great.	Demonstrates a compelling modesty, shunning public adulation; never boastful.
Demonstrates an unwavering resolve to do whatever must be done to produce the best long-term results, no matter how difficult.	Acts with quiet, calm determination; relies principally on inspired standards, not inspiring charisma, to motivate.
Sets the standard of building an enduring great company; will settle for nothing less.	Channels ambition into the company, not the self; sets up successors for even greater success in the next generation.
Looks in the mirror, not out the window, to apportion responsibility for poor results, never blaming other people, external factors, or bad luck.	Looks out the window, not in the mirror, to apportion credit for the success of the company—to other people, external factors, and good luck.

From *Good to great* (p. 36), by J. Collins, 2001. New York: HarperCollins Publishing, Inc. Copyright 2001 by Jim Collins. Reprinted with permission

Studer (2008) also recognizes that leaders need education, but he believes it is equally important to have promotions that reflect desired leadership behaviors. When a vice president is allowed to type on a Blackberry or edit reports during a meeting, it encourages a lack of attention and a lack of respect for others in attendance. Leaders need to be accountable; they need to meet performance expectations and hold others accountable. Without the skill to hold employees accountable, greatness will never be achieved. When the leadership training in core competencies is aligned with the organizational mission and focuses on the skills needed in the *present* environment, then the business, according to Drucker, will be successful.

Emily Friedman (2001) has been an outspoken advocate for change in health care and for a return to the social and moral aspects of health care, which society has entrusted to healthcare professionals and leaders. The future leader she desires will be characterized by: (1) an acute understanding of the realities of the field; (2) sensitivity to the country's changing demographics; (3) a sense of honesty; (4) accountability; (5) the courage to act; (6) a profound sense of community; (7) flexibility; and (8) a striving to be a force for change. In this list are three key points on the moral compass—honesty, accountability, and courage.

Conclusion

Unfortunately, there is no consensus as to the required competencies for effective leadership education. Many studies have looked at competencies, but no agreement between academics and healthcare executives has been reached. This chapter indicates some of the knowledge, skills, and traits required for effective leadership. Since benchmarks for success have been given throughout this book, the benchmark for successful organizations by Collins (2001) was used to describe *Level 5 leadership*. Will and humility are not a combination we normally attribute to successful leaders, but, on reflection, they make sense if you want to build a lasting and outstanding organization. Moral leadership requires many communication skills.

Key Points to Remember

1. The Healthcare Leadership Alliance produced the *Competency Directory* for executives/managers, which lists 300 competencies and categorizes them into five domains: (1) leadership, (2) communications and relationship management, (3) professionalism, (4) business knowledge and skills, and (5) knowledge of the healthcare environment.
2. This list of competencies is criticized in its lack of "knowledge competencies" and lack of focus on important ability of implementation.
3. The focus of the "professional and managerial ethics" domain was organizational business and personal ethics; professional standards and codes of ethics; conflict of interest situations as defined by organizational bylaws, policies, and procedures; and ethics committee's roles, structure, and functions.
4. Strategy implementation skills were seen as more important than strategy formulation.
5. Leaders need to be strategic thinkers, flexible and able to read the signs of the times, so they can continuously adjust course.
6. Leaders need both "real-life" experience supplemented with mentoring and solid business education, especially finance.
7. Executives and the managers must repeatedly strike a balance between profits and investing to meet community needs.
8. Mentors can help developing leaders gain a "real world" perspective, where they recognize that leadership is a marathon, not a sprint.
9. IOM has given leaders rules to help them redesign healthcare system (Exhibit 19.2).
10. Jim Collins affirms there are seven crucial components in the breakthrough process of going from good to great organization; one of these focuses specifically on leadership.
11. Collins states there are five levels of leadership, but level 5 is needed for the transformation—"building enduring greatness through a paradoxical blend of personal humility and professional will."
12. When the leadership training in core competencies is aligned with organizational mission and focuses on the skills needed in the *present* environment, then the business will be successful.
13. Freidman describes the characteristics of the type of future leaders she desires as: 1) having an acute understanding of the realities of the field; 2) sensitivity to the country's changing demographics; 3) a sense of honesty; 4) accountability; 5) courage to act; 6) a profound sense of community; 7) flexibility; and 8) striving to be a force for change.

14. Obvious in the lists of many leadership studies are the communication skills of conflict resolution and negotiation.
15. If you want a moral organization then you need to hire people with integrity and then help them develop their leadership skills.

References

Bennis, W.G., & O'Toole, J. (2005). How business schools lost their way. *Harvard Business Review, 85*(5), 96–104.

Collins, J. (2001). *Good to great.* New York: HarperCollins.

Corrigan, J.M., Donaldson, M., & Kohn, L. (2000). *To err is human: Building a safer health system.* Washington, DC: National Academy Press.

Drucker, P. (1994). The theory of business. *Harvard Business Review, 72*(5), 95–104.

Friedman, E. (2001). The healthcare executive as a singular presence. Special Issue: The future of education and practice in health management and policy. *Journal of Health Administration Education, 19*(4), 68–80.

Garman, A.N., & Johnson, M.P. (2006). Leadership competencies: An introduction. *Journal of Healthcare Management, 49*(5), 307–321.

Griffith, J.R. (2007). Improving preparation for senior management in healthcare. *Journal of Health Administration Education, 24*(1), 11–32.

Hartman, S.J., & Crow, S.M. (2002). Executive development in healthcare during times of turbulence. *Journal of Management in Medicine, 16*(5), 359–370.

Healthcare Leadership Alliance (HLA). *HLA competency directory.* Retrieved September 9, 2008, from http://www.healthcareleadershipalliance.org/

Lanser, E.G. (2000). Lessons from the business side of healthcare. *Healthcare Executive, 15*(5), 4–19.

Shewchuk, R.M., O'Conner, S.J., & Fine, D.J. (2006). Bridging the gap: Academic and practitioner perspectives to identify early career competencies needed in healthcare management. *Journal of Healthcare Administration, 23*(4), 367–392.

Studer, Q. (2008). *Results that last: Hardwiring behaviors that will take your company to the top.* Hoboken, NJ: John Wiley and Sons.

Welton, W.E. (2006). Managing today's complex healthcare business enterprise: Reflections on distinctive requirements of healthcare management education. *Journal of Health Administration, 21*(4), 391–418.

White, K.R., Clement, D.C., & Nayar, P. (2006). Evidence-based healthcare management competency evaluation: Alumni perception. *Journal of Health Administration Education, 23*(4), 335–349.

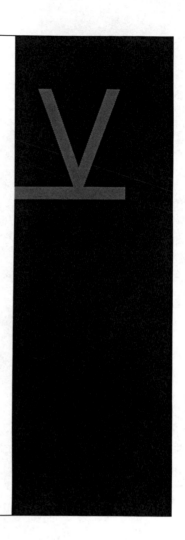

Further Opportunities for Moral Courage

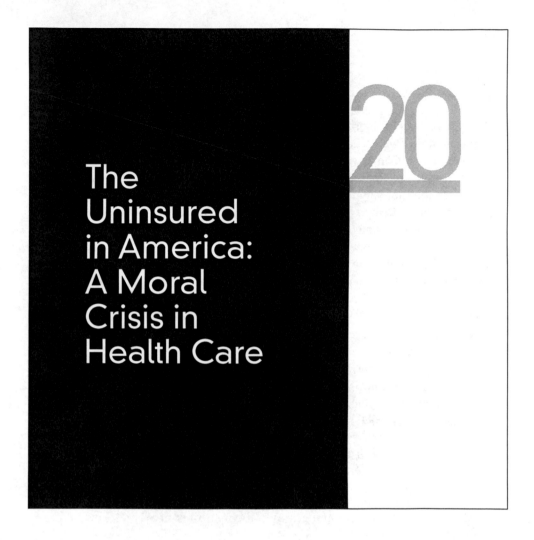

The Uninsured in America: A Moral Crisis in Health Care

20

I . . . believe that every American has the right to affordable health care. I believe that the millions of Americans who can't take their children to a doctor when they get sick have that right . . . We now face an opportunity—and an obligation—to turn the page on the failed politics of yesterday's health care debates. It's time to bring together businesses, the medical community, and members of both parties around a comprehensive solution to this crisis, and it's time to let the drug and insurance industries know that while they'll get a seat at the table, they don't get to buy every chair.

—Barack Obama, President of the United States, Speech in Iowa City, IA, May 27, 2007

There are many stories from uninsured Americans that can be told. This one from Cathy Davis is a true story.

Case 20.1

Cathy Davis, age 56, is from Lancaster, Pennsylvania. She is a divorced mother of two children, Rachel, 20, and Fran, 15. Until she was laid off in February of last year, she worked on an assembly line in a candy company. She was unable to take the option of continuing health coverage with COBRA, because she could not afford the monthly payments. Her only source of income was her unemployment check. Cathy's two children have coverage under their father's policy. Though she was formally terminated by the company in September, she recently returned to the assembly line as a temporary employee. In this position, she is ineligible for benefits. Cathy suffers from multiple sclerosis which causes difficulty in standing for long periods and she has significant fatigue. It makes working long hours very difficult. As the disease progresses, it will likely prevent her from living a normal life. While she is able to receive some care at a local healthcare clinic, she is not receiving the level of treatment required for the medical management of this disease.

Cathy is not the only member of her family who has been affected by the devastating effects of being uninsured. Her sister, 59, died last month after suffering from ulcerative colitis and liver cancer. She was uninsured and was unable to receive the treatments she needed to survive.

Cathy Davis is one of the 18.1% of women who are uninsured, as compared with 22% for men (Facts and Research on the Uninsured, 2006). People from the ages of 25 to 44 account for 50% of uninsured nonelderly adults. Although Cathy is older than the individuals in this largest group of uninsured people, she is a non-Hispanic White person, the group that constitutes nearly 66% of the uninsured nonelderly population.

Cathy's story is just one of the 50 million stories I could share with you. While each has its own narrative, all are the result of a system that has failed to provide healthcare to the neediest Americans. Like Cathy, many have relied on employer-based healthcare and, through no fault of their own, have lost this healthcare insurance because of layoffs, downsizing, or mergers. A just government has the responsibility to protect with the most vulnerable of its people.

With the economic downturn in 2008, an increasing number of people have been left without health insurance. The effects are devastating. For example, Massachusetts has witnessed a huge increase in the number of people without jobs and without affordable health insurance. The unemployment rate rose from 4.1% to 5.9% in 8 months. As a result, there has been 73% increase in applications for the state's Medical Security Program, a lifeline that aids middle- and lower-income unemployed residents pay their health insurance premiums (Lazar, 2008). This 20-year-old Medical Security Program is the only one of its type in the nation. The $71.8 million left in the program's reserves will likely be sufficient for another year, but then the medical security of Massachusetts unemployed citizens will be absent. Like Cathy, most of these unemployed people can not afford the COBRA premiums.

This chapter lays out the key problems with our healthcare policies and discusses common healthcare reform myths that many patients and healthcare providers believe (Pipes, 2008a,b; Sarpel, Vladeck, Divino, & Klotman, 2008). After reviewing the state of U.S. health care, the discussion will move to the costs of the present system. Comparisons to other countries will be offered. The State Children's Health Insurance Program (SCHIP) will receive a special focus because children are our future. The chapter then analyzes the anticipated cost of changing to universal health care and what can be done to contain cost. Finally, the chapter concludes with President Barack Obama's proposed healthcare plan.

Millions of Americans in service industries do not receive healthcare benefits from their employers because the company has made a survival decision or profit-motivated decision not to offer healthcare benefits. As the United States is the *only* developed country that does not offer universal healthcare benefits, many Americans and their children do not receive the health care that they need to survive, thrive, and contribute to their country, their communities, and their families. From both a policy and ethics perspective, I find this policy to be wrong. Many of the other moral issues discussed in this book need to be addressed on the healthcare policy stage. It is time for all Americans to understand the truth about the present system.

This chapter informs you about the problem; maybe the statistics and comparisons will stimulate your moral outrage. My hope is that you will realize that the issue of the uninsured is a serious moral problem. Most of the uninsured adults are working Americans who have been forced to choose among the necessities of food, clothing, and healthcare. Moreover, the lack of universal healthcare affects not only the uninsured, but businesses as well.

Were you angry at the 2008 Big Three auto bailout? Why is the industry in such trouble? How else could the government have helped? The truth is that universal health care would make automakers more competitive. The auto industry's problems underscore the need for a government-backed system of universal health care, which would relieve companies of some of the costs that make them less competitive.

What can each individual do to remedy this moral problem? Covertheun insured.org provides guidance for many activities and events that you can organize and host, such as a news conference, campus event, faith event, letter to your local newspaper, working with the media, and health and enrollment fairs.

Comparison Between the United States and Other Countries

Myth #1: The U.S. healthcare system is the best in the world. The disparity between myth and reality is captured in many studies. In the World Health Organization (WHO) (2000) report, the United States ranked 32nd in infant survival, 24th in life expectancy, and 54th for fairness (justice). Overall, WHO ranked the United States 37th in the world.

A recent international study by Schoen, Osborn, Doty, Bishop, Peugh, and Murukutla (2007) pointed to the effects of the cost of health insurance in United States. The study surveyed people in Australia, Canada, Germany, the Netherlands, New Zealand, the United Kingdom, and the United States. According to this study, U.S. adults are more likely than adults in six other countries to go without health care because of cost. In addition, 34% of U.S. adults (the highest among the seven countries) think that the healthcare system needs to be completely rebuilt. This may be the result of anxiety about the lack of affordable health insurance. Country patterns mirror underlying insurance policy choices. This survey also reported that U.S. adults reported the highest overall healthcare error rates. Finally, the issue of access to care—the long waits, even the rationing of care, was not an issue for over half of the patients in Germany, the Netherlands, and New Zealand. Only 30% of U.S. adults said they could get same-day appointments with their doctors when sick. In both the United States and Canada, approximately 40% of those with an emergency room visit said the condition could have been treated by their regular doctor if available. Even though the United States spends double what other countries spend for medical care—$6,697 per capita in 2005—this study across countries reveals a number of benefits that universal health insurance offers. Americans will soon be spending $1 out of every $5 of national income for health care. We deserve a better return on this investment.

The U.S. Healthcare System

The lack of health insurance results in a lower quality of life, increased morbidity and mortality, and increased financial burdens. In 2002, the Institute of Medicine (IOM) estimated that 18,000 Americans died in 2000 because they were uninsured (Dorn, 2008). Because the number of uninsured has grown, estimates indicate for 2006 reached 22,000 deaths (Dorn, 2008).

Myth #2: The uninsured have equal access to medical care through the emergency room. The Institute of Medicine (2002) reports:

> *that working-age Americans without health insurance are more likely to receive too little care and receive it to late; be sicker and die sooner; receive poorer care when they are in the hospital, even for acute situations, like vehicle crash (p. 8).*

When the uninsured are cared for in emergency rooms, they fail to develop the patient-physician link that leads to regular screening and checkups that result in disease prevention and early detection of problems. It also means that people who come to the emergency room with legitimate emergencies experience longer waits and possibly delays in treatment. A number of studies draw a strong correlation between the lack of insurance and poor health.

The evidence paints a dramatic portrait of the U.S. healthcare system, as it is experienced by low- and moderate-income families. Health insurance is often too expensive or unavailable, healthcare costs require an increasing share of household budgets, and the result is that a growing number of Americans are underinsured. Once diagnosed, they cannot afford care and treatment. Medical debt accumulates, and people hold back on purchasing prescription drugs and following up on required care. With so many working families in crisis, the time has never been more critical for policymakers to develop answers to the nation's deteriorating health insurance problem.

The State of U.S. Health Care in 2008

A virtual storm of pessimistic financial trends is battering working families all over the United States. The federal minimum wage is now three dollars an hour lower, in real terms, than it was 40 years ago. Food prices are soaring, home values are declining, and healthcare costs are increasing much faster than income. Nearly 9 million Americans have lost their health insurance since 2000 (Collins, Kriss, Doty, & Rustgi, 2008).

Myth #3: A certain segment of the population will always be uninsured.

In 2007, 28% of U.S. adults, or an estimated 50 million people, were reported as uninsured during the previous year (Collins et al., 2008). This is an increase of 24% since 2001, an increase that is projected to reach 56 million by 2013. In addition, an estimated 16 million more are "underinsured" because they have high out-of-pocket costs in comparison to their incomes (Collins et al., 2008). These gloomy statistics often lead people to believe in Myth #3.

The reasons for these statistics are complex, but most are the result of the increasing cost of insurance, the growing share of insurance that employers expect employees to pay, and the declining number of employers who offer insurance. Even this shifting of costs does not decrease national healthcare expenditures (Sarpel et al., 2008). These expenditures are expected to double to $4 trillion, or 20% of national income, over the next decade, while millions of U.S. residents continue on the road to becoming uninsured or underinsured.

In addition, the quality of health care is declining. In its first health system scorecard released two years ago, the Commonwealth Fund Commission on a High Performance Health System (2007) found that the United States fell far short of benchmarks for access, quality, efficiency, and other key measures of health system performance. The 2008 scorecard paints an even more discouraging picture. An analysis of trends for the dimensions of health system performance, as well as for individual indicators, validates that the U.S. healthcare system persists in falling far short of what is possible, especially given its resources. The scorecard contains 37 indicators in five dimensions of health system performance: healthy lives, quality, access, efficiency, and equity (see Figure 20.1). With a general score of 65 (out of a possible 100), the United States now ranks *last* out of 19 industrialized countries on a measure of mortality amenable to medical care, falling from 15th as other countries raised the bar on performance.

Therefore, on the whole, U.S. performance did not improve from 2006 to 2008.

1. Access to health care has appreciably declined.
2. The number of uninsured or underinsured adults between 19 and 64 years of age increased 35% between 2003 and 2007.
3. The U.S. also failed to keep up with advances in health outcomes, falling from 15th to 19th among industrialized nations in terms of the number of premature deaths that could possibly have been prevented by well-timed access to care.

20.1

Results of the National Scorecard on U.S. Health System

Scores: Dimensions of a High Performance Health System

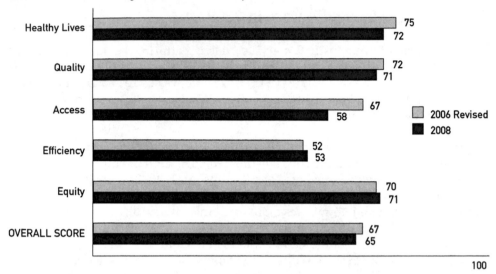

From "Why Not the Best? Results from the National Scorecard on U.S. Health System Performance," by The Commonwealth Fund Commission on High Performance Health System (July 17, 2008). 2008, p. 97. Retrieved September 9, 2008, from http://www.commonwealthfund.org/publications/publications_show.htm?doc_id =692682. Copyright 2008 by Commonwealth Fund. Reprinted with permission.

Is there any good news in this scorecard report? Based on the Institute for Healthcare Improvement's "100,000 Lives Campaign," there are some bright spots:

1. Mortality ratios, a key measure of safety, improved by 19 percent from 2000–2002 to 2004–2006 (Davis, 2008, July).
2. Hospitals are increasingly meeting evidence-based treatment guidelines based on data collected and described on a Medicare Web site.
3. Management of two familiar chronic conditions, diabetes and high blood pressure, has also improved considerably.

These measures are widely reported by health plans, and physician groups are rewarded for improving treatment of these conditions. These results indicate that improvement is possible, but it requires committed leadership, a focus on the goal, concentrated action, and constant follow-up.

Costs of the Present U.S. Healthcare System

Employer-sponsored insurance coverage has long formed the backbone of the U.S. health insurance system. As this type of insurance becomes more expensive and less available, costs have increased and access to health care has decreased.

In the end, the lack of employer-based coverage increases public costs, as taxpayers finance public insurance or uncompensated care programs that would otherwise be paid for through insurance. The report from Commonwealth Fund uses data from the Medical Expenditure Panel Surveys to approximate public program expenditures and uncompensated care costs (Glied & Mahato, 2008). In 2004, uninsured and publicly insured workers and their dependents cost $45 billion in public money. This included $32.5 billion linked with public program insurance costs and $12 billion in uncompensated care costs.

This Commonwealth Fund report, which describes four years of survey data (2001, 2003, 2005, and 2007), also indicated that 41 percent of working-age Americans—or 72 million people—have problems paying medical bills or are paying off medical debt. This is an increase of 34 percent between 2005 and 2007 (Collins, Kriss, Doty, & Rustgi, 2008). In 2007, nearly two-thirds of U.S. adults struggled to pay medical bills, went without needed care because of cost, were uninsured for a time, or were underinsured (Collins, Kriss, Doty, & Rustgi, 2008). For adults 65 and older, 7 million reported problems with medical bills or debt. Because of the decline in insurance coverage and rising health care costs, 45 percent of people reported that they did not receive needed care in 2007. Of the adults who experienced problems paying medical bills, 29% could not pay for basic necessities; 39% used savings to pay medical bills; and 30% acquired credit card debt related to their medical bills. In addition, both insured and uninsured adults spent larger shares of their income on out-of-pocket medical expenses and on increasing premiums between 2001 and 2007.

The proportion of insured adults who expended more than 5% to 10% of their income on health care and insurance increased across all income groups between 2001 and 2007 (Collins, Kriss, Doty, & Rustgi, 2008). As a result, the number of underinsured adults climbed to 25 million people in 2007, up from 16 million in 2003.

These facts speak volumes about the state of the U.S. healthcare system. What was a small problem has become mammoth. Americans are not getting the needed preventive services they or their children need and are using emergency departments as a healthcare provider of last resort.

The State Children's Health Insurance Program (SCHIP)

The State Children's Health Insurance Program (SCHIP) is a joint federal-state program enacted in 1997 to cover children in families that earned too much income to qualify for Medicaid, but could still not afford private insurance. Two-thirds (68%) of all uninsured children come from families in which a parent or guardian works full time (SCHIP: Overview, 2008). They are more than three times as likely as insured children not to visit a doctor in the course of a year (SCHIP: Overview, 2008). In addition, more than half of all uninsured children did not have a "well-child" checkup. This is more than double the rate of children with insurance.

According to the latest Commonwealth Fund/"Modern Healthcare" Health Care Opinion Leaders survey, SCHIP has been successful in increasing access to health care for low-income children and in decreasing the rate of uninsured, low-income children. This broad group of 170 peer-nominated opinion leaders in health policy and innovators in healthcare delivery and finance was positive about the increase in access to health care, but only 34 percent of these health-care leaders felt that SCHIP was successful in motivating state innovation in designing delivery models for children. Overall, more than 20 million children were covered by either Medicaid or SCHIP in 2007, but that still leaves nine million uninsured children across the nation. This is more than the total number of children enrolled in the first and second grades in all of U.S. public schools.

This report illustrates that programs like SCHIP are a true lifeline for at-risk children. Making sure they have insurance helps preserve their health and, eventually, the strength of our nation. While many working parents do not realize it, most are eligible for Medicaid or SCHIP. Enrolling these children must become a major moral focus for healthcare organizations.

The Children's Health Insurance Program (CHIP) Reauthorization Act of 2007 was passed in the House of Representatives by a vote of 265 to 159 on September 25, 2007 and in the Senate by a vote of 67 to 29 two days later. It was an amendment to a Senate amendment to a House revenue bill. However, President Bush vetoed this legislation on October 3, 2007. Unfortunately, a vote to override the President's veto failed in the House on October 18, 2007 by a vote of 273 to 156. President Bush signed an extension of the program to cover current enrollment levels through March 2009, so that problematic issues in the program could be fixed. SCHIP has cost the federal government $40 billion during its first 10 years, and the debate over its fiscal impact reflects the larger debate in the United States over the government's role in health care.

The President's Health Care Tax Proposal did not serve as an effective substitute for expansion of SCHIP (Blumberg, 2007). Blumberg's study found that the financial burden for families of four earning between approximately $32,000 to 65,000 would rise dramatically more under the tax-deduction approach than under SCHIP. Therefore, the potential to decrease the number of uninsured children would be substantially greater under an expansion of SCHIP than under the proposed tax deductions.

Children with health insurance receive needed care, while uninsured children go without (Needed Lifeline: Chronically Ill Children and Public Health Insurance Coverage, 2008). SCHIP and Medicaid provide a significant safety net for America's families, in particular for families with chronically ill children. More than one in three chronically ill children nationwide is enrolled in one of these programs. As a result, they have constant access to needed care. As long as politicians keep backing away from universal coverage for Americans, they at need to at least exercise their moral courage and reaffirm their commitment to children. Finally, politicians stepped up and passed the Children's Health Insurance Program Reauthorization Act of 2009 (CHIPRA). It was signed into law in February 2009. The Act extends and expands the State Children's Health Insurance Program (now referred to as CHIP, not SCHIP).

Is Universal Health Care the Answer?

Research by Hadley et al. (2008) suggests a significant financial burden for uninsured. People who were uninsured for any part of 2008 spent approximately $30 billion out of pocket and received approximately $56 billion in uncompensated care. Government programs finance about 75% of uncompensated care. If all uninsured people were fully covered, their medical spending would increase by $122.6 billion, which represents 5 percent of current national health spending and .8 percent of gross domestic product.

Providing full-year coverage to all Americans currently uninsured for any fraction of the year would have increased medical spending in 2008 by $122.6 billion (Hadley et al., 2008). For comparison purposes, a recent analysis estimated that the tax subsidy received by privately insured workers with employer-sponsored insurance was more than $200 billion in 2006. The estimate implicitly assumes that the uninsured's new coverage and medical care use would reflect current distributions of public and private coverage and benefits held by lower-income and lower middle-income insured people. Therefore, many believe in *Myth #4: we just cannot afford to cover everyone.* But every other industrialized nation in the world offers universal coverage at a lower cost than United States currently spends. What Americans do not want to acknowledge is that much of the cost goes to administrative personnel as a result of our multipayer system.

However, a recent report from the Commonwealth Fund estimates that a menu of fifteen savings options could reduce health spending by $1.55 trillion over ten years (Commonwealth Fund Commission on a High Performing Health System, 2007). For example, Americans pay more for medications than do patients in other countries; this cost could have been dealt with in Medicare Part D, but the Federal government's bargaining opportunity was missed. Reducing the number of unnecessary medical procedures, such as coronary angioplasty and Cesarean sections, could be another cost control. It is also estimated that approximately half the cost of universal coverage is already in the system, but the government is already spending it on the uninsured (Hadley & Holahan, 2003).

Unquestionably, covering all of uninsured people/families could have major cost repercussions for the federal government, no matter how the reform is designed. If the cost of the additional care is added to current spending by or for the uninsured, the total medical care costs for newly insured people would be approximately $208.6 billion (roughly $3,800 per full-year-equivalent newly insured person), consisting of $122.6 billion in new spending on top of the $86 billion already in the system (Commonwealth Fund Commission on a High Performing Health System, 2007). Although this is substantial, not all of this money necessarily represents new government spending. Of the $86 billion, the uninsured now pay $30 billion themselves. Some of the total costs of covering the uninsured could be counterbalanced by redirecting the nearly $43 billion that we estimate government programs now spend on the uninsured. Recognizing the political difficulties of eliminating existing subsidies to hospitals, most actual reform plans look to savings or increased efficiencies in other parts of the system (e.g., greater use of information technology, better care management, and increased use of medical effectiveness research) to fund increased coverage. Another source of savings might accrue from the improved health of the uninsured. Numerous studies have shown that the uninsured delay seeking care for treatable conditions that often require more costly care when they progress to an advanced state (Hadley, 2003).

Some still believe that capitalistic system of competition for goods and services is a better option than a universal healthcare system. They believe in *Myth #5: a free market is the best way to get the highest quality health insurance at the lowest cost.* But the consumer can not influence the price of goods, as 70% of healthcare insurance is purchased by third parties (e.g., employers). At present, the United States has hundreds of private insurers whose high administrative costs are spent on aggressive marketing and billing, as well as utilization review programs to further trim services. This leaves little attention to the low-yield issues, such as chronic mental and physical illness and preventative care.

The goal should be a 2010 National Scorecard that lives up to American resourcefulness and promise. Aspiring higher and traveling on a more positive path will necessitate new strategies. The strategies recommended by The Commonwealth Fund Commission on High Performance Health System (2008) include:

- universal and well-designed coverage.
- coverage that ensures affordable access and continuity of care, with low administrative costs.
- incentives aligned to promote higher quality and more efficient care.
- care that is designed and organized around the patient, not providers or insurers.
- widespread implementation of health information technology with information exchange.
- explicit national goals to meet and exceed benchmarks and monitor performance.
- national policies that promote private-public collaboration and high performance.

Many of these goals will be found in President Obama's healthcare plan.

Obama Healthcare Plan

The Obama-Biden healthcare plan (2008) has several components that addressed the uninsured. The general approach begins with ensuring that all children have health insurance by expanding both Medicaid and SCHIP. President Obama proposes to establish a National Health Insurance Exchange through which individuals could buy a public plan or a qualified private insurance plan. This proposal requires participating insurers to offer coverage on a guaranteed basis and charge a fair and stable premium that is not related to health status. This would be important to Cathy Davis and millions of other Americans with pre-existing conditions.

The plan will improve efficiency and lower costs through three major actions. First, the administration proposes to invest $10 billion a year for five years to adopt a standards-based electronic health information system, including electronic health records. It estimates a $77 billion savings through reduced hospital stays, avoidance of duplicative and unnecessary testing, more appropriate drug utilization, and other efficiencies (Obama-Biden healthcare plan, 2008).

Second, Obama and Biden want to advance medical practice by improving access to prevention and proven disease management programs. All plans that participate in the new public plan will be required to utilize these evidence-based plans for chronic disease management. With more than 133 million Americans having at least one chronic disease, slowing the progression or even halting the disease will yield billions in savings (Obama-Biden healthcare plan, 2008). Incentives will be offered for excellence, as an independent institute will research comparative effectiveness. In addition, they propose to tackle the well-known health disparities by implementing evidence-based interventions, such as patient navigator programs.

Third, they will lower costs by taking on anticompetitive actions in the drug and insurance companies. As reported earlier, the Commonwealth Fund Commission on High Performance Health Systems reported exorbitant administrative overhead. Obama and Biden will deal with the second fastest growing type of medical expense of prescription drugs by (1) allowing consumers to import safe drugs from other countries; (2) preventing drug companies from blocking generic drugs from consumers; and (3) allowing Medicare to negotiate for cheaper drug prices (Obama Biden healthcare plan, 2008).

This plan will guarantee affordable, accessible health coverage for all Americans. There are a number of requirements for the health insurance options, including guaranteed eligibility and tax credits for families and small businesses. This refundable tax credit of up to 50% of premiums will entice small businesses to offer health plans to their employees.

Our history on healthcare reform indicates that whatever plan is finally brought to vote will be vetted in a number of public and political forums. Opportunities will abound to test out the skills of moral courage in addressing this and other healthcare issues, such as the warehousing of the elderly. Moral courage becomes a habit with practice; the vulnerable uninsured population is a good place to start.

Politics will stalk Obama's plan for access, quality, and efficiency, as well as his recent executive order concerning stem cell research. But even with this significant controversy, progress will be made because citizens and business alike know change is needed.

Members of the Business Roundtable—encompassing executives of top U.S. companies that jointly provide healthcare to 35 million people—assured President Obama that business wanted to work with him in this moment in time to reform the healthcare system (Walker, 2009c). Obama's plan will necessitate that employers purchase insurance for their employees or to provide them with money to do so on their own. But it would not require individuals who are not covered by employers to buy their own insurance, except to cover their children. However, the Business Roundtable would like the existing employer-based system to stay in place.

Obama's plan would not abandon the employer-based system, but it would fashion a national insurance plan to compete with the private plans. People could select to keep their plans or to purchase low-cost coverage through the government-run plan. Critics of the comparable public plan declare it would give the government an unreasonable advantage over private plans, making true competition unattainable.

The Business Roundtable, which has been a long-time supporter of improvements in electronic health records, praised the president's $18 billion health information technology upgrade proposal, which was incorporated in the economic stimulus bill (Walker, 2009b). The health provisions in the stimulus bill are only a small step toward the healthcare reform that both Democrats and Republicans have promised.

What is the view of the American Medical Association (AMA) on Obama's plan? The president of the AMA, Nancy Nielsen, MD, warned Ezekiel Emanuel, MD, a special adviser for healthcare at the Office of Management and Budget, that the Obama administration should not treat physicians as the adversary in the healthcare reform process (Walker, 2009a).

Dr. Emanuel—chairman of the National Institutes of Health's bioethics department and brother of White House chief of staff Rahm Emanuel—told the audience of AMA members that they would ultimately be reimbursed based on how successfully they can keep a certain patient from being readmitted to the hospital within 30 days. This focus on prevention of hospitalization was met with multiple voices of concern, especially for older and sicker patients.

What about the accusations that the Obama plan supports socialized universal health care? A national health insurance system as personified in the single-payer health plan was reintroduced as legislation this year by Representative John Conyers, Jr. (D-Mich.) (Wharton, 2009). That bill would supply comprehensive coverage, offer a complete range of choice of doctors and services, and eliminate the primary cause of personal bankruptcy—healthcare bills. Obama's plan would do the opposite. By mandating that every person be insured, ObamaCare would grant private health insurance companies license to systematically underinsure policyholders, while cashing in on the moral currency of universal coverage (Wharton, 2009). If Obama is a socialist, then on health care, he is doing a reasonably good job of obscuring it. I wonder if he can sell a healthcare reform package that will only end up enriching a private health insurance industry.

Finally, what other law has he changed that potentially affects health care? President Obama cleared the way on March 9, 2009, for the National Institutes of Health (NIH) and other federal agencies to fund research using all kinds of human embryonic stem cells (Kaplan, 2009). Funding restrictions imposed by previous President George W. Bush were removed, making hundreds of newer lines eligible for NIH funding. The new policy also eliminates red tape in laboratories; this will reduce duplicate labs that researchers set up so they could work on human embryonic stem cells with money from state and private sources. But federal funds can not be used to make new human embryonic stem cell lines. Under the Dickey-Wicker Amendment, it is illegal to use federal money on research that involves the creation or destruction of human embryos.

Conclusion

I consider the lack of healthcare coverage for every American a moral outrage. It demonstrates to the world that America's moral compass has become unhinged. The effect on the physical, emotional, and financial well-being of citizens and their families is immeasurable pain and suffering. According to the IOM, 22,000 people died in 2006 because they lacked health insurance. One-third of U.S. adults in 2007 spent 10% or more of their income on health insurance and health care. Multiple reports by nationally recognized and well-respected organizations have repeatedly documented these healthcare financial bankruptcy consequences. Even though we spend twice as much as other nations, we clearly do not reap the reduction in mortality and morbidity statistics one would expect.

The new presidential administration will have a historic opportunity to change direction. A wide-ranging strategy that aims to concurrently guarantee health insurance for all, improve quality, and achieve better efficiency is needed. It is time to address this moral crisis that the whole world can see. What remains to be seen is if U.S. politicians have the moral courage to finally right this wrong.

Key Points to Remember

1. Facts show that 18.1% of women are uninsured, as compared with 22% of men. People from the ages of 25 to 44 account for 50% of uninsured nonelderly adults; non-Hispanic White people constitute nearly 66% of the uninsured nonelderly population.
2. Almost 50 million Americans do not have health insurance, and an estimated 16 million more are measured as "underinsured" because they have high out-of-pocket costs comparative to their income.
3. National Scorecard shows that the United States now ranks *last* out of 19 industrialized countries on a measure of mortality amenable to medical care, falling from 15th as other countries raised the bar on performance.
4. In 2007, nearly two-thirds of U.S. adults struggled to pay medical bills, went without needed care because of cost, were uninsured for a time or were underinsured.
5. An international study surveyed people in Australia, Canada, Germany, the Netherlands, New Zealand, the United Kingdom, and the United States. According to this study, U.S. adults are more probable than adults in six other countries to go without health care because of the cost; 34% stated they thought the system needed to be entirely rebuilt.
6. "Working-age Americans without health insurance are more likely to receive too little care and receive it too late; be sicker and die sooner; receive poorer care when they are in the hospital, even for acute situations, like vehicle crash."
7. Remedy this moral problem of uninsured by hosting an event such as a news conference, campus event, faith event or health and enrollment fair or writing a letter to the editor of your local newspaper and working with the media. Covertheuninsured.org provides guidance for all of these activities.
8. The State Children's Health Insurance Program (SCHIP) is a joint federal-state program enacted in 1997 to cover children in families with too much income to qualify for Medicaid, but who still could not afford private insurance.
9. SCHIP and Medicaid provide a significant safety net for America's families, in particular for families with chronically ill children.
10. It is also estimated that approximately half the cost of universal coverage is already in the system and is being spent by government on uninsured people.
11. The Obama-Biden healthcare plan's (2008) general approach begins with ensuring that all children have health insurance by expanding both Medicaid and SCHIP.
12. The Obama-Biden healthcare plan proposes to invest $10 billion a year for five years to adopt a standards-based electronic health information system, including electronic health records.

13. The Obama-Biden healthcare plan advances medical practice by improving access to prevention and proven disease management programs.
14. The Obama-Biden healthcare plan will lower costs by allowing competitive actions in the drug and insurance companies.

References

Anderson, G.F., & Hussey, P.S. (1999). *Health and population aging: A multinational comparison.* New York: The Commonwealth Fund.

Blumberg, L. J. (October, 2007). *Can the president's health care tax proposal serve as an effective substitute for SCHIP expansion?* Retrieved September 9, 2008, from http://covertheuninsured .org/pdf/SCHIPReauthorization1007.pdf

Collins, S.R., Kriss, J.L., Doty, M., & Rustgi, S.D. (August 20, 2008). *Losing ground: How the loss of adequate health insurance is burdening working families: Findings from the Commonwealth Fund Biennial Health Insurance Surveys, 2001–2007.* The Commonwealth Fund, 99. Retrieved September 8, 2008, from http://www.commonwealthfund.org/topics/topics _list.htm?attrib_id=15309

Commonwealth Fund/"Modern healthcare" Health care opinion leaders survey: Assessing SCHIP. Retrieved September 9, 2008, from http://www.commonwealthfund.org/surveys/surveys _show.htm?doc_id=479133

Commonwealth Fund Commission on High Performance Health System. (July 17, 2008). *Why not the best? Results from the national scorecard on U.S. health system performance, 2008,* 97. Retrieved September 9, 2008, from http://www.commonwealthfund.org/publications/ publications_show.htm?doc_id=692682

Commonwealth Fund Commission on a High Performing Health System. (December, 2007). *Bending the curve: Options for achieving savings and improving value in U.S. health spending.* New York: Commonwealth Fund.

Davis, K. (2008, July). *Headed in the wrong direction: The 2008 National Scorecard on U.S. health system performance.* Commonwealth Fund. Retrieved January 3, 2009, from http://www .commonwealthfund.org/aboutus/aboutus_show.htm?doc_id=693648

Dorn, S. (2008). *Uninsured and dying because of it: Updating the Institute of Medicine analysis on the impact of uninsurance on mortality.* Urban Institute. Retrieved September 9, 2008, from http://www.urban.org/publications/411588.html

Facts and Research on the Uninsured. (2006). *Cover the uninsured.* Retrieved September 9, 2008, from http://covertheuninsured.org/factsheets/display.php?FactSheetID=102

Glied, S., & Mahato, B. (May 2, 2008). *Who pays for health care when workers are uninsured?* Commonwealth Fund, 37, 1–16. Retrieved September 8, 2008, from http://www .commonwealthfund.org/publications/publications_show.htm?doc_id=683563

Hadley, J. (2003). Sicker and poorer: The consequences of being uninsured. *Medical Care Research and Review, 60*(2), 3S-75S.

Hadley, J., & Holahan, J. (2003). How much medical care do the uninsured use, and who pays for it? *Health Affairs,* suppl Web exclusives, W3-66–W3-81.

Hadley, J., Holahan, J., Coughlin, T.A., & Miller, D.M. (2008). Covering the uninsured in 2008: Current costs, sources of payment, and incremental costs. *Health Affairs, 27*(5), 399–415.

Institute of Medicine. (2002). *Care without coverage: Too little, too late.* Washington, DC: Institute of Medicine.

Kaplan, K. (March 10, 2009). What Obama's executive order on stem cells means. *Los Angeles Times.* Retrieved March 13, 2009, from http://www.latimes.com/news/printedition/asection/ la-na-obama-stem-cell-qanda10-2009mar10,0,6387848.story

Lazar, K. (December 28, 2008). Jobless turn to health lifeline. *Boston Globe.* Retrieved January 3, 2009, from http://www.boston.com/news/local/massachusetts/articles/2008/12/28/ jobless_turn_to_health_lifeline/

A needed lifeline: Chronically ill children and public health coverage. (August, 2008). Princeton, NJ: Robert Wood Johnson. Retrieved September 9, 2008, from http://covertheuninsured .org/pdf/ANeededLifeline.pdf

Obama Biden healthcare plan. (2008). Retrieved January 3, 2009, from http://www.barackobama .com/pdf/issues/HealthCareFullPlan.pdf

Pipes, S.C. (2008a). Five myths about health care. *Forbes.* Retrieved January 3, 2009, from http://www.forbes.com/opinions/2008/10/31/obama-health-care-oped-cx_scp_1101pipes .html?partner=relatedstoriesbox

Pipes, S.C. (2008b). *The top ten myths of American health care: A citizen's guide.* San Francisco: Pacific Research Institute.

Sarpel, U., Vladeck, B.C., Divino, C.M., & Klotman, P.E. (2008). Fact and fiction: Debunking myths in the US healthcare system. *Annals of Surgery, 247*(4), 563–569.

Schoen, C., Osborn, R., Doty, M.M., Bishop, M., Peugh, J., & Murukutla, N. (2007). *International health policy survey in seven countries.* The Commonwealth Fund. http://www.common wealthfund.org/surveys/surveys_show.htm?doc_id=568326

Schoen, C., Osborn, R., How, S.K.H., Doty, M.M., & Peugh, J. (2008). In chronic condition: Experiences of patients with complex health care needs, in eight countries. *Health Affairs,* Web Exclusive, Nov. 13, 2008, w1-w16.

SCHIP: Overview of the State Children's Health Insurance Program (SCHIP). (2008). *Cover the uninsured.* Retrieved September 9, 2008, from http://covertheuninsured.org/factsheets/ display.php?FactSheetID=126

Walker, E.P. (March 11, 2009a). Despite disagreements, AMA to work toward health reform. *Washington Post.* Retrieved March 13, 2009, from http://www.medpagetoday.com/Washington-Watch/Washington-Watch/13232?impressionId=1237072271990

Walker, E.P. (February 11, 2009b).Senate passes stimulus bill with $19 billion for health IT. *Washington Post.* Retrieved March 13, from http://www.medpagetoday.com/Washington-Watch/Washington-Watch/12843

Walker, E.P. (March 13, 2009c). Business leaders offer Obama healthcare support. *Washington Post.* Retrieved March 13, 2009, from http://www.medpagetoday.com/Washington-Watch/ Washington-Watch/13267

World Health Organization (WHO). (2000). *The world health report 2000—Health systems: Improving performance.* Geneva: WHO.

Index